TCM Case Studies: Internal Medicine

Project Editors: Zeng Chun, Harry F. Lardner & Liu Shui
Copy Editor: Ye Xiao
Book Designer: Li Xi
Cover Designer: Li Xi
Typesetter: Shan Si

TCM Case Studies:
Internal Medicine

Liu Bai-yan
Hunan University of Chinese Medicine
Suzanne Robidoux
Beijing University of Chinese Medicine
Ye Xiao
Zhejiang Chinese Medical University

Reviewers
Chinese reviewed by
Cai Guang-xian
Hunan University of Chinese Medicine
Wang Ming-qiang
First Affiliated Hospital of Guiyang College of Chinese Medicine

English reviewed by
Or Shampanier
Beijing University of Chinese Medicine

Associate Editors
Hu Xue-jun
Chief Physician and Director, Emergency Department of Integrated Chinese and Western Medicine, Affiliated Hospital of Hunan Institute of Chinese Medicine
Zhu Ying
Chief Physician, Professor, Director of Internal Medicine Department of the 2nd Affiliated Hospital of Hunan University of Traditional Chinese Medicine, and Director of the Teaching and Research Section of Internal Medicine
Kim Jong Youp
Beijing University of Chinese Medicine

人民卫生出版社
PMPH PEOPLE'S MEDICAL PUBLISHING HOUSE

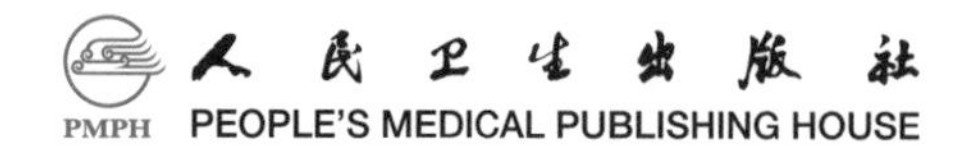

Website: http://www.pmph.com/en

Book Title: TCM Case Studies: Internal Medicine
中医病案教育系列：内科学

Contact address: No. 19, Pan Jia Yuan Nan Li, Chaoyang District, Beijing 100021, P.R. China, phone/fax: 8610 5978 7584, E-mail: pmph@pmph.com

For text and trade sales, as well as review copy enquiries, please contact PMPH at pmphsales@gmail.com

First published: 2014
ISBN: 978-7-117-20003-5/R·20004

Cataloguing in Publication Data:
A catalogue record for this book is available from the CIP-Database China.

Printed in The People's Republic of China

Contributors

Yu Zheng-ke
Professor, Chief Physician, Famous Expert and Director of the Internal Medicine Department, Affiliated Hospital of Hunan Institute of Chinese Medicine

Fan Wen-tao
Affiliated Hospital of Shaanxi College of Chinese Medicine

Zhou Ke
First Affiliated Hospital of Hunan University of Chinese Medicine

He Hai-xia
First Affiliated Hospital of Hunan University of Chinese Medicine

Tang Li-wen
Associate Professor and Associate Chief Physician, First Affiliated Hospital of Hunan University of Chinese Medicine

Lin Xiao-yuan
First Affiliated Hospital of Hunan University of Chinese Medicine

Xie Yong
Hunan University of Chinese Medicine

Translator-in-Chief

Ye Xiao
Zhejiang Chinese Medical University

English Editors

Suzanne Robidoux
Beijing University of Chinese Medicine

Kim Jong Youp
Beijing University of Chinese Medicine

Or Shampanier
Beijing University of Chinese Medicine

About the Authors

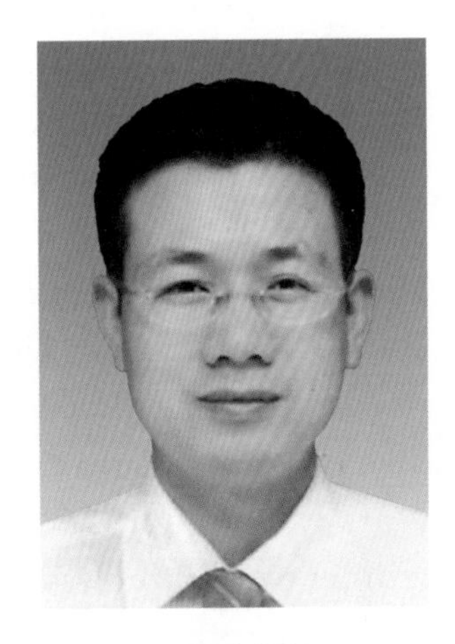

刘柏炎教授

Liu Bai-yan was born in 1970 and is currently the president of Yiyang Medical Junior College. He is a professor, a doctoral supervisor and specializes his clinical practice in the prevention and treatment of the digestive and cardiovascular diseases as well as insomnia. He completed his doctoral program from the Central South University in 2002 and then undertook post-doctoral work in the Hunan College of Traditional Chinese Medicine from 2002 to 2004. He was a visiting scholar in the Chinese University of Hong Kong in 2006 and has served as presidency and secretary of CPC General Branch of the Postgraduate Education Department. He has also been the Director of Tertiary Research Lab of Vascular Biology of the State Administration of Traditional Chinese Medicine and the Director of Chinese Internal Medical Lab of the Key Lab of Hunan Colleges and Universities. He has acted as the vice chairman of Neurology Specialized Committee of Hunan Institute of the Integrated Chinese and Western Medicine, as well as vice chairman of Hunan Health Management Specialized Committee. He has undertaken 13 scientific research projects supported by the National Natural Science Foundation of China, State Branch Program, Ministry of Education, and provincial and bureau sources. He has been awarded with the 1st Prize of the Science and Technology of Hunan Province and 7 other provincial awards. Up to date, he has published over 40 medical papers including 4 in SCI cited journals.

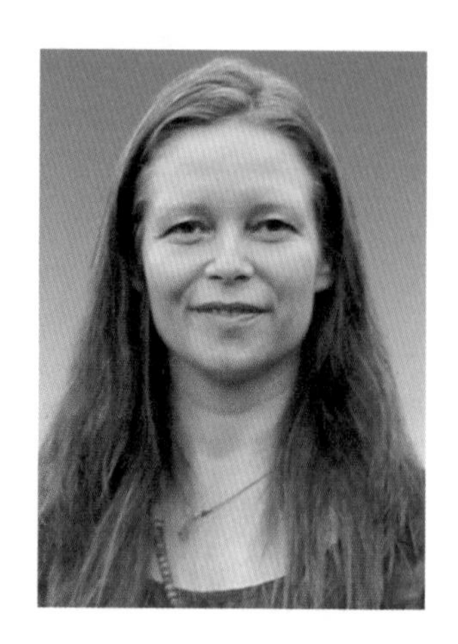

Suzanne Robidoux

Suzanne Robidoux is a Canadian licensed practitioner as well as an international speaker, author and researcher. Dr. Robidoux has spent over 14 years living and practicing Chinese medicine in China after completing her Master's at the International Institute of Chinese Medicine, US. She is presently a fellow laureate at the Beijing University of Chinese Medicine conducting a post-doctoral clinical research on the application of the classical understanding of Zhang Zhong-jing's medical system of Six Syndromes and Classical formulas recorded in the Shang Han Lun and Jin Gui Yao Lue. She completed her doctorate in 2007 at the Nanjing University of Chinese Medicine researching the efficacy in the treatment of various neurological and psychosomatic diseases and disorders with acupuncture and moxibustion. She spent over 6 years working for the People's Medical Publishing House, managing, editing and writing over 20 professional Chinese medicine books on acupuncture, moxibustion, medicinal formulas, health cultivation and martial arts. She has been published in English, French, German and Portuguese. Dr. Robidoux now teaches in conference and academic institutions all over Europe, Asia and North America advanced acupuncture, moxibustion and classical medicine techniques. She has founded ChineseMedicineTraveller.com which is an English platform to join practitioners from around the world to learn rare and effective clinical skills from masters in China in hopes to defy the challenges of cultural differences, language barriers, distance and time limitations in the goals of bringing people with similar goals and passion together.

Ye Xiao is a teacher and translator of Chinese medicine for the Humanities and Social Sciences College, Zhejiang Chinese Medical University. He is currently a council member of the Specialty Committee of Translation of World Federation of Chinese Medicine Societies and a member of Translation Branch of China Association of Chinese Medicine. He has been involved in teaching English translation of Chinese medicine for undergraduates and postgraduates for more than seven years. He has translated about 10 books on Chinese medicine including *Three Character Scripture School Pediatric Massage, The Clinical Practice of Chinese Medicine—Postpartum Hypogalactia & Breast Hyperplasia, Herpes Zoster—Help From Chinese Medicine, Pediatric Tuina, Five-Animal Exercise, Acupuncture and Moxibustion For Obesity*, and *Chinese Medicine For Hepatitis C and Cirrhosis.*

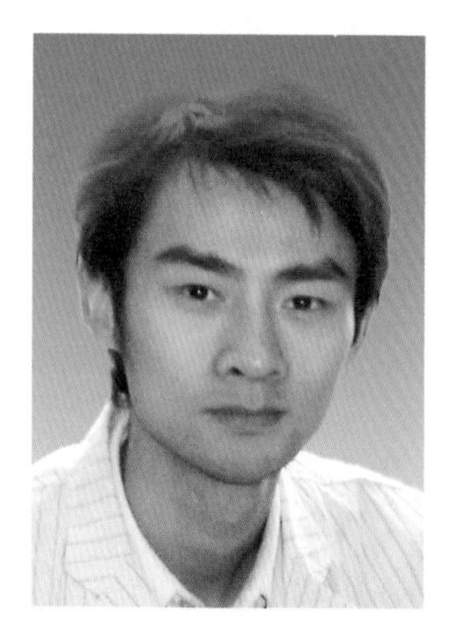

叶晓

Editorial Board for *the TCM Case Studies in the International Standard Library of Chinese Medicine*

Cara O. Frank, L.OM. Dipl. OM.
Educational Director of the Department of Chinese Herbology, Won Institute of Graduate Studies, Glenside, PA, USA

Chen Yun-hui (陈云慧) , Ph.D. TCM
Lecturer of Chinese Materia Medica, School of International Education, Chengdu University of TCM, Chengdu, China

He Qing-hu (何清湖), Ph.D. TCM
Professor and Doctoral Supervisor of Chinese External Medicine, and Vice President of Hunan University of CM, Changsha, China

Hu You-ping (胡幼平)
Professor and Doctoral Supervisor, Acupuncture and Tuina College, The Third Affiliated Hospital, Chengdu University of TCM, Chengdu, China

Huang Ying (黄莺)
Chief Physician, Professor and Vice-Director of the Department of Dermatology, Teaching Hospital of Chengdu University of TCM, Chengdu, China

Jake Paul Fratkin, OMD, L.Ac.
Continuing Education Faculty, American College of Traditional Chinese Medicine, San Francisco; Continuing Education Faculty, Oregon College of Oriental Medicine, Portland; Continuing Education Faculty, Austin College of Oriental Medicine, Austin, Texas, USA

James Flowers
PhD Candidate, College of Oriental Medicine, Wonkwang University, South Korea; Secretary General, International Association for the Study of Traditional Asian Medicine

Lei Lei (雷磊), Ph.D. TCM
Chief Physician, Professor & Doctoral Supervisor, Department of Gynecology and Obstetrics, School of Integrated Chinese and Western Medicine, Hunan University of CM, Changsha, China

Lei Yu-e (雷玉娥)
Associate Professor, Hunan University of CM, Changsha, China

Liu Bai-yan (刘柏炎), Ph.D. Integrative Medicine
Professor and Doctoral Supervisor of TCM Internal Medicine, Hunan University of CM; Director of Hunan Provincial Key University Laboratory of TCM Internal Medicine, Changsha, China

Ma Xi-tao (马喜桃)
Resident Physician, Teaching Hospital of Chengdu University of TCM, Chengdu, China

Misha R. Cohen, OMD, L.Ac.
Clinic Director, Chicken Soup Chinese Medicine; Research Specialist in Integrative Medicine, UCSF Institute for Health and Aging; Associate Member, UCSF Comprehensive Cancer Center; Director, MRCE Foundation

Pär Rufus Scott, MOAM, Lic. Ac.

Peng Qing-hua (彭清华), Ph.D. TCM
Chief Physician, Professor and Doctoral Supervisor of TCM Ophthalmology, the First Hospital Affiliated to Hunan University of Chinese Medicine; President of the School of International Education, Hunan University of CM, Changsha, China

Portia Barnblatt, DAOM, L.Ac. Dipl.Ac.
Portia Chan Acupuncture Clinic, San Francisco, U.S.A.; Clinical supervisor for American College of Traditional Chinese Medicine, San Francisco, U.S.A

Suzanne Robidoux (苏璇), Ph.D, DOM, L.Ac.
Post Doctor Laureates of Beijing University of Chinese Medicine, Specialized in Classical Medicine and Neurology, Beijing, China

Wan Peng (万鹏), M.S. TCM
Lecturer and Attending Physician of Chinese External Medicine, School of Clinical Medicine/Teaching Hospital of Chengdu University of TCM, Chengdu, China

Wang Jing (王静), Ph.D. TCM
Lecturer of TCM Gynecology, Chengdu University of TCM, Chengdu, China

Wang Meng-qing (王孟清), Ph.D. TCM
Professor and Chief physician of TCM Pediatrics, the First Hospital Affiliated to Hunan University of Chinese Medicine; Director of TCM Pediatrics Department and TCM Pediatrics Teaching Office, Hunan University of CM, Changsha, China

William R. Morris, PhD, DAOM, L.Ac.
President, AOMA Graduate School of Integrative Medicine, Austin, Texas, USA

Wu Jun-mei (吴俊梅), Ph.D. of Acupuncture and Moxibustion
Professor and Master Supervisor, Acupuncture and Tuina College/The Third Affiliated Hospital, Chengdu University of TCM, Chengdu, China

Wu Qian-zhi (吴潜智), M.S. TCM
Vice President of Faculty, Professor and Licensed Acupuncturist, AOMA Graduate School of Integrative Medicine, Austin, Texas, USA

Ye Xiao (叶晓) , M.S. TCM
Lecturer, Humanities and Social Sciences College, Zhejiang Chinese Medical University, Hangzhou, China

Zeng Chun (曾纯), M.S. TCM
Editor and Projector Manager of International Publication Center, People's Medical Publishing House, Beijing, China

Zeng Sheng-ping (曾升平), M.S. TCM
Chief Physician and Professor of TCM Rheumatology and Immunology, Chengdu University of TCM, Chengdu, China

Zhang Yan-hong (张艳红)
Associate Professor, English Teaching and Research Office, Hunan University of CM, Changsha, China

Zheng Qi (郑琦)
Freelance Translator/Interpreter, Beijing, China

Sponsored by

World Federation of Chinese Medical Societies

Preface

Chinese medicine, as an important part of Chinese culture, is a great benefit for the well being and health of all human kind. Its principles are based upon the natural laws of the eight guiding principles and six syndromes and hold thousands of years of clinical efficacy. In the combination of medical classics and the priceless clinical expertise, practitioners all over the world use this medical science and system to treat and cure diseases. There is a common saying in Chinese medicine which says: "What is the essence of being a good medical practitioner? The essence lies in the powder of understanding differentiation and the refining of clinical practice!" Therefore, the key to cultivating and enhancing our ability as medical practitioner is completely based on understanding the classical teachings and proficient clinical practice.

Medical case studies have been recorded throughout history by multiple ancient masters handing down their precious knowledge and experience. These authentic records of disease condition, causes, mechanisms, clinical manifestations, as well as their analysis, pattern differentiation and treatment methods are gems to our medical society. In the spirit of keeping this priceless tradition alive we have recorded over 100 different cases studies by clearly illustrating their treatment methods with medicinals, acupuncture and moxibustion. With these clear reviews of medical cases, practitioner can capture the experts' thought process and earn a deeper understanding of the chosen medicinals and acupuncture points. Furthermore, by reviewing other experts' approach to complex diseases, practitioners will move into a deeper understanding and maybe even learn a new approach to some diseases.

Chinese internal medicine is the foundation of clinical practice of Chinese medicine and covers a large variety of diseases and symptoms. Developing expertise in every internal disease requires a lot of practice and extensive studies. However, after mastering the theory of Chinese classical medicine etiology and pathomechanism of diseases, the practitioner must acquire many years of practice. One could spend years accumulating first hand experience, however since there are ample information collected from successful cases studies available, it is highly profitable for the practitioner to analyze and grasp the knowledge through the experience of the masters that came before them. In this approach, medicine itself will continue to evolve and improve.

This collection of clinical case in internal medicine contains typical medical cases of commonly seen diseases recorded by Chinese medical experts in modern times. These medical cases are concrete and informational, and with full medical analysis on the theory, treatment principles with medicinals, formula, acupuncture and moxibustion. In addition, to deepen the level of understanding of the diseases, comprehension questions have been added at the end of each chapter with detailed answers.

We hope these clinical case reviews will help practitioners of Chinese classical medicine all over the world and bring a deeper understanding of the possible patterns and treatments. We welcome anyone to contact us if you wish to offer your comments.

The Authors

August, 2014

Contents

Part I

Lung Conditions

1.1 Cough & Wheezing

Cough, wheezing and panting are very commonly seen symptoms in clinic which can be either acute or chronic secondary symptoms associated to upper respiratory track diseases or primary symptoms caused by an external invasion of a pathogen. In TCM, these symptoms are viewed as the inability of lung qi to descend either due to the invasion of an external or an internal pathogen, or due to an internal weakness of the lung, spleen or kidney.

If we first analyze the cause of these symptoms due to the invasion of external pathogen such as pathogenic wind, cold, heat or damp heat, we understand that they are related to the weather conditions. However, these exterior pathogens can only invade the body once the body's natural defense is weakened. This internal weakness is also important to address when treating the external pathogen. As for the blockage of the lung qi due to internal pathogen causing cough and wheezing, we can notice that the retention of internal dampness or phlegm in the lungs will inhibit the lungs natural descending function and cause the symptoms of cough and wheezing.

When we see there is an internal deficiency syndrome causing cough or wheezing, we need to consider that the function of the lungs themselves of descending is impaired to the lack of qi or to the lack of body fluid causing lung dryness. The secondary organs we need to consider when the symptoms of cough is seen in a deficient pattern, is the weakness of the spleen qi not being able to transform and transport the fluids appropriately and having the phlegm and dampness stagnate in the lungs causing the cough. The kidneys are also to be considered when we are treating cough with weakness of taking deep inhales. In this case the body shows us that the ability of the kidney to grasp the lung qi downward is impaired causing cough and wheezing.

In Western medicine, the symptom of cough is a natural bodily reflex to expectorate whether a foreign pathogen, irritant, or secretions. Coughing can be either voluntary or involuntary. Wheezing is seen as a continuous coarse, whistling sound produced in the airways while breathing. Wheezing occurs when there is obstruction or narrowing of the bronchi. A frequent cough is the sign of a virus or a bacteria, most of the time a cough and wheezing are due to upper respiratory tract infections, but some other diseases and conditions can also cause coughing such as smoking, air pollution, asthma, gastroesophageal reflux disease, post nasal drip, bronchitis, heart failure just to name the most important ones.

Cough is classified by its duration, quality and timing. It is considered an acute cough when the duration is less than three weeks. It is considered subacute when it has lasted from three to eight weeks, and chronic when it has lasted over eight weeks. The most common western medication given for coughs are cough suppressants like codeine, anti-inflammation or mucus expectoration medication. However, in most cases suppressing the cough might be harmful.

Wheezing occurs in different portions of the breathing cycle. Identifying which portion is affected is one of the most important aspects to diagnose which aspect of the lungs is obstructed and can prove important to monitor the treatment efficacy or the progression of the disease.

CLINICAL PATTERNS DIFFERENTIATION AND TREATMENTS

As mentioned above, the commonly known etiopathologies for the symptoms of cough and wheezing are divided in two groups: due to external pathogens, and due to internal damage. These patterns are identified according to the presenting symptoms. These following treatments are recommended for each pattern.

1. Cough and Wheezing due to External Pathogens

A. Wind-cold Attacking the Lung

Symptoms: Acute cough or wheezing which is frequent and loud, with thin and white sputum, simultaneous chills and fever, no sweating, headache, muscles and body aches and pains, stiffness of the neck and shoulders, blocked or runny nose, frequent sneezing, normal tongue with thin white coating, and a floating and tight pulse.

Treatment Principle:

- Expel wind and dissipate cold
- Redirect lung qi downward and stop cough

Main Acupuncture Points:

- LI 4 (*hé gŭ*) and LU 7 (*liè quē*): Combination of the large intestine's *yuan*-source point and the *luo*-connecting point of the lung to clear the upper and dispel external wind attacking the lung
- SJ 5 (*wài guān*), GB 20 (*fēng chí*), and BL 12 (*fēng mén*): To expel the external wind
- BL 13 (*fèi shù*): Back-*shu* point of the lung to support the lung and support its natural function of descending and expanding
- ST 36 (*zú sān lĭ*): To support the middle qi

Supporting Points:

- EX-HN 3 (*yìn táng*): To unblock the nose and calm the mind
- EX-HN5 (*tài yáng*): To treat headache

Recommended Formula: Combined *Sān Ào Tāng* (三拗汤, Rough and Ready Three Decoction) from the *Beneficial Formulas from the Taiping Imperial Pharmacy* (*Tài Píng Huì Mín Hé Jì Jú Fāng*, 太平惠民和剂局方) and *Zhǐ Sòu Sǎn* (止嗽散, Cough-Stopping Powder) from the *Medical Revelations* (*Yī Xué Xīn Wù*, 医学心悟).

Formula Modifications:

- For severe external wind-cold: Add *fáng fēng* (Radix Saposhnikoviae) and *qiāng huó* (Rhizoma et Radix Notopterygii) to increase the effect of removing wind and dissipating cold
- For severe sore throat: Add *niú bàng zǐ* (Fructus Arctii) and *chán tuì* (Periostracum Cicadae) to remove wind and treat sore throat
- For nasal obstruction: Add *xīn yí* (Flos Magnoliae) and *cāng ěr zǐ* (Fructus Xanthii) to open the orifice of the nose
- For chest oppression and pain: Add *bàn xià* (Rhizoma Pinelliae), *hòu pò* (Cortex Magnoliae) and *fú líng* (Poria) to dry dampness and resolve phlegm

B. Wind-heat Attacking the Lung

Symptoms: Acute cough with hacking sound, or cough with a yellow sticky sputum which is difficult to expectorate, fever with little or no chills, nasal obstruction, yellow and sticky nasal discharge, sore, dry and scratchy throat, thirst, headache, a red tongue with thin white or thin yellow coating, a floating and rapid pulse.

Treatment Principle:

- Expel wind and clear heat
- Transform phlegm and redirect lung qi downward to treat cough

Main Acupuncture Points:

- LI 4 (*hé gǔ*) and LU 7 (*liè quē*): Combination of the large intestine's *yuan*-source point and the *luo*-connecting point of the lung to clear the upper and dispel external wind attacking the lung
- SJ 5 (*wài guān*), GB 20 (*fēng chí*), and BL 12 (*fēng mén*): To expel the external wind
- LI 11 (*qū chí*) and DU 14 (*dà zhuī*): To expel heat
- KI 6 (*zhào hǎi*) and LU 11 (*shào shāng*): To clear lung heat and nourish yin
- BL 13 (*fèi shù*): Back-*shu* point of the lung to support the lung and support its natural function of descending and expanding
- LU 5 (*chǐ zé*): *He*-sea point of the lung area to support lung and support its natural function of descending and expanding, and expel the pathogens

Supporting Points:

- RN 22 (*tiān tū*): To open the throat and relieve sore and scratchy throat
- EX-HN3 (*yìn táng*): To unblock the nose and calm the mind
- EX-HN5 (*tài yáng*): To treat headache

Recommended Formula: *Sāng Jú Yǐn* (桑菊饮, Mulberry Leaf and Chrysanthemum Beverage) from the *Systematic Differentiation of Warm Diseases* (*Wēn Bìng Tiáo Biàn*, 温病条辨).

Formula Modifications:

- For severe cough: Add *yú xīng cǎo* (Herba Houttuyniae) and honey fried *pí pá yè* (Folium Eriobotryae)
- For blood streaked sputum: Add *bái máo gēn* (Rhizoma Imperatae Cylindrecae) and *ǒu jié* (Nodus Nelumbinis Nuciferae)

C. Wind-dryness Attacking the Lung

Symptoms: Dry hacking cough which is non-productive or with scant mucus which is difficult to expectorate, chest pain, dryness of the mouth and throat, headache, mild fever and chills, normal or red tongue with scant coating and a thready and rapid pulse.

Treatment Principle:

- Clear lung heat and moisten dryness
- Redirect lung qi downward and stop cough

Main Acupuncture Points:

- LI 4 (*hé gǔ*) and LU 7 (*liè quē*): Combination of the large intestine's *yuan*-source point and the *luo*-connecting point of the lung to clear the upper and dispel external wind attacking the lung
- SJ 5 (*wài guān*) and BL 12 (*fēng mén*): To expel the external wind
- LU 5 (*chǐ zé*) and DU 14 (*dà zhuī*): To expel lung heat
- KI 6 (*zhào hǎi*) and KI 7 (*fù liū*): To clear heat and nourish yin
- BL 13 (*fèi shù*): Back-*shu* point of the lung to support the lung and support its natural function of descending and expanding
- LU 9 (*tài yuān*): *Yuan*-source point of the lung to nourish the lung qi and its natural function of descending and expanding

Supporting Points:

- RN 22 (*tiān tū*): Open the throat and relieve sore and scratchy throat
- EX-HN 3 (*yìn táng*): To unblock the nose and calm the mind
- EX-HN 5 (*tài yáng*): To treat headache

Recommended Formula: *Sāng Xìng Tāng* (桑杏汤, Mulberry Leaf and Apricot Kernel Decoction) to remove wind, moisten dryness and redirect lung qi downwards to stop cough.

Formula Modifications:

- For severe damage to the fluid: Add *mài mén dōng* (Radix Ophiopogonis), *yù zhú* (Rhizoma Polygonati) and *shí hú* (Caulis Dendrobii) to nourish lung yin
- For severe heat symptoms: Add *shēng shí gāo* (Gypsum) and *zhī mǔ* (Rhizoma Anemarrhenae) to clear lung heat
- For blood-streaked sputum: Add *shēng dì huáng* (Radix Rehmanniae) and *bái máo gēn* (Rhizoma Imperatae) to clear heat, cool blood and stop bleeding

Summary Chart for Cough and Wheezing due to External Patterns

External Patterns	Main Points	Supporting Points	Formulae
Wind-cold Attacking the Lung	LI 4, LU 7, SJ 5, GB 20, BL 12, BL 13, ST 36	EX-HN 3 for unblocking the nose and calming the mind EX-HN 5 for headache	Combined *Sān Ào Tāng* and *Zhǐ Sòu Sǎn*
Wind-heat Attacking the Lung	LI 4, LU 7, SJ 5, GB 20, BL 12, LI 11, DU 14, KI 6, LU 11, BL 13, LU 5	RN 22 for opening the throat and relieving sore and scratchy throat EX-HN 3 for unblocking the nose and calming the mind EX-HN 5 for headache	*Sāng Jú Yǐn*
Wind-dryness Attacking the Lung	LI 4, LU 7, SJ 5, BL 12, LU 5, DU 14, KI 6, KI 7, BL 13, LU 9	RN 22 for opening the throat and relieving sore and scratchy throat EX-HN 3 for unblocking the nose and calming the mind EX-HN 5 for headache	*Sāng Xìng Tāng*

2. Cough and Wheezing due to Internal Causes

A. Phlegm-dampness Accumulating in the Lung

Symptoms: Chronic or recurrent cough with profuse thin or thick white or clear mucus, rattling sound in the chest with cough which tends to worsen in the morning, fullness and stuffiness in the chest, poor appetite, nausea or vomiting, lethargy and lassitude, pale and swollen tongue with teeth marks and a soft and slippery pulse.

Treatment Principle:

- Strengthen the spleen and dry dampness
- Transform phlegm and stop cough

Main Acupuncture Points:

- LU 7 (*liè quē*): *Luo*-connecting point of the lung to open the lung
- BL 13 (*fèi shù*) and BL 43 (*gāo huāng*): To support the lung and support its natural function of descending and expanding
- LU 9 (*tài yuān*): *Yuan*-source point of the lung to nourish the lung qi and its natural function of descending and expanding
- BL 20 (*pí shù*) and SP 3 (*tài bái*): To support the function of the spleen in transforming internal fluid
- ST 36 (*zú sān lǐ*): To support the middle qi
- EX-B 1 (*dìng chuǎn*): To stop wheezing, panting and cough

Supporting Points:

- RN 22 (*tiān tū*): To open the throat and relieve sore and scratchy throat

- EX-HN 3 (*yìn táng*): To unblock the nose and calm the mind
- PC 6 (*nèi guān*): To treat fullness of the chest

Recommended Formula: Combine *Èr Chén Tāng* (二陈汤, Two Matured Substances Decoction) and *Sān Zǐ Yǎng Qīn Tāng* (三子养亲汤, Three-Seed Filial Devotion Decoction)

Formula Modifications:

- For severe cold phlegm with white sticky sputum: Add *gān jiāng* (Rhizoma Zingiberis) and *xì xīn* (Herba Asari) to warm the lung and resolve phlegm
- For poor appetite due to spleen deficiency: Add *dǎng shēn* (Radix Codonopsis), *bái zhú* (Rhizoma Atractylodis Macrocephalae) and *fú líng* (Poria)
- For difficult expectoration of phlegm: Add *guā lóu rén* (Semen Trichisanthis), *chuān bèi mǔ* (Bulbus Fritillariae Cirrhosae) and *hǎi fú shí* (Pumex) to resolve phlegm and regulate qi

B. Retention of Phlegm-heat in the Lung

Symptoms: Hacking cough with profuse thick, yellow or green, hard to expectorate mucus, fullness and stuffiness in the chest, wheezing which worsens at night, poor appetite, nausea, loose stools or constipation, bitter taste in the mouth, thick yellow tongue coating with a slippery and rapid pulse.

Treatment Principle:

- Support the spleen and transform phlegm
- Clear heat and stop cough

Main Acupuncture Points:

- LU 7 (*liè quē*): *Luo*-connecting point of the lung to open the lung
- BL 13 (*fèi shù*) and BL 43 (*gāo huāng*): To support the lung and its natural function of descending and expanding
- LU 9 (*tài yuān*): *Yuan*-source point of the lung to nourish the lung qi and its natural function of descending and expanding
- BL 20 (*pí shù*), SP 6 (*sān yīn jiāo*) and SP 9 (*yīn líng quán*): To support the function of the spleen in transforming internal fluid and clear damp heat stagnation
- EX-B 1 (*dìng chuǎn*): To stop wheezing, panting and cough

Supporting Points:

- RN 22 (*tiān tū*): To open the throat and relieve sore and scratchy throat
- EX-HN 3 (*yìn táng*): To unblock the nose and calm the mind
- PC 6 (*nèi guān*): To treat fullness of the chest

Recommended Formula: *Qīng Jīn Huà Tán Tāng* (清金化痰汤, Metal-Clearing and Phlegm-Transforming Decoction)

Formula Modifications:

- For yellow pus like sputum or foul smelling sputum: Add *yú xīng cǎo* (Herba Houttuynia), *dōng guā zǐ* (Semen Benincasae) and *yì yǐ rén* (Semen Coicis) to clear heat and resolve phlegm

• For chest fullness and constipation: Add *tíng lì zǐ* (Semen Lepidii seu Descurainiae) and *dà huáng* (Radix et Rhizoma Rhei) to resolve phlegm and promote bowel movement

• For fever and restlessness: Add *shēng shí gāo* (Gypsum) and *zhī mǔ* (Rhizoma Anemarrhenae) to clear heat and calm the mind

C. Liver Fire Attacking the Lung

Symptoms: Paroxysmal severe cough which comes in bursts, cheat and hypochondriac pain, often aggravated or provoked by stress or emotional outbursts, accompanied by heat raising to the head, flushed complexion, red sore eyes, bitter taste in the mouth, irritability and restlessness, rib-side pain, red and dry tongue with a wiry or slippery and wiry pulse.

Treatment Principle:

• Clear liver fire and moisten the lung

• Transform phlegm and stop cough

Main Acupuncture Points:

• LU 7 (*liè quē*): *Luo*-connecting point of the lung to open the lung

• BL 13 (*fèi shù*) and BL 43 (*gāo huāng*): To support the lung and support its natural function of descending and expanding

• LU 9 (*tài yuān*): *Yuan*-source point of the lung to nourish the lung qi and its natural function of descending and expanding

• BL 18 (*gān shù*), LV 2 (*xíng jiān*) and GB 34 (*yáng líng quán*): To clear liver fire heat and subdue the liver

• EX-B 1 (*dìng chuǎn*): To stop wheezing, panting and cough

Supporting Points:

• RN 22 (*tiān tū*): Open the throat and relieve sore and scratchy throat

• EX-HN 3 (*yìn táng*): To unblock the nose and calm the mind

• PC 6 (*nèi guān*): To treat fullness of the chest

Recommended Formula: Combine *Dài Gé Sǎn* (黛蛤散, Natural Indigo and Clam Shell Powder) and *Xiè Bái Sǎn* (泻白散, White-Draining Powder)

Formula Modifications:

• For severe liver fire: Add *zhī zǐ* (Fructus Gardeniae) and *dān pí* (Cortex Moutan) to clear liver fire

• For chest oppression and reversed flow of lung qi: Add *tíng lì zǐ* (Semen Lepidii seu Descurainiae), *zhǐ qiào* (Frutus Aurantii) and *guā lóu* (Frutus Trichosanthis) to redirect the upsurging qi and clear the lung

• For sticky sputum with expectoration: Add *hǎi fú shí* (Pumex), *zhè bèi mǔ* (Bulbus Fritillariae Verticillatae) and *dǎn nán xīng* (Arisaema Cun Bile)

D. Lung-yin Deficiency

Symptoms: Chronic cough with no or scant sputum, dry mouth and throat, low grade fever, malar flush, night sweat, heat sensation in the palms and feet, emaciation, lethargy, red tongue with no coating, thready and rapid pulse.

Treatment principle:

- Nourish the lung yin and stop cough
- Moisten the lung and transform phlegm

Main Acupuncture Points:

- LU 1 (*zhōng fŭ*), LU 9 (*tài yuān*) and LU 7 (*liè quē*): To nourish and open the lung
- BL 13 (*fèi shù*) and BL 43 (*gāo huāng*): To support the lung and support its natural function of descending and expanding
- BL 20 (*pí shù*) and SP 3 (*tài bái*): To support the function of the spleen in transforming internal fluid
- KI 6 (*zhào hăi*), KI 3 (*tài xī*), SP 6 (*sān yīn jiāo*): To nourish root yin and clear empty heat
- EX-B 1 (*dìng chuăn*): To stop wheezing, panting and cough

Supporting Points:

- RN 22 (*tiān tū*): Open the throat and relieve sore and scratchy throat
- EX-HN 3 (*yìn táng*): To unblock the nose and calm the mind
- PC 6 (*nèi guān*): To treat fullness of the chest

Recommended Formula: *Shā Shēn Mài Mén Dōng Tāng* (沙参麦门冬汤, Adenophora and Ophiopogon Decoction)

Formula Modifications:

- For chronic fever due to lung dry heat: Add *dì gŭ pí* (Cortex Lycii Radicis) and *sāng bái pí* (Cortex Mori Radicis) to clear lung heat
- For blood streaked phlegm: Add *dān pí* (Cortex Moutan), *zhī zĭ* (Frustuc Gardeniae) and *bái máo gēn* (Rhizoma Imperatae) to clear heat
- For night sweats: Add raw *mŭ lì* (Conchae Ostreae) and *fú xiăo mài* (Fructus Tritici Levis)

E. Lung and Spleen Qi Deficiency

Symptoms: Chronic or recurrent cough with thin watery sputum usually accompanied by wheezing and panting which worsens with exertion, generalized edema, fatigue, low or poor appetite, aversion to cold, dizziness and palpitation, swollen tongue with teeth marks with a moist coating and a deep and slippery pulse.

Treatment Principle:

- Nourish qi and disperse cold and fluid
- Strengthen the spleen and lung
- Nourish the lung and stop cough

Main Acupuncture Points:

- LU 7 (*liè quē*): *Luo*-connecting point of the lung to open the lung
- BL 13 (*fèi shù*) and BL 43 (*gāo huāng*): To support the lung and its natural function of descending and expanding

- LU 9 (*tài yuān*): *Yuan*-source point of the lung to nourish the lung qi and its natural function of descending and expanding
- BL 20 (*pí shù*), BL 23 (*shèn shù*), KI 3 (*tài xī*) and SP 3 (*tài bái*): To support the function of the spleen and kidney qi
- ST 36 (*zú sān lǐ*): To support the middle qi
- EX-B 1 (*dìng chuǎn*): To stop wheezing, panting and cough

Supporting Points:

- RN 22 (*tiān tū*): Open the throat and relieve sore and scratchy throat
- EX-HN 3 (*yìn táng*): To unblock the nose and calm the mind
- PC 6 (*nèi guān*): To treat fullness of the chest

Recommended Formula: *Zhēn Wǔ Tāng* (真武汤, True Warrior Decoction) or *Jīn Guì Shèn Qì Wán* (金匮肾气丸, Golden Cabinet's Kidney Qi Pill)

Formula Modifications:

- For severe cough: Add *gān jiāng* (Rhizoma Zingiberis Officinale) and *xì xīn* (Herba Cun Rhizoma Asari)
- For sever fluid accumulation in the lung: Add *tíng lì zǐ* (Semen Sinapsis Albae)
- For severe shortness of breath: Add *dǎng shēn* (Radix Codonopsis Pilosulae)

Summary Chart for Cough and Wheezing due to Internal Patterns

Internal Patterns	Main Points	Supporting Points	Formulae
Phlegm-dampness Accumulating in the Lung	LU 7, BL 13, BL 43, LU 9, BL 20, SP 3, EX-B 1, ST 36	LU 6 and ST 40 for unblocking excessive phlegm PC 6 for treating fullness of the chest	Combined *Èr Chén Tāng* and *Sān Zǐ Yǎng Qīn Tāng*
Retention of Phlegm-heat in the Lung	LU 7, BL 13, BL 43, LU 9, BL 20, SP 6, SP 3, SP 9, DU 14, EX-B 1	EX-HN 3 for unblocking the nose PC 6 for treating fullness of the chest	*Qīng Jīn Huà Tán Tāng*
Liver Fire Attacking the Lung	LU 7, BL 13, BL 43, LU 9, BL 18, LV 2, GB 34, EX-B 1	RN 22 for sore and scratchy throat EX-HN 3 for unblocking the nose	Combined *Dài Gé Sǎn* and *Xiè Bái Sǎn*
Lung Yin Deficiency	LU 1, LU 9, LU 7, BL 13, BL 20, BL 43, SP 3, KI 3, SP 6, EX-B 1	RN 22 for sore and scratchy throat PC 6 for treating fullness of the chest	*Shā Shēn Mài Mén Dōng Tāng*
Lung and Spleen Qi Deficiency	LU 7, BL 13, BL 43, LU 9, BL 20, BL 23, KI 3, SP 3, ST 36, EX-B 1	RN 22 for sore and scratchy throat PC 6 for treating fullness of the chest	*Zhēn Wǔ Tāng* or *Jīn Guì Shèn Qì Wán*

CASE STUDY 1: Common Cold

Ms Li, a 30-year-old female, first consultation on July 10th, 2013.

Chief Complaint: Cough and sore throat for 2 days.

Medical History: She was previously in good health and had no history of smoking or drinking alcohol.

Presenting Symptoms: Cough with sticky and yellow sputum, low grade fever the day prior to consultation, aversion to wind, spontaneous sweating, sore and swollen throat, difficulty to speak loudly, yellow nasal discharge, thirst and headache.

Tongue and Pulse: Thin and yellow tongue coating, and floating and rapid pulse.

Physical Examination: Temperature: 37.5 ℃, pulse: 80 bpm, respiration: 22 bpm, blood pressure: 120/85 mmHg.

Observation: The patient was mentally active and cooperative. The complexion and sclera were non-icteric. Lymph nodes were not enlarged and the breath sound of both lungs was rough. There was no enlargement of the heart and there was a regular rhythm. No heart murmur was heard. The liver and spleen were not palpable. No percussion pain over the kidney region.

Other Medical Test Results:

Blood and urine routine test: Normal.

Chest X-ray: Increased lung markings.

Pattern Differentiation

This is a wind-heat invading the lung pattern leading to the failure of the lung to perform its natural functions of clearing and purifying causing cough with coarse breath sounds. The heat in the lung consumes the healthy fluids manifesting as thirst and sore throat. This heat also causes the healthy fluids to congeal and transform into pathogenic phlegm leading to the presentation of sticky and yellow sputum which are difficult to expectorate as well as yellow nasal discharge. The invasion of wind-heat in the exterior layer of the body harms the exterior *wei* qi and results in symptoms of aversion to wind, perspiration, headache and fever. Thin and yellow tongue coating and floating and rapid pulse are signs of wind-heat in the exterior layer.

Diagnosis

TCM Diagnosis: Cough due to wind-heat invasion

Western Medicine Diagnosis: Acute tracheobronchitis

Treatment

The pathomechanism of this case is wind-heat invading the lung which leads to failure of lung qi to clear and descend the uprising qi manifested as cough.

Principles:

- Remove wind and clear exterior heat
- Diffuse the lung and relieve cough

Formula: *Sāng Jú Yǐn* (Mulberry Leaf and Chrysanthemum Beverage) recorded in *Systematic Differentiation of Warm Diseases* (*Wēn Bìng Tiáo Biàn*, 温病条辨)

Ingredients:

桑叶	*sāng yè*	7.5 g	Folium Mori
菊花	*jú huā*	3 g	Flos Chrysanthemi
杏仁	*xìng rén*	6 g	Semen Armeniacae Amarum
连翘	*lián qiáo*	5 g	Fructus Forsythiae
薄荷	*bò hé*	2.5 g	Herba Menthae
桔梗	*jié gěng*	6 g	Radix Platycodonis
甘草	*gān cǎo*	2.5 g	Radix et Rhizoma Glycyrrhizae
芦根	*lú gēn*	6 g	Rhizoma Phragmitis

Formula Analysis

In this formula, *sāng yè* is the chief medicinal as it is sweet and cool and it can disperse wind-heat in the upper *jiao*. Moreover, it specially enters the lung to clear lung heat and relieve cough. *Jú huā* disperses wind heat, clears heat from the head and eyes and purifies the lung. *Xìng rén* and *jié gěng* soothe lung qi to relieve cough. These three medicinals are used as deputy medicinals. *Lián qiáo* clears heat and removes toxins, *bò he* scatters wind heat, and *lú gēn* clears heat and promotes fluid production to relieve thirst, all of which are used as assistant medicinals. *Gān cǎo* harmonizes the actions of all medicinals in the formula and combines with *jié gěng* to benefit the throat. The combination of these ingredients removes wind heat from the upper *jiao* and soothes lung qi, consequently relieving the exterior and soothing the cough.

Follow-up Consultations

After taking 3 days of the formula, the headache and swelling and sore throat were relieved. The cough with expectoration reduced. After another 2 days of the same formula, all the symptoms subsided.

Clinical Analysis

Since this was an acute case of common cold due to invasion of external wind heat on the exterior layers of the body, we can also understand it as a *Tai Yang* syndrome as listed in the *Treatise on Cold Damage* (*Shāng Hán Lùn*, 伤寒论). Since the case is presenting with aversion to wind and sweating, we notice that there is already weakness of the *wei* qi and the exterior layer is deficient. The sweating causes a deficiency of internal body fluid causing internal heat presenting as dry mouth. The scant yellow sputum is also a sign that there is disturbance in the natural body fluid absorption and internal heat intermingling with the stagnated phlegm.

In this case we can also consider a substitute formula *Guì Zhī Jiā Hòu Pò Xìng Zi Tāng* (Cinnamon Twig Plus Magnolia and Armeniaca Decoction) from the *Treatise on Cold Damage*. We can see in Clause 18 where it says: "For any form of wheezing, *Guì Zhī Tāng* plus *hòu pò* (Cortex Magnoliae Officinalis) and *xìng rén* (Semen Armeniacae Amarum) is appropriate." *Guì Zhī Tāng* (*桂枝汤, Cinnamon Twig Decoction*) formula is often used for a *Tai Yang Zhong Feng* pattern with symptoms of cough, headache, aversion to wind and sweating. However *hòu pò* (Cortex Magnoliae Officinalis) and *xìng rén* (Semen Armeniacae Amarum) are added in this case to relieve the soreness and swelling of the throat as well as the coarse breathing.

CLINICAL KEY POINTS

According to the TCM understanding, it is necessary to clarify the state of healthy qi and pathogenic factors, and deficiency or excess as well as if it is an external or internal pattern. In the case of externally contracted cough, it is usually consulted while still in the primary and acute stage and it tends to have a short course of disease. It is often caused by an exterior pattern of pathogenic excess of wind, heat, cold or dampness in the lung-*wei* layer as seen in the Pattern Differentiation Section. In these cases the pattern is treated by dispelling pathogens and clearing the lung. On the other hand, if the cough is due to an internal damage to the organs, it is often seen in a chronic stage with a long course of disease. In these cases, the patient might show various signs demonstrating that other organs besides the lung are also affected and need attention. In chronic patterns we often identify a combination of excess of pathogens with a weak healthy qi which is unable to expel the pathogen. However, in both acute and chronic cases, we must always remember to support the healthy qi while dispelling the pathogens to relieve cough. Even if the symptom of cough might be the main presenting symptom, it is necessary to take into consideration both the root of the disease being the underlining weakness as well as the branch being the presenting symptoms to treat the syndrome completely and correctly.

COMPREHENSION QUESTIONS

1. Name the 3 external patterns of cough as well as their recommended formulas.
2. How do we diagnose an externally contracted cough?
3. Multiple choice questions:

1) Mr. Li, 23 years old. His clinical manifestations are cough with scanty expectoration, dry throat and nose, aversion to co1d with fever, headache, no sweating, thin and white tongue coating, and floating pulse. What pattern does this case belong to?

A. Wind-cold cough

B. Wind-heat cough
C. Wind-dryness cough
D. Cool-dryness cough
E. Yin deficiency cough

2) Mr. Li, 18 years old. His clinical manifestations are cough with yellow and sticky expectoration, sweating, thirst and fever, aversion to wind, with a thin and yellow tongue coating, and floating and rapid pulse. The treatment method for this case is to:
A. Expel wind and dissipate cold, diffuse the lung and relieve cough
B. Fortify the spleen and dry dampness, dissolve phlegm and relieve cough
C. Clear lung heat and dissolve phlegm, purify the lung and redirect qi downward
D. Expel wind and clear heat, diffuse the lung and dissolve phlegm
E. Expel wind and clear heat, moisten dryness and relieve cough

3) Mr. Zhang, 32 years old. His clinical manifestations are cough with excessive white and sticky phlegm, coarse breathing, distention, fullness and pain in the chest and rib-side, flushed face, fever, dry mouth with desire to drink, yellow, thick and greasy tongue coating, red tongue, and a rapid pulse. The treatment method for this case is to:
A. Clear lung heat, pacify the liver and subdue fire
B. Clear heat, dissolve phlegm and purify the lung
C. Expel wind, clear heat and purify the lung
D. Fortify the spleen, dry dampness and dissolve phlegm
E. Warm and remove phlegm-dampness and diffuse the lung

4) Mr. He, 18 years old. His clinical manifestations are cough with scanty sputum streaked with blood that is difficult to expectorate, dry nose and throat, aversion to wind, fever, red tongue with scanty fluid, and a floating and rapid pulse. This pattern is:
A. Yin deficiency cough
B. Wind-dryness cough
C. Lung abscess at the initial stage
D. Wind-heat cough
E. Phlegm-heat cough

Answers

1. For wind-cold invading the lung, the formula is *Sān Ào Tāng* (Rough and Ready Three Decoction) together with *Zhĭ Sòu Săn* (Cough-Stopping Powder).

For wind-heat invading the lung, the formula is *Sāng Jú Yĭn* (Mulberry Leaf and Chrysanthemum Beverage).

For warm dryness impairing the lung, the formula is *Sāng Xìng Tāng* (Mulberry Leaf and Apricot Kernel Decoction).

2. We must diagnose the externally contracted cough from the symptoms

presentation, such as heat sensation or fever, aversion to cold, aversion to wind, spontaneous sweating, floating and tight or a floating and moderate pulse. The medical history of upper respiratory tract infection, frequent dry cough with scanty and sticky sputum or aggravated cough with gradual increase amount of sputum which might be blood-streaked.

The course of disease will have an acute onset while the disease will not last over a month with the symptoms of cough with sputum usually only lasting from 2 to 3 weeks.

Further tests might also show signs of coarse breathing sounds or occasional audible moist rales in the lungs, while chest X-ray might show a thickened and disorganized lung markings.

3. 1) A, 2) D, 3) B, 4) B.

CASE STUDY 2: Chronic Panting

Ms. Li, 50 years old. First consultation on December 9th, 2009.

Main Complaint: Repeated cough, chest oppression, and panting for over 8 years with relapse for a month.

Medical History: The patient suffered from cough from a common cold 8 years ago. At that time, there were gurgling sounds of sputum in the throat that was aggravated by exertion. When panting occurred, she was unable to lie supine and suffered from chest oppression. She took some Chinese patent medicines, which brought a slight relief. One week ago, she caught a common cold and showed symptoms of cough, chest oppression, panting, and gurgling sound of sputum in the throat. It was aggravated after exertion and occurred sporadically.

Presenting Symptoms: Cough with massive white and loose sputum which is difficult to expectorate, gurgling sound of sputum in the throat, unable to lie in the supine position due to panting, chest fullness and oppression, slightly aversion to cold, bitter taste in the mouth, poor appetite, poor sleep and normal urine and stools.

Physical Examination: Temperature: 36.5 ℃, pulse: 76 bpm, respiration: 24 bpm, blood pressure: 120/85 mmHg.

The patient was active, conscious and cooperative. The skin and sclera were non-icteric. No significant lymph nodes were enlarged. The breath sounds of both lungs were rough with obvious rhonchi and moist rales. The edge of the heart was not enlarged. The heart beat rhythm was regular without heart murmur. The liver and spleen were not palpable. No percussion pain over the kidney region. There was a pale tongue with white and glossy coating, and a slippery and wiry pulse.

Other Medical Test Results:

Blood Routine Test: WBC 8.9×10^9/L, N 78%.

Pattern Differentiation

Due to the symptoms of aversion to cold and white sputum we can differentiate that the symptom of wheezing is caused by external wind-cold attacking the lung. When pathogenic wind-cold stagnates in the lung, the lung qi fails to distribute body fluids which accumulate as phlegm and become the cause of the wheezing. There are various causes of internal phlegm stagnating in the lung which can be external contraction of pathogens or an unhealthy habit of improper diet, emotional excess, and fatigue. This internal phlegm obstructs the natural flow of lung qi or opening and descending and causes spasmodic and difficult breathing with symptoms of cough, wheezing and panting. In this case, the signs of a pale tongue with white and glossy coating, and slippery and wiry pulse are also signs of internal retention of cold phlegm.

Diagnosis

TCM Diagnosis: Wheezing due to cold invasion

Western Diagnosis: Chronic panting

Treatment

This is a case of internal cold phlegm retention in the lungs causing cough and panting.

Principles:

- Diffuse the lung and disperse cold
- Warm the lung and dissolve rheum
- Dissolve phlegm and relieve panting

Formula: Five doses of a combination of *Xiǎo Qīng Lóng Tāng* (Two Matured Substances Decoction) and *Èr Chén Tāng* (Two Matured Substances Decoction) were given.

Ingredients:

麻黄	*má huáng*	8 g	Herba Ephedrae (liquid-fried)
桂枝	*guì zhī*	8 g	Ramulus Cinnamomi
干姜	*gān jiāng*	3 g	Rhizoma Zingiberis
细辛	*xì xīn*	3 g	Radix et Rhizoma Asari
法半夏	*fǎ bàn xià*	10 g	Rhizoma Pinelliae Praeparatum
甘草	*gān cǎo*	6 g	Radix et Rhizoma Glycyrrhizae
白芍	*bái sháo*	15 g	Radix Paeoniae Alba
五味子	*wǔ wèi zǐ*	10 g	Fructus Schisandrae Chinensis
苦杏仁	*kǔ xìng rén*	10 g	Semen Armeniacae Amarum (crushed)
薤白	*xiè bái*	10 g	Bulbus Allii Macrostemi
桔梗	*jié gěng*	12 g	Radix Platycodonis
陈皮	*chén pí*	6 g	Pericarpium Citri Reticulatae
紫菀	*zǐ wǎn*	15 g	Radix et Rhizoma Asteris
茯苓	*fú líng*	20 g	Poria
麦芽	*mài yá*	15 g	Fructus Hordei Germinatus
谷芽	*gǔ yá*	15 g	Fructus Setariae Germinatus

Formula Analysis

As this is a case of cold-damp phlegm retention in the lung, the formulas *Xiǎo Qīng Lóng Tāng* (Two Matured Substances Decoction) and *Èr Chén Tāng* (Two Matured Substances Decoction) were combined to dry dampness and dissolve phlegm, warm the lung and dissolve rheum. In this formula, the effect of diffusing the lung, calming panting, and warming qi to move water of the liquid-fried *má huáng* is reinforced by *guì zhī,* both acting as of chief medicinals. The *gān jiāng, xì xīn,* and *fǎ bàn xià* warm the lung, dissolve rheum, correct the counterflow of qi and calm panting. *Zǐ wǎn* dissolves phlegm and relieves cough. *Bái sháo* and *wǔ wèi zǐ* both have a dispersing and astringing effect. *Gǔ yá* and *mài yá* fortify the spleen and tonify qi to dissolve the accumulated water qi. As the patient has chest oppression, *xiè bái* is added to soothe the chest and disperse masses.

Follow-up Consultations

2nd consultation on December 14th.

The symptoms of cough resolved and the chest oppression and panting were significantly relieved. By removing *xiè bái* and adding *zǐ sū yè* 12 g to the previous formula in order to expel the external pathogenic cold, 7 more doses were prescribed. One week later, the symptoms were significantly resolved and the patient had a good quality of life. However, she came back in the future when contracting a common cold since it reactivated the previous symptoms. The new attacks were easily resolved with more Chinese medicine.

Clinical Analysis

Wheezing is a paroxysmal disease with sputum gurgling and panting, characterized by abnormal sounds when breathing, shortness of breath, panting, or in severe cases unable to lie on the back due to the difficulty in breathing. There are many diseases with these manifestations in Western medicine, such as bronchial asthma, asthmatic bronchitis, chronic obstructive emphysema, pulmonary heart disease, cardiac asthma, and other respiratory allergic diseases.

When treating a chronic pattern in clinic, we must consider that the long standing pathogen has created a weakness in one or many organs in the body and address this deficiency in the treatment approach. When there is qi deficiency of the spleen with internal retention of phlegm in the lung, it might manifest as spasm and narrowing of respiratory tract causing wheezing and panting. The main pattern differentiation of this disease is listed above and depends on the symptom presentation. It is also necessary to notice if the presenting case is a reoccurring case or an acute case. Patterns which are most commonly seen in clinic are wheezing due to cold or heat excess, and lung, spleen and kidney deficiency.

CLINICAL KEY POINTS

The treatment principle of wheezing is to treat the branch during the occurrence stage and treat the root during the remission stage. In addition, the treatment should be based on differentiating the cold from heat pathogens, and deficiency from excess. During the occurring stage, the treatment method to cold-type wheezing is warming the lung and dissipating cold, dissolving phlegm and relieving panting, while to treat heat-type wheezing is clearing heat and diffusing the lung, dissolving phlegm and relieving panting. During the remission stage, the treatment method to lung deficiency is supplementing the lung to consolidate *wei* qi, to spleen deficiency is fortifying the spleen to dissolve phlegm, and to kidney deficiency is boosting kidney and qi. It is essential to boost kidney, because the kidney is the foundation of congenital constitution. If kidney essence is sufficient, the root can be secured. However, in the course of reinforcing the healthy qi, it is necessary to add herbs for directing qi downward and dissolving phlegm, the purpose of which is to reduce relapse by eliminating obstinate phlegm lurking in the internal.

BRIEF SUMMARY

Asthma is a commonly seen disease which affects a large portion of society. It is a recurrent disease caused by the pathological retention of internal phlegm and dampness which affect the function of the lungs making it difficult to breathe with ease and causing wheezing and panting. Children often develop asthma after contracting a common cold, while adults usually suffer from asthma in results from a chronic cough.

Asthma belongs to various differentiations and we can identify them clearly through observing the symptoms carefully. Knowing the correct pattern will lead us to apply the appropriate treatment principle. As a quick summary we will review the important patterns and treatment principles. If the asthma is due to internal retention of cold phlegm, we need to warm the lung and spleen and disperse cold while draining the internal fluids to relieve the symptoms of wheezing and panting. When asthma is due to phlegm-heat accumulation in the lung, we need to clear internal stagnation of heat while removing the phlegm retention. We will also moisten the lung to restore the natural function of the lung and stop panting. If asthma is due to lung and kidney yin deficiency, we will nourish yin and moisten the lung, to restore the function of the lung and stop panting. If asthma is due to a combination of lung and spleen qi deficiency, we will need to tonify the spleen and fortify the lung. In Chinese medicine, we say fortifying the spleen-earth element will strengthen the lung-metal element. If the syndrome of asthma is due to heart and kidney yang deficiency, we will need to nourish the heart and strengthen the kidney, warm yang and check the panting. Acupuncture and moxibustion can also bring relief from asthma. The main points include point from the lung and spleen channels as well as the back-*shu* and front-*mu* points of the lung. For more specific points please check the Treatment Summary Chart section listed above.

COMPREHENSION QUESTIONS

1. What are the pattern differentiation and formulas for wheezing?
2. How do we differentiate the symptoms of wheezing from panting?
3. What are the 2 main key clinical points and some daily recommendations for patients with chronic wheezing and excessive internal phlegm?
4. Mutiple choice questions:

1) Male, 56 years old. He suffered from wheezing for ten years. It relapsed 15 days ago and has been relieved a little after treatment, but he is still presenting with the following symptoms and signs: chest oppression, shortness of breath which worsen after exertion, difficult to inhale, weakness of the back, lack of strength, easily tired, irritability, heat sensation, dry mouth, red tongue with scanty coating and a thin and rapid pulse. The presenting pattern is:

A. Turbid phlegm obstructing the lung
B. Deficiency in the lower and excess in the upper
C. Deficiency of the lung and kidney
D. Heart yang depletion
E. Deficiency of both the spleen and kidney

2) Male, 62 years old. The patient suffered from asthma for years and it relapsed 2 months ago. The asthma is sometimes mild and sometimes severe. In recent two days, the cough and panting have worsened and it is accompanied by bluish complexion during panting, restlessness, spontaneous sweating, cold limbs, pale and bluish tongue, and a thin pulse. The appropriate treatment principle is to:

A. Tonify qi, restore yang to rescue from counterflow of qi
B. Nourish yin and boost qi to rescue from depletion
C. Tonify the spleen and qi to rescue from depletion
D. Tonify the lung and kidney to rescue from depletion
E. Warm the kidney and calm panting to rescue from depletion

3) Mr. Sun, 66 years old. The patient suffered from poor appetite, stuffiness sensation in the stomach area, wheezing usually induced by improper diet, fatigue, shortness of breath, pale tongue with white coating and slippery and thin pulse. The appropriate formula for this case is:

A. *Shēng Mài Săn* (Pulse-Engendering Powder)
B. *Sì Jūn Zĭ Tāng* (Four Gentlemen Decoction)

C. *Liù Jūn Zĭ Tāng* (Six Gentlemen Decoction)
D. *Xiāng Shā Liù Jūn Zĭ Tāng* (Costusroot and Amomum Six Gentlemen Decoction)
E. *Bŭ Zhōng Yì Qì Tāng* (Center-Supplementing and Qi-Boosting Decoction)

4) Ms. Yang, 62 years old. The patient suffered from chronic panting and shortness of breath which worsened after exertion, difficult inhalation, malar flush, dizziness, tinnitus, back and knee weakness, and easily suffered from asthma attacks when exhausted. The appropriate treatment principle is to:
A. Warm and supplement kidney yang
B. Boost the spleen and kidney
C. Nourish yin and boost the kidney
D. Fortify the lung and the kidney
E. Supplement the essence and blood

5) Mr. Zhang, 52 years old. The patient suffered from rough breathing with sputum gurgling sounds in the throat, white and sticky sputum which is difficult to be expectorated, restlessness, bitter taste in the mouth, thirst with desire to drink, red tongue with yellow coating, and slippery and rapid pulse. The optimal formula for treatment is:
A. *Shè Gān Má Huáng Tāng* (Arrest Wheezing Decoction)
B. *Dìng Chuăn Tāng* (Arrest Wheezing Decoction)
C. *Xiăo Qīng Lóng Tāng* (Minor Green Dragon Decoction)
D. *Sū Zĭ Jiàng Qì Tāng* (Perilla Fruit Qi-Descending Decoction)
E. *Kòng Xián Wán* (Drool-Controlling Pill)

6) Mr. Li, 62 years old. The patient presents with symptoms of hasty breathing, wheezing sound in the throat, fullness and oppression of the chest, dull bluish complexion, no thirst, aversion to cold, white and slippery tongue coating, and a wiry and tight pulse. It is a pattern of exterior cold and interior fluid retention with serious cold manifestations. The optimal formula for treatment is:
A. *Shè Gān Má Huáng Tāng* (Belamcanda and Ephedra Decoction)
B. *Dìng Chuăn Tāng* (Wheezing-Arrest Decoction)
C. *Xiăo Qīng Lóng Tāng* (Minor Green Dragon Decoction)
D. *Sū Zĭ Jiàng Qì Tāng* (Perilla Fruit Qi-Descending Decoction)
E. *Sān Zĭ Yăng Qīn Tāng* (Three-Seed Filial Devotion Decoction)

Answers

1. A. During the acute stage:
- For heat wheezing, use *Dìng Chuăn Tāng* (Arrest Wheezing Decoction)
- For cold wheezing, use the combination of *Èr Chén Tāng* (Two Matured Substances Decoction) and *Sān Zĭ Yăng Qīn Tāng* (Three-Seed Filial Devotion

Decoction).

B. During the remission stage:

- For the lung deficiency, use *Yù Píng Fēng Săn* (*Yù Píng Fēng Săn*)
- For the spleen deficiency, use *Liù Jūn Zĭ Tāng* (Six Gentlemen Decoction)
- For the kidney deficiency, use *Jīn Guì Shèn Qì Wán* (Golden Cabinet's Kidney Qi Pill) or *Qī Wèi Dū Qì Wán* (Seven Ingredients for Restraining Qi Pill).

2. We recognize the symptom of wheezing while observing breath sounds which resemble a gurgling or stifling sound and occur repeatedly. The symptom of panting on the other hand refers to the act of taking repeated shallow breaths. Both symptoms can be seen in acute and chronic diseases of the respiratory system and both symptoms demonstrate a difficulty and shortness of breath; however, we will always show the sign of panting when there is wheezing, while panting is not necessarily accompanied by wheezing.

3. 1) The key clinical points or the treatment principle for treating chronic wheezing with internal phlegm retention is to reinforce the healthy qi and expel the pathogenic phlegm retention in the acute stage.

2) Another clinical key factor is to take notice of the seasonal and climate changes. For example, in the spring and autumn, tell your patient to avoid staying out in the wind or being exposed to many allergens. In the summer, take some health nourishing medicinals to avoid the acute stage of respiratory diseases in the winter. In the winter, stay warm and avoid being exposed to extreme cold for long periods of time.

3) Make it a good habit to have a healthy and appropriate diet. For infants who suffer from asthma, it is best to reduce the intake of protein. For elderly patients with respiratory diseases, avoid phlegm inducing foods such as fatty, sweet, artificially flavoured, sea food and acrid types of food. Additionally, take food which nourishes the lung and kidney according to the constitution of patient, such as ginkgo nut, ginseng, porridge, walnut and lotus nut.

4) Maintain a positive and healthy frame of thought and avoid extreme emotions especially anger and sadness. Encourage the patient to have a positive outlook during their recuperation stage.

5) Practice daily physical exercise to build the body's resistance to diseases and prevent from contracting a common cold. Recommend to your patient to practice soft physical activities such as *tai chi chuan*, *qi gong*, *ba gua zhang*, jogging, and walking. Also maintain a balanced schedule between work and rest to avoid overly exhausting the mind and the body.

4. 1) C, 2) E, 3) C, 4) D, 5) B, 6) B.

CASE STUDY 3: Bronchitis

Mr. Tang, male, age 60.

Main Complaint: Recurrent chronic cough and shortness of breath for over 30 years with a severe relapse in the last 7 days.

Medical History: The patient suffered from chronic bronchitis for more than 30 years, and he also had hypertension for 20 years. He caught a cold 7 days prior which triggered cough and panting with sticky, yellow and fish-smelling sputum which was difficult to expectorate. The patient also felt distending pain and heat sensation in the chest for over a week.

Presenting Symptoms: Cough with yellow and excessive sputum, panting, oppression and heat sensation in the chest, flushed face, profuse sweating, dry throat, thirst with desire for cold drinking, yellow urine, constipation, red tongue with yellow coating and a slippery and rapid pulse.

Physical Examination: Temperature: 37.0 ℃; pulse: 80 bpm; respiration: 22 bpm; blood pressure: 140/85 mmHg. The patient showed an active and conscious mind and was cooperative. The skin and sclera were non-icteric. No significant lymph nodes were enlarged. Scattered rhonchi and moist rales were heard at the base of the lung. There was no enlargement of the heart and there was a regular rhythm. No heart murmur was heard. The liver and spleen were not palpable. No percussion pain over the kidney area.

Other Medical Test Results:

Blood Routine Test: WBC 12.0×10^9/L.

Urine routine test: Normal.

Chest X-ray: Thickened and disarranged lung markings which are net-shaped, cord-like or spotted plaques.

Pattern Differentiation

Sticky smelly profuse phlegm from the lung as well as the yellow tongue coating are symptoms and signs which show that the cough in this case is due to phlegm-heat obstructing the lung qi. This phlegm-heat retention in the lung is causing failure of lung qi to perform its natural function of descending and opening manifesting as cough with massive sticky and yellow sputum. The symptoms of heat sensation and oppression in the chest are demonstrating that there is internal excessive heat retention in the chest. This heat is also causing the internal fluids to transform in thick phlegm which is difficult to expectorate giving it a strong fishy smell. This heat in the lung also burns up the natural body fluids which causes dryness and thirst with desire for cold drinks. If we further observe the red tongue with yellow coating as well as the slippery and rapid pulse we can confirm the internal retention of excessive phlegm-heat.

Diagnosis

TCM Diagnosis: Cough due to phlegm-heat obstructing the lung

Western Medicine Diagnosis: Chronic bronchitis with acute recurrence

Treatment

We need to treat this cough according to the presenting pattern.

Principles:

- Clear lung heat
- Dissolve phlegm and relieve panting

Formula: *Qīng Jīn Huà Tán Tāng* (Metal-Clearing and Phlegm-Transforming Decoction) recorded in *General Guideline of Formulas* (*Tǒng Zhǐ Fāng*, 统旨方).

Ingredients:

黄芩	*huáng qín*	12 g	Radix Scutellariae
山栀	*shān zhī*	12 g	Fructus Gardeniae
桔梗	*jié gěng*	10 g	Radix Platycodonis
麦冬	*mài dōng*	10 g	Radix Ophiopogonis
桑白皮	*sāng bái pí*	18 g	Cortex Mori
贝母	*bèi mǔ*	15 g	Bulbus Fritillaria
知母	*zhī mǔ*	10 g	Rhizoma Anemarrhenae
瓜蒌	*guā lóu*	10 g	Fructus Trichosanthis
橘红	*jú hóng*	10 g	Exocarpium Citri Rubrum
茯苓	*fú líng*	10 g	Poria
甘草	*gān cǎo*	6 g	Radix et Rhizoma Glycyrrhizae

Formula Analysis

Sāng bái pí, huáng qín, shān zhī, and *bèi mǔ* are included in the formula to clear lung heat. *Bèi mǔ, guā lóu* and *jié gěng* are used to clear lung heat and resolve phlegm to relieve cough. *Mài dōng, jú hóng, fú líng* and *gān cǎo* are used to nourish yin to clear the empty heat while resolving phlegm.

Follow-up Consultations

After 7 days of the treatment, the cough and panting were relieved and there was no more sputum. However, there were still some chest oppression and dry stools which indicated lingering internal phlegm-heat that blocked the natural movement of qi. The same formula was prescribed again to clear heat, dissolve phlegm and relieve cough. The patient was cured and there was no relapse within the following year.

Clinical Analysis

Chronic bronchitis is a long-term non-specific inflammation in the trachea, bronchial mucosa, and surrounding tissues. Its clinical manifestations are characterized by chronic cough with sputum production or shortness of breath. In Chinese medicine, it is classified in the cough and panting syndromes. The pattern differentiation of the bronchitis is also very similar to ones of cough and panting that include affliction of external or internal pathogens or can be due to internal damage of organs causing the failure of lung qi to diffuse and descend.

If we observe this case according to the philosophy of the *Treatise on Cold Damage*, we notice that the symptoms of cough with excessive sputum and spontaneous sweating demonstrate that the *Tai Yang* syndrome is effected. However, we also notice severe internal heat signs with the heat sensation in the chest, thirst with desire for cold drinks, yellow urine, constipation and rapid and slippery pulse. These symptoms are clear signs of internal *Yang Ming* heat. Clause 63 of the treatise on Cold Damage says: "After the promotion of sweat, one should not give *Guì Zhī Tāng* (Cinnamon Twig Decoction). If there is sweating and wheezing with no severe fever, one can give *Má Xìng Shí Gān Tāng* (Ephedra, Apricot Kernel, Gypsum and Licorice Decoction)". In this case, as a secondary option we can also consider using *Má Xìng Shí Gān Tāng* to treat this *Tai Yang Yang Ming* concurrent pattern. Since there is a clear presence of yellow and excessive sputum we can also add *Bàn Xià Hòu Pò Tāng* (Pinellia and Officinal Magnolia Bark Decoction) which is often clinically used for cough with sputum which is difficult to expectorate.

CLINICAL KEY POINTS

Externally contracted cough is usually easily treated, but if the treatment is delayed and incorrect, it can render weakness in the internal organs and create a deficiency causing the cough to linger or reoccur frequently and further damage the healthy qi. Cough due to internal damage is often a chronic disease and relapses often. As the pathogen is located in the deeper layers of the body, it is also comparatively more stubborn to treat. In case of elderly patients with productive cough, they usually have a prolonged illness which has impaired both the lung and spleen causing an internal retention of dampness and phlegm. Besides these main internal causes, chronic cough due to internal damage can also involve weakness of the kidney qi depletion which may result in phlegm stagnation, blood stasis, and water retention later developing into panting, dyspnea, lung distention, deficiency-consumption (*xū láo*, 虚劳) syndrome and so on. Consequently, the disease course becomes more complicated to treat.

BRIEF SUMMARY

Bronchitis is seen under the categories of cough and wheezing in Chinese medicine. To understand these symptoms fully, we need to comprehend the causes of the disease. The important pathomechanisms to understand are due to exogenous pathogens, internal excesses and internal damage. When cough and wheezing are due to exogenous pathogens, the pathogens create an excessive stagnation on the exterior layers of the body affecting the free flow of the *wei* qi and inhibiting the lung to freely disperse and descend. When cough and wheezing are due to internal excess of dampness and phlegm or phlegm-heat, the internal rheum prohibits the lung to perform the function of dispersing and descending causing the symptoms of cough, panting and wheezing. When patients suffer from a long standing disease or have a deficient constitution, there is an inner damage of organs which easily causes the symptoms of cough and wheezing when the lung, spleen and kidney are affected.

The general understanding for treating these symptoms is to open the lung, unblock qi, expel pathogens from the exterior layer for cough due to exogenous pathogens. As for cough due to internal damage, we need to fortify the lung, nourish the spleen and strengthen the kidney, clear liver heat, resolve phlegm and treat cough and wheezing.

COMPREHENSION QUESTIONS

1. What are the formulas for other patterns of this disease?
2. How to diagnose chronic bronchitis (cough due to internal damage)?
3. How do we differentiate "acute" from "chronic" bronchitis?
4. Multiple choice questions:

1) Mr. Wang, 35 years old. His symptoms are cough with sticky sputum which is difficult to expectorate, panting, fever, body ache, no sweating, dry mouth, red tongue with yellow coating and a floating rapid pulse. The primary formula for treatment is:

A. *Má Huáng Tāng* (Ephedra Decoction)
B. *Má Xìng Shí Gān Tāng* (Ephedra, Apricot Kernel, Gypsum and Licorice Decoction)
C. *Qīng Jīn Huà Tán Tāng* (Lung-Clearing and Phlegm-Transforming Decoction)
D. *Èr Chén Tāng* (Two Matured Substances Decoction) and *Sān Zǐ Yǎng Qín Tāng* (Three-Seed Filial Devotion Decoction)
E. *Bǔ Fèi Tāng* (Lung-Supplementing Decoction)

2) Ms. Han, 63 years old. Her symptoms are panting, shortness of breath, low voice, wheezing sound in the throat, cough in a low pitch, thin and loose sputum, spontaneous sweating, aversion to wind, extremely susceptible to catching a cold, pale red tongue, and soft and weak pulse. The primary treatment principle is to:

A. Diffuse the lung with acrid and cool medicinals, purge heat to calm panting
B. Dissolve phlegm and redirect the qi downward to treat panting
C. Supplement the lung qi and nourish yin to dissolve phlegm
D. Tonify kidney yang to improve the reception of qi and relieve panting
E. Diffuse the lung to treat panting, induce sweating to release the exterior

3) Ms. Tian, 47 years old. She suffered from a deep and harsh cough with profuse white sticky sputum for 7 years with panting, chest fullness and oppression, pale

tongue with a thick, greasy and white coating and a slippery pulse. The primary formula is:

A. *Jīn Guì Shèn Qì Wán* (Golden Cabinet's Kidney Qi Pill)
B. *Má Xìng Shí Gān Tāng* (Ephedra, Apricot Kernel, Gypsum and Licorice Decoction)
C. *Qīng Jīn Huà Tán Tāng* (Lung-Clearing and Phlegm-Transforming Decoction)
D. *Èr Chén Tāng* (Two Matured Substances Decoction) and *Sān Zĭ Yāng Qīn Tāng* (Three-Seed Filial Devotion Decoction)
E. *Bŭ Fèi Tāng* (Lung Supplementing Decoction)

4) Mr. Yi, 40 years old. His symptoms are cough with massive loose and white sputum, panting, shortness of breath, chest distention and oppression, headache, nasal congestion, sneezing, runny nose, no sweating with aversion to cold. The primary formula is:

A. *Má Huáng Tāng* (Ephedra Decoction)
B. *Má Xìng Shí Gān Tāng* (Ephedra, Apricot Kernel, Gypsum and Licorice Decoction)
C. *Jīn Guì Shèn Qì Wán* (Golden Cabinet's Kidney Qi Pill) and *Shēn Gé Tāng* (Ginseng and Gecko Decoction)
D. *Èr Chén Tāng* (Two Matured Substances Decoction) and *Sān Zĭ Yăng Qīn Tāng* (Three-Seed Filial Devotion Decoction)
E. *Bŭ Fèi Tāng* (Lung Supplementing Decoction)

5) Mr. Xia, 70 years old. His symptoms include dry cough, chronic panting with more expiration than inspiration, aggravated by exertion, emaciation, lethargy, occasional urinary incontinence due to severe cough, sweating, cold limbs, swelling lower limbs, pale tongue with a black and moist coating and a slightly thin pulse. The primary formula is:

A. *Qīng Jīn Huà Tán Tāng* (Lung-Clearing and Phlegm-Transforming Decoction)
B. *Má Xìng Shí Gān Tāng* (Ephedra, Apricot Kernel, Gypsum and Licorice Decoction)
C. *Jīn Guì Shèn Qì Wán* (Golden Cabinet's Kidney Qi Pill) and *Shēn Gé Tāng* (Ginseng and Gecko Decoction)
D. *Èr Chén Tāng* (Two Matured Substances Decoction) and *Sān Zĭ Yăng Qīn Tāng* (Three-Seed Filial Devotion Decoction)
E. *Bŭ Fèi Tāng* (Lung Supplementing Decoction)

Answers

1. There are various external and internal patterns to treat cough and panting. Here are a few of the commonly seen patterns with their primary treatment formula:

- For wind-cold obstructing the lung, we need to diffuse the lung to relieve panting and induce sweating to release the exterior with *Má Huáng Tāng* (Ephedra Decoction).

- For exterior cold affecting the *Tai Yang* syndrome with interior heat in the *Yang Ming* syndrome, we need to diffuse the lung with acrid and cool medicinals, and purge internal heat to relieve panting with *Má Xìng Shí Gān Tāng* (Ephedra, Apricot Kernel, Gypsum and Licorice Decoction).
- For phlegm-heat obstructing the lung, we need to clear lung heat and dissolve phlegm to relieve panting, and prescribe *Qīng Jīn Huà Tán Tāng* (Lung-Clearing and Phlegm-Transforming Decoction).
- For turbid phlegm obstructing the lung, we need to dissolve phlegm and redirect the qi downward to relieve panting with *Èr Chén Tāng* (Two Matured Substances Decoction) and *Sān Zǐ Yǎng Qīn Tāng* (Three-Seed Filial Devotion Decoction).
- For lung qi deficiency, we need to supplement the lung qi and nourish yin to dissolve phlegm with *Bǔ Fèi Tāng* (Lung Supplementing Decoction) in combination with *Yù Píng Fēng Sǎn* (Jade Wind-Barrier Powder).
- For spleen and kidney yang deficiency, we need to strengthen kidney yang to improve its function of reception of qi and relieve panting with *Jīn Guì Shèn Qì Wán* (Golden Cabinet's Kidney Qi Pill) in combination with *Shēn Gé Tāng* (Ginseng and Gecko Decoction).

2. There are many ways to diagnose chronic bronchitis. First, we can observe the symptoms of repeated occurrence of cough with sputum, panting, and chest oppression which have lasted over 3 months. Then, there will be signs of scattered rhonchi and moist rales at the lung base during acute episode. For asthmatic type of bronchitis there will also be wheezing sounds which can be heard after the cough or deep breaths and there will be wide-spread moist rales and wheezing sound during an acute onset. During the physical examination, we will notice thickened and disarranged lung markings, net-shaped or cord-like or spotted plaques on the lungs without any obvious abnormality seen in the chest X-ray.

3. To differentiate chronic bronchitis from the acute type, we need to take the following 3 characteristics into account:

A. Disease History: Acute bronchitis usually has no past history of bronchitis, cough with expectoration, or panting. However, chronic bronchitis has a history of the above 3 symptoms which have lasted over 3 months.

B. Course of disease and symptoms: The course of disease for acute bronchitis is very short and manifests as dry cough in the beginning while the presence of sticky or purulent sputum is often accompanied by oppression and pain behind the sternum and fever develops eventually. The general symptoms of acute bronchitis, such as fever, often reduce within 3 to 5 days, but the symptoms of cough with sputum will last for about 2 to 3 weeks before recovery. However, the course of disease in chronic bronchitis is characterized by long-standing and progressive recurrent cough with sputum with a history lasting from 3 months to many years.

C. The productive cough is relevant to the severity of the infection and can be either mild or severe and might be accompanied by panting. In addition, it is important to notice that chronic bronchitis is usually accompanied by obstructive emphysema which is not the case in acute bronchitis.

4. 1) B, 2) C, 3) D, 4) A, 5) C.

1.2 Sweating Syndrome

The symptoms of spontaneous sweating, night sweating, yellow sweat and lack of sweating are very interesting syndromes to analyze and understand in Chinese medicine. We have placed these sweating syndromes in the chapter of lung conditions. However, it is important to notice that sweating syndromes are not only associated to the disorder of the lung in Chinese medicine, but can also be caused by disorders of the liver, heart, spleen and kidney. If we observe etiopathologies of abnormal sweating we know that external contraction of pathogenic wind, cold or heat with a disharmony between *ying* and *wei* qi causing spontaneous sweating with fever and aversion to cold, heat sensation and floating pulse. If the sweating occurs frequently in the daytime regardless of environmental influence and aggravates after exertion, it is called spontaneous sweating and is normally caused by deficiency. If profuse sweating occurs during the night and stops after waking up, it is called night sweats and is normally due to yin deficiency or internal excessive heat. If we observe Western diseases related to the last two sweating disorders, we know that both spontaneous sweating and night sweats are commonly seen in diseases of hyperthyroidism, vegetative nerve functional disturbance, rheumatic fever, tuberculosis, menopausal syndrome and many more.

Chinese medicine philosophy categorizes "sweat" as the category of body fluids which has a close relationship to blood since they both have the same original source. Consequently, deficiency of one will cause deficiency of the other. Similarly, tonifying the blood will also increase the body fluids. There are both internal and external causes for the symptoms of pathological sweating which include disharmony between *ying* and *wei* qi, deficiency of *wei* qi due to lung qi deficiency, internal excessive heat and deficient fire raising due to kidney yin deficiency. We can classify the correct differentiation according to the presenting symptoms and the eight guiding principles.

Patterns commonly seen in clinical practice are following four types: lung-*wei* insecurity, disharmony between *ying* and *wei* qi, yin deficiency resulting in vigorous fire, and heat constraint and steaming.

CLINICAL PATTERNS DIFFERENTIATION AND TREATMENTS

1. Disharmony between *Ying* and *Wei*

Symptoms: Sweating with aversion to wind, general discomfort, headaches, alternating fever and chills, uni-lateral sweating or sweating from specific body parts, thin and white tongue coating and a floating and moderate pulse.

Treatment Principle:

- Harmonize the *ying* and *wei* qi
- Expel the pathogen in the external layer
- Strengthen the middle

Main Acupuncture Points:

- LI 4 (*hé gǔ*) and DU 14 (*dà zhuī*): To secure the exterior and regulate sweating
- KI 7 (*fù liū*): To treat febrile diseases and regulate fluid passages
- GB 12 (*wán gǔ*): To expel pathogenic wind and relieve headaches
- SP 6 (*sān yīn jiāo*): To nourish the *ying* qi and invigorate blood
- ST 36 (*zú sān lǐ*): To tonify the immune system and *wei* qi

Supporting Points:

- BL 12 (*fēng mén*): To tonify *wei* qi
- HT 6 (*yīn xì*): *Xi*-cleft point of the heart, to clear heat and calm the spirit

Recommended Formula: *Guì Zhī Tāng* (桂枝汤, Cinnamon Twig Decoction) from the *Treatise on Cold Damage* (*Shāng Hán Lùn*, 伤寒论)

Substitute Formula: *Guì Zhī Jiā Huáng Qí Tāng* (桂枝加黄芪汤, Cinnamon Twig Plus Astragalus Decoction)

2. Lung Qi Deficiency

Symptoms: Aversion to wind, spontaneous sweating, susceptible to contracting common colds, sallow complexion, poor appetite, thin white tongue coating and a thready and weak pulse.

Treatment Principle:

- Tonify lung qi
- Secure the exterior *wei* qi and arrest abnormal sweating

Main Acupuncture Points:

- DU 14 (*dà zhuī*): To secure the exterior and regulate sweating
- DU 20 (*bǎi huì*): To supplement and raise the qi
- LU 9 (*tài yuān*): *Yuan*-source point of the lung, to tonify lung qi and invigorate the spleen
- BL 12 (*fēng mén*): To tonify *wei* qi
- BL 13 (*fèi shù*): Back-*shu* point of the lung, to tonify lung qi and yin, release the exterior
- ST 36 (*zú sān lǐ*): To tonify the immune system and *wei* qi

Supporting Points:

- KI 1 (*yǒng quán*): To help anchor and strengthen inhalation
- BL 42 (*pò hù*): To tonify lung and nourish yin, alleviate cough and dyspnea
- EX-HN 15 (*jǐng bǎi láo*): To nourish lung qi and yin, relieve asthmatic and whooping cough with profuse phlegm

Recommended Formula: *Yù Píng Fēng Sǎn* (玉屏风散, Jade Wind-Barrier Powder) from the *Effective Formulas from Generations of Physicians* (*Shì Yī Dé Xiào Fāng*, 世医得效方)

Substitute Formula:

- *Mǔ Lì Sǎn* (牡蛎散, Oyster Shell Powder)
- *Shēng Mài Sǎn* (生脉散, Pulse-Engendering Powder)

Patent Formula: *Yù Píng Fēng Jiāo Náng* (玉屏风胶囊, Jade Wind-Barrier Capsule)

3. Heart Blood Deficiency

Symptoms: Spontaneous sweating or night sweats, palpitations, brittle hair and nails, poor sleep, fatigue, pale complexion, shortness of breath, palpitations, pale tongue body and wiry pulse.

Treatment Principle:

- Nourish the heart qi
- Tonify blood and arrest sweating

Main Acupuncture Points:

- LV 3 (*tài chōng*): *Yuan*-source point of the liver, to nourish blood and yin
- ST 36 (*zú sān lǐ*): To nourish blood and support the healthy qi
- BL 17 (*gé shù*): Influential point of the blood, to activate the blood circulation, dispel stasis
- BL 15 (*xīn shù*): Back-*shu* point of the heart, to nourish the heart and unbind the chest
- HT 3 (*shào hǎi*): *He*-sea point of the heart, to regulate the qi and calm the spirit
- HT 7 (*shén mén*): *Yuan*-source point of the heart, to regulate and tonify the heart's original qi

Supporting Points:

- EX-HN 3 (*yìn táng*) and EX-HN 24 (*ān mián*): To calm the mind and resolve insomnia
- SP 6 (*sān yīn jiāo*) and SP 8 (*dì jī*): To harmonize blood and resolve poor appetite

Recommended Formula: *Guī Pí Tāng* (归脾汤, Spleen-Restoring Decoction) from the *Formulas to Aid the Living* (*Jì Shēng Fāng*, 济生方)

Substitute Formula: *Shí Quán Dà Bǔ Tāng* (十全大补汤, Perfect Major Supplementation Decoction)

Patent Formula: *Guī Pí Wán* (归脾丸, Spleen-Restoring Pill)

4. Yin Deficiency with Empty Fire

Symptoms: Night sweats, irritability, heat sensation in the five centers, afternoon tidal fever, malar flush and thirst, red tongue body with a scanty coating and thready and rapid pulse.

Treatment Principle:

- Nourish yin and nourish body fluid
- Clear deficient fire and arrest abnormal sweating

Main Acupuncture Points:

- LI 6 (*piān lì*): *Luo*-connecting point of the large intestine, to clear heat and dredge the channel
- LV 3 (*tài chōng*): *Yuan*-source point of the liver, to clear fire, nourish yin and blood and treat insomnia
- KI 7 (*fù liū*): To regulate sweating and the fluid passages, clear deficient fire
- SP 6 (*sān yīn jiāo*): To nourish yin and invigorate blood
- KI 3 (*tài xí*): *Yuan*-source point of the kidney, to nourish yin and resolve insomnia
- HT 6 (*yīn xì*): *Xi*-cleft point of the heart, to clear heat and calm the spirit, alleviate night sweats and irritability
- BL 13 (*fèi shù*): Back-*shu* point of the lung, to nourish lung yin, clear heat and alleviate night sweats

Supporting Points:

- LU 5 (*chǐ zé*): To nourish lung yin
- BL 43 (*gāo huāng*): To nourish yin and resolve asthmatic cough

Recommended Formula: *Dāng Guī Liù Huáng Tāng* (当归六黄汤, Chinese Angelica Center-Fortifying Decoction) from the *Secrets from the Orchid Chamber* (*Lán Shì Mì Cáng*, 兰室秘藏)

Substitute Formula: *Liù Wèi Dì Huáng Tāng* (六味地黄汤, Six Ingredients Rehmannia Decoction)

Patent Formula: *Liù Wèi Dì Huáng Wán* (六味地黄丸, Six Ingredients Rehmannia Pill)

5. Accumulation of Excessive Heat

Symptoms: Sticky sweat, a red face, restlessness, a bitter taste in the mouth, dark yellow urine, thin and yellow tongue coating and a wiry and rapid pulse.

Treatment Principle:

- Clear heat and resolve dampness
- Harmonize the *ying* and *wei* qi

Main Acupuncture Points:

- LI 11 (*qū chí*): *He*-sea point of the large intestine, to clear damp-heat and cool blood, regulate qi and blood, reduce fever
- PC 6 (*nèi guān*): *Luo*-connecting point of the pericardium, to clear heat and regulate qi
- KI 7 (*fù liū*): To regulate night sweating and clear heat, resolve edema and regulate fluid passages
- ST 40 (*fēng lóng*): To clear damp-heat, nourish the spleen and calm the spirit
- BL 19 (*dǎn shù*): To resolve bitter taste in the mouth and expel damp-heat
- GB 20 (*fēng chí*): To clear heat, benefit the head and eyes
- LV 2 (*xíng jiān*): To clear liver fire and cool the blood

- GB 43 (*xiá xī*): To clear gallbladder damp-heat, alleviate headache

Supporting Points:

- ST 37: To clear intestinal damp-heat
- BL 28 : To clear damp-heat in the lower *jiao*

Recommended Formula: *Lóng Dǎn Xiè Gān Tāng* (龙胆泻肝汤, Gentian Liver-Draining Decoction) from the *Medical Formulas Collected and Analyzed* (*Yī Fāng Jí Jiě*, 医方集解)

Substitute Formula: *Bái Hǔ Tāng* (白虎汤, White Tiger Decoction)

Patent Formula: *Lóng Dǎn Xiè Gān Wán* (龙胆泻肝丸, Gentian Liver-Draining Pill)

Summary Chart for Sweating Disorders

External Patterns	Main Points	Supporting Points	Formulae
Disharmony Between *Ying* and *Wei*	LI 4, DU 14, KI 7, GB 12, SP 6, ST 36	BL 12 for *wei* qi insufficiency HT 6 for night sweats	*Guì Zhī Tāng* or *Guì Zhī Jiā Huáng Qí Tāng*
Lung Qi Deficiency	DU 14, DU 20, LU 9, BL 12, BL 13, ST 36	KI 1 for difficult inhalation BL 42 for cough and dyspnea EX-HN 15 for asthma and cough with phlegm	*Yù Píng Fēng Sǎn*
Heart Blood Deficiency	LV 3, ST 36, BL 17, BL 15, HT 3, HT 7	EX-HN 3, EX-HN 24 for insomnia SP 6, SP 8 for poor appetite	*Guī Pí Tāng* or *Shí Quán Dà Bǔ Tāng*
Yin Deficiency with Empty Fire	LI 6, LV 3, KI 7, SP 6, KI 3, HT 6, BL 13	LU 5 for lung yin deficiency BL 43 for yin deficiency with asthmatic cough	*Dāng Guī Liù Huáng Tāng* or *Liù Wèi Dì Huáng Wán*
Accumulation of Excessive Heat	LI 11, PC 6, KI 7, ST 40, BL 19, GB 20, LV 2, GB 43	ST 37 for intestinal damp-heat BL 28 for damp-heat in the lower *jiao*	*Lóng Dǎn Xiè Gān Tāng* or *Bái Hǔ Tāng*

CASE STUDY 1: Spontaneous Sweating
By Dr. He Ming-jing

Ms. Li, 30 years old, 1st consultation on November 8th, 1996.

Main Complaint: Frequent spontaneous sweating for 2 weeks.

Medical History: The patient experienced general weakness, fatigue, shortness of breath and easily contracted common cold since she had an abortion 5 years prior. Three weeks prior to consultation, she caught a cold with symptoms of headache, fever, aversion to cold, and nasal congestion.

Presenting Symptoms: The symptoms of headache and nasal congestion were gone within a week with medication, but the profuse sweating persisted and occurred frequently though the weather was not hot. She also had a slight aversion to wind, slightly pale complexion and emaciation.

Tongue and Pulse: The patient had a pale tongue and a weak pulse.

Pattern Differentiation

The chief complaint of the patient is spontaneous sweating that is more often in the day than the night. According to her medical history, the patient has lost a considerable amount of qi, blood and essence during her abortion causing a residual weakness and deficiency of the constitution presenting shortness of breath, lack of strength, prone to contracting a common cold and weakness of the *wei* qi to consolidate the exterior causing the spontaneous sweating. Recently an external contraction of pathogenic cold on the exterior layer shown in the symptoms of headache, fever, aversion to cold and nasal congestion has further damaged her lung qi and caused a disharmony between *ying* and *wei* qi. The depletion of lung qi has caused a severe depletion of *wei* qi causing the symptoms of spontaneous sweating and aversion to wind.

Diagnosis

TCM Diagnosis: Spontaneous sweating due to disharmony between *ying* and *wei* qi

Western Medicine Diagnosis: Abnormal sweating

Treatment

The pathomechanism of the spontaneous sweating in this case is due to a deficiency of qi combined with a disharmony between *ying* and *wei* qi.

Principles:

- Harmonize *ying* and *wei* qi
- Strengthen qi and consolidate the exterior

Formula: Modified *Guì Zhī Tāng* (Cinnamon Twig Decoction)

Ingredients:

桂枝	*guì zhī*	20 g	Ramulus Cinnamomi
白芍	*bái sháo*	20 g	Radix Paeoniae Alba
生姜	*shēng jiāng*	3 pieces	Rhizoma Zingiberis Recens
浮小麦	*fú xiǎo mài*	15 g	Fructus Tritici Levis
大枣	*dà zǎo*	5 pieces	Fructus Jujubae
麻黄根	*má huáng gēn*	15 g	Radix et Rhizoma Ephedrae
黄芪	*huáng qí*	15 g	Radix Astragali
炙甘草	*zhì gān cǎo*	10 g	Radix et Rhizoma Glycyrrhizae Praeparata cum Melle

Formula Analysis

In the formula, *guì zhī* is the chief medicinal and releases the exterior layer, scatters the exterior wind and dissipates cold. *Bái sháo* supplements yin and astringes to arrest sweating. The combination of *guì zhī* and *bái sháo* harmonizes *ying* and *wei* levels.

Huáng qí supplements lung and *wei* qi, strengthens qi and secures the exterior. *Fú xiăo mài* and *má huáng gēn* astringe to arrest sweating. These three ingredients serve as deputy medicinals.

Shēng jiāng is acrid and warm and assists *guì zhī* in releasing the exterior layer while warming the stomach to stop nausea. *Dà zăo* is sweet and neutral and can strengthen qi and fortify the middle *jiao*. They are considered assistant medicinals in this formula.

Zhì gān căo is an assistant and envoy medicinal and strengthens qi and harmonizes the middle. Combined with *guì zhī* it can release the exterior layer and combines with *bái sháo* to nourish yin.

As a whole, this formula serves to harmonize the *ying* and *wei* levels, secure the exterior layer and arrest sweating.

Follow-up Consultations

After taking 3 days of the formula, the spontaneous sweating and aversion to cold resolved. A modified *Yù Píng Fēng Săn* (Jade Wind-Barrier Powder) was administrated for one more week to strengthen the lung qi and consolidate the treatment to prevent a reoccurrence of the external contraction of pathogens.

The ingredients and dosages of the formula given are:

黄芪	*huáng qí*	25 g	Radix Astragali
白术	*bái zhú*	15 g	Rhizoma Atractylodis Macrocephalae
防风	*fáng fēng*	10 g	Radix Saposhnikoviae
浮小麦	*fú xiăo mài*	15 g	Fructus Tritici Levis
党参	*dăng shēn*	15 g	Radix Codonopsis
饴糖	*yí táng*	15 g	Saccharum Granorum
炙甘草	*zhì gān căo*	10 g	Radix et Rhizoma Glycyrrhizae Praeparata cum Melle

Clinical Analysis

In clause 12 of the Treatise on Cold Damage, it reads: "*Tai Yang Zhong Feng* (wind strike), the yang is floating and the yin is weak. When the yang is floating, there is spontaneous heat; when the yin is weak, there is spontaneous sweating. [In case of] chills with aversion to cold, aversion to wind, intermittent heat sensation, with snuffling nose and dry vomiting, use *Guì Zhī Tāng* (Cinnamon Twig Decoction)." This clause illustrates the symptoms demonstrated in a *Tai Yang Zhong Feng* pattern when the exterior layer is weak and the *wei* qi is not consolidating the exterior and the pathogenic cold is able to enter the external layer. At that time the healthy qi tries to contract with the pathogen causing spontaneous sweating and aversion to wind. In this clause the "yin" refers to the body fluids. By nourishing the healthy qi and releasing the exterior pathogen while consolidating the exterior layer the patient recovered in 3 days. Because of the long standing history of weakness and shortness of breath due to lung qi deficiency the formula *Yù Píng Fēng Săn* (Jade Wind-Barrier Powder) was given to strengthen the lung qi and facilitate breathing.

CASE STUDY 2: Chronic Abnormal Sweating
By Dr. Zhang Qi

Mr. Li, 23 years old. 1st consultation on March 6th, 1980.

Medical History: The patient suffered from spontaneous sweating for over a year which triggered when nervous. Other symptoms included dizziness, restless and dreamful sleep and forgetfulness. It was diagnosed with vegetative nerve functional disturbance and was prescribed diazepam and oryzanol which did not alleviate the symptoms.

Presenting Symptoms: Continuous and persistent sweating especially at the head and face. The patient also suffered from vertigo, weakness and lethargy. He once had taken *Chái Hú Jiā Lóng Gŭ Mŭ Lì Tāng* (Bupleurum Decoction With Keel and Oyster Shell) with *huáng qí* for 8 days which slightly relieved the dizziness but sweating remained the same. The patient felt irritable and helpless. With careful observation, the doctor noticed there was a cold sensation of the body together with constant trembling of the four extremities.

Tongue and Pulse: His tongue was pale with a white coating, and he had a slippery and deep pulse.

Diagnosis

TCM diagnosis: Spontaneous sweating due to yang and *wei* qi deficiency

Western medicine diagnosis: Vegetative nerve functional disturbance

Treatment

This is a case of spontaneous sweating due to *wei* qi deficiency and yang depletion. The chronic yang depletion has affected the exterior *wei* qi layer which is incapable to secure the exterior and astringe the body fluid causing spontaneous sweating.

Principles:

- Warm yang and tonify qi
- Harmonize *ying* and *wei* levels
- Secure the exterior and arrest sweating

Formula: Modified *Guì Zhī Jiā Lóng Gŭ Mŭ Lì Tāng* (桂枝加龙骨牡蛎汤, Cinnamon Twig Decoction With Keel and Oyster Shell)

Ingredients:

桂枝	*guì zhī*	20 g	Ramulus Cinnamomi

白芍	*bái sháo*	20 g	Radix Paeoniae Alba
甘草	*gān cǎo*	10 g	Radix et Rhizoma Glycyrrhizae
大枣	*dà zǎo*	5 pieces	Fructus Jujubae
生姜	*shēng jiāng*	10 g	Rhizoma Zingiberis Recens
附子	*fù zǐ*	10 g	Radix Aconiti Lateralis Praeparata
龙骨	*lóng gǔ*	20 g (calcined)	Os Draconis
牡蛎	*mǔ lì*	20 g (calcined)	Concha Ostreae
麻黄根	*má huáng gēn*	15 g	Radix et Rhizoma Ephedrae
党参	*dǎng shēn*	15 g	Radix Codonopsis
黄芪	*huáng qí*	50 g	Radix Astragali
五味子	*wǔ wèi zǐ*	15 g	Fructus Schisandrae Chinensis

Follow-up Consultations

- 2nd consultation, May 8th

There was a significant reduction of the spontaneous sweating and dizziness and the patient had experienced more strength. However, the symptoms of cold and trembling extremities persisted. These changes indicated that the formula was appropriate. However, the remaining symptoms also indicated there was a severe yang deficiency, hence 15 g to 25 g of *fù zǐ* was added gradually to the original formula in a period of 20 days.

- 3rd consultation, June, 1st

The symptom of sweating was resolved and the extremities were warm. The sleep had improved and all the other symptoms were completely resolved. Another 10 doses of the same formula were prescribed to consolidate the treatment. Follow-up visits continued during the following year and the patient reported there was no reoccurrence of spontaneous sweating.

Clinical Analysis

Observing the medical history of this case, we see that the Western medication given to treat the previous diagnosis of vegetative nerve functional disturbance was ineffective. On the other hand, in the first prescription of the Chinese formula tending to the *ying* and *wei* disharmony with a deficiency of the exterior listed as a *Tai Yang Zhong Feng* pattern in the Treatise on Cold Damage Clause 13 listed as: "*Tai Yang* diseases, with headaches, fever, sweating, and aversion to wind, *Guì Zhī Tāng* governs." However when a *Guì Zhī Tāng* pattern presents itself with irritability, insomnia, and restlessness due to deficiency of body fluids we can apply the formula *Guì Zhī Jiā Lóng Gǔ Mǔ Lì Tāng* as it is listed in Clause 118 of the Treatise on Cold Damage. The medicinals *lóng gǔ* and *mǔ lì* are added to clear heat in the chest and calm the spirit as well as astringe the body fluid to prevent excessive sweating, which relieved both the sweating and dizziness symptoms. However, since there was a severe cold sensation and trembling of the extremities we needed to also add *fù zǐ* to support and warm the root yang.

The Inner Classic states "Yang circles in the exterior as the envoy of yin, while yin resides in the interior as the support of yang." If the yang qi in the *wei* level fails to secure the exterior, the yin qi in the *ying* level is unable to remain inside which manifests as profuse sweating. As the yang qi is deficient, it fails to reach the extremities and keep them warm which is reflected in the symptom of cold limbs. The deficiency of yang qi and loss of body fluids also lead to fatigue and lethargy as well as the trembling extremities. Clear yang qi failing to reach the upper parts of the body is seen in the symptom of headache and restlessness. Sweat is the fluid of heart and profuse sweating impairs the body fluids which results in empty heat causing insomnia and excessive dreaming. Therefore, administering a modified *Guì Zhī Jiā Lóng Gǔ Mǔ Lì Tāng* is effective in relieving the syndrome.

CLINICAL KEY POINTS

When we are faced with the sweating syndrome in clinic, it is important to begin by categorizing it between an excessive and deficient syndrome. If the sweating is aggravated by exertion it is generally a qi deficiency syndrome not securing the exterior while the body fluids leak outward. However, if the sweating occurs with fever and other severe heat sign we can categorize it in an excessive or deficient heat pattern. Furthermore, it is important to remember that if the sweating has occurred for a long period of time there will be deficiency of body fluid as well as some possible deficient heat symptoms that might need to be addressed. Long standing sweating might also cause deficiency of qi, blood, yin and yang. We need to address the syndrome correctly as listed above in the pattern differentiation as well as astringe body fluids and arrest sweating with medicinals such as *fú xiǎo mài* and *mǔ lì* added to the formula.

COMPREHENSION QUESTIONS

1. What are the different and common clinical presentations of spontaneous sweating and night sweat?

2. List the different syndromes of sweating accompanied by their corresponding treatment principles, representative formulas.

3. Multiple choice questions:

1) Ms. Zhang, 32 years old. The patient easily contracts common colds and presents with spontaneous sweating which worsens with exertion, aversion to wind, fatigue, weakness, lustreless complexion, thin and white tongue coating and a thin and feeble pulse.

The primary formula is:
A. *Yù Píng Fēng Săn* (Jade Wind-Barrier Powder)
B. *Dāng Guī Liù Huáng Tāng* (Chinese Angelica Six Yellow Decoction)
C. *Guì Zhī Tāng* (Cinnamon Twig Decoction)
D. *Liù Wèi Dì Huáng Wán* (Six-Ingredient Rehmannia Pill)

2) Mr. Li, 56 years old. The patient presents with excessive sweating at night which stops after waking up, hot sensation in the palms and soles, vexation, insomnia, red tongue with scanty coating, and a thin and rapid pulse. The diagnosis is:
A. Spontaneous sweating due to disharmony between *ying* and *wei* qi
B. Night sweats due to heart blood insufficiency
C. Night sweats due to yin deficiency resulting in empty fire
D. Night sweats due to excessive heat stagnation

Answers

1. The pathological symptoms of abnormal sweating are due to disharmony between *ying* and *wei* qi due to external or internal, deficiency or excessive syndromes. It is classified as spontaneous sweating when the sweating occurs frequently during the daytime and it is unrelated to the surrounding environment and aggravates with exertion. It is called night sweats when it happens at night and stops after waking up. Spontaneous sweating is usually due to deficiency of *wei* qi and night sweats belongs to yin deficiency and internal heat.

2. Abnormal sweating is mainly manifested as deficiency of the *wei* qi on the external layer causing profuse sweating and it is classified in various syndromes according to their clinical manifestations. In clinic, it can be seen as spontaneous sweating, night sweats, sweating with aversion to cold, deficient sweating and yellow sweat. It can either be deficient or excess and it is closely related to the lung, heart and kidney. The various syndrome and treatment approaches are listed as:

- Disharmony between *ying* and *wei* qi treated by harmonizing the *ying-wei* with the recommended formula *Guì Zhī Tāng* (Cinnamon Twig Decoction);
- Deficiency of lung qi treated by tonifying lung qi to consolidate the exterior with the recommended formula *Yù Píng Fēng Săn* (Jade Wind-Barrier Powder);
- Heart blood deficiency treated by nourishing blood and strengthening heart and spleen qi with the recommended formula *Guī Pí Tāng* (Spleen-Restoring Decoction);
- Yin deficiency with empty fire treated by nourishing yin and subduing fire with the recommended formula *Dāng Guī Liù Huáng Tāng* (Chinese Angelica Six Yellow Decoction);
- Accumulation of excessive heat treated by clearing the liver and purging heat, removing dampness and harmonizing *ying* level with *Lóng Dăn Xiè Gān Tāng* (Gentian Liver-Draining Decoction).

3. 1) A, 2) C.

1.3 *Xiāo Kě* Disorder

Xiāo kě (消渴) is mainly translated as "wasting and thirsting disorder" in English and it is characterized by excessive thirst and hunger that is not satisfied by eating and drinking, profuse urine, or turbid urine with sweet taste and emaciation. It is usually a chronic syndrome which occurs predominantly among people above 40 years old. In Western medicine, it is usually attributed to diabetes.

The major etiology of *xiāo kě* is yin deficiency with pathogenic dryness and heat in the beginning stage, while the later stages include blood stasis and yang deficiency. The main pathomechanism of *xiāo kě* can be categorized by syndrome affecting upper, middle or lower *jiao*. *Xiāo kě* affecting the upper *jiao* is the excessive pathogenic factor of dryness and heat attacking the lung causing dry mouth, vexation and frequent and profuse urination. *Xiāo kě* affecting the middle *jiao* is the excessive pathogenic heat in the stomach manifesting as severe and urgent hunger. *Xiāo kě* affecting the lower *jiao* manifests as kidney yin, yang and essence deficiency manifesting as weakness and soreness of the lumbar and knees, insomnia and fatigue. Simultaneous occurrence of lung dryness, stomach heat and kidney deficiency is also possible. The treatment principle is to clear heat and moisten dryness, nourish yin and promote fluid production. At the later stages, the treatment will also need to move blood stasis and nourish yang and essence.

CLINICAL PATTERNS DIFFERENTIATION AND TREATMENTS

1. Dry Heat in the Lung

Symptoms: Excessive thirst with a strong desire for drinking large amount of water, drinking does not relieve the thirst, dry mouth and tongue, profuse and frequent urination, restlessness, a red tongue with a thin and yellow coating and a surging and rapid pulse.

Treatment Principle:

- Clear heat and nourish body fluid
- Nourish the lung and calm the spirit

Main Acupuncture Points:

- RN 12 (*zhōng wǎn*): To invigorate the spleen and harmonize the stomach
- LU 5 (*chǐ zé*): *He*-sea point of the lung to clear heat and regulate fluids
- ST 36 (*zú sān lǐ*): To tonify the spleen and nourish the healthy qi

• PC 6 (*nèi guān*): *Luo*-connecting point of the pericardium to regulate the heart, unbind the chest and treat heart pain

• LU 11 (*shào shāng*): To revive consciousness, clear heat, relieve sore throat

• SP 6 (*sān yīn jiāo*): To invigorate spleen, liver and kidney, tonify yin and harmonize lower *jiao*

• LI 11 (*qū chí*): *He*-sea point of the large intestine, to resolve stagnation, expel dampness, alleviate diarrhea and stop pain

Supporting Points:

• LU 7 (*liè quē*): Confluent point of the *ren mai* to harmonize *ren mai* and unbind the chest, regulate upper fluid passage, promote lung descending function, release exterior and expel wind

• HT 7 (*shén mén*): *Yuan*-source point of the heart to tonify the original qi of the heart, stop palpitations and calm the spirit

Recommended Formula: *Xiāo Kě Fāng* (消渴方, Consumptive Thirst Formula) from the *Teachings of [Zhu] Dan-xi* (*Dān Xī Xīn Fǎ*, 丹溪心法)

Substitute Formula: *Yù Yè Tāng* (玉液汤, Jade Humor Decoction)

Patent Formula: *Xiāo Kě Wán* (消渴丸, Diabetes-Relieving Pill)

2. Severe Heat in the Stomach

Symptoms: Hunger soon after eating, even after overeating, weight loss, dry stool, a red tongue with a yellow coating and a rapid and surging pulse.

Treatment Principle:

• Clear stomach fire and nourish body fluid

• Nourish essence and expel stool

Main Acupuncture Points:

• BL 21 (*wèi shù*): Back-*shu* point of the stomach to regulate digestion and harmonize the middle qi

• SP 6 (*sān yīn jiāo*): To nourish yin, invigorate blood, treat hypertension, insomnia and various gynaecological disorders

• ST 36 (*zú sān lǐ*): To tonify spleen, support the correct qi and tonify deficiency

• ST 34 (*liáng qiū*): *Xi*-cleft point of the stomach to harmonize the stomach and regulate the qi

• KI 6 (*zhào hǎi*): To clear deficient fire and regulate the *yin qiao* vessel

• PC 6 (*nèi guān*): *Luo* point of the pericardium to unbind the chest and calm the spirit

• SP 4 (*gōng sūn*): To invigorate spleen, harmonize middle *jiao* and regulate qi

Supporting Points:

• HT 9 (*shào chōng*): To clear heat, calm the spirit, stop heart pain, treat fever, stroke and loss of consciousness

• LI 11 (*qū chí*): *He*-sea point of the large intestine to resolve stagnation, expel dampness, alleviate diarrhea and stop pain

Recommended Formula: *Yù Nǚ Jiān* (玉女煎, Jade Lady Decoction) from *The Complete Works of [Zhang] Jing-yue* (*Jǐng Yuè Quán Shū*, 景岳全书)

Substitute Formula:

- *Bái Hǔ Jiā Rén Shēn Tāng* (白虎加人参汤, White Tiger Decoction Plus Ginseng)
- *Zēng Yè Chéng Qì Tāng* (增液承气汤, Fluid-Increasing and Qi-Guiding Decoction)

3. Deficiency Both Qi and Yin

Symptoms: Thirst and a large intake of fluids, simultaneous polyphagia and loose stool, fatigue, shortness of breath, dry red tongue, and fine rapid pulse without strength or weak pulse.

Treatment Principle:

- Replenish qi and nourish yin
- Promote fluid production and quench thirst

Main Acupuncture Points:

- BL 13 (*fèi shù*): Back-*shu* point of the lung to nourish lung, descend qi, release exterior, regulate sweating and harmonize breathing
- BL 20 (*pí shù*): Back-*shu* point of the spleen to regulate middle *jiao* qi, invigorate spleen, resolve hemoptysis
- BL 21 (*wèi shù*): Back-*shu* point of the stomach to regulate digestion and harmonize the middle qi
- BL 23 (*shèn shù*): Back-*shu* point of the kidney to benefit the original qi and kidney yin
- ST 44 (*nèi tíng*): To clear toxic heat and dampness, regulate *yangming* channels
- RN 6 (*qì hǎi*): To support the original qi, tonify kidney and treat general weakness
- RN 12 (*zhōng wǎn*): To regulate qi and invigorate spleen
- ST 36 (*zú sān lǐ*): To tonify spleen, support the correct qi and tonify deficiency
- KI 3 (*tài xī*): *Yuan*-source point of the kidney to nourish kidney yin and yang
- SP 6 (*sān yīn jiāo*): To nourish the yin, invigorate blood, treat hypertension, insomnia and various gynecological disorders

Supporting Points:

- SP 4 (*gōng sūn*): To invigorate spleen, harmonize middle *jiao* and regulate qi
- RN 4 (*guān yuán*): To tonify the original qi, nourish kidney, supplement deficiencies and treat general weakness

Recommended Formula: *Shēng Mài Yǐn* (生脉饮, Pulse-Engendering Beverage) from the *Important Formulas Worth a Thousand Gold Pieces for Emergency* (*Bèi Jí Qiān Jīn Yào Fāng*, 备急千金要方)

Substitute Formula:

- *Shēn Líng Bái Zhú Sǎn* (参苓白术散, Ginseng, Poria and Atractylodes Macrocephalae Powder)
- *Liù Wèi Dì Huáng Wán* (六味地黄丸, Six Ingredients Rehmannia Pill)

Patent Formula: *Shēng Mài Yǐn* (生脉饮, Pulse-Engendering Beverage)

4. Kidney Yin Deficiency

Symptoms: Frequent urination with profuse, thick turbid urine containing sugar, five-center heat, insomnia, dry mouth and lips, a red tongue with a scanty coating and a deep thready and rapid pulse.

Treatment Principle:

- Nourish kidney and supplement yin
- Clear empty fire and calm the spirit

Main Acupuncture Points:

- KI 3 (*tài xī*): *Yuan*-source point of the kidney to nourish kidney yin and yang
- HT 7 (*shén mén*): *Yuan*-source point of the heart to regulate and tonify the heart, stop heart pain and palpitations
- LV 3 (*tài chōng*): To relieve chest congestion and irritability
- BL 23 (*shèn shù*): Back-*shu* point of the kidney to benefit the original qi and kidney yin
- SP 6 (*sān yīn jiāo*): To nourish the yin, invigorate blood, treat hypertension, insomnia and various gynaecological disorders
- LI 3 (*sān jiān*) : To expel wind, clear heat, benefit the throat and teeth, dispel fullness, regulate qi of the large intestine and treat diarrhea

Supporting Points:

- PC 7 (*dà líng*): *Yuan*-source point of the pericardium to tonify heart qi and blood, promote circulation, unbind the chest and treat palpitations
- HT 5 (*tōng lǐ*): To treat heart pain with arrhythmia

Recommended Formula: *Liù Wèi Dì Huáng Wán* (六味地黄丸, Six Ingredients Rehmannia Pill) from the *Key to Diagnosis and Treatment of Children's Diseases* (*Xiǎo Ér Yào Zhèng Zhí Jué*, 小儿药证直诀)

Substitute Formula: *Dì Huáng Yǐn Zǐ* (地黄饮子, Rehmannia Drink)

Patent Formula: *Yù Quán Wán* (玉泉丸, Stream-Reducing Pill)

5. Kidney Yin and Yang Deficiency

Symptoms: Frequent urination with profuse, thick turbid urine containing glucose, dark complexion, dizziness, fatigue, lethargy, soreness and weakness of the lower back and knees, impotence, infertility, aversion to cold, cold limbs, a pale tongue with a white coating and a deep thready and weak pulse.

Treatment Principle:

- Tonify kidney yin and warm yang
- Strengthen spleen and nourish essence

Main acupuncture points:

- BL 20 (*pí shù*): Back-*shu* point of the spleen to regulate middle *jiao* qi, invigorate spleen, resolve hemoptysis

- RN 12 (*zhōng wǎn*): To regulate qi and invigorate spleen
- ST 36 (*zú sān lǐ*): To tonify the spleen, nourish the healthy qi, nourish blood and resolve insomnia
- KI 3 (*tài xī*): *Yuan*-source point of kidney to tonify spleen and kidney yin, clear deficient heat and resolve hemoptysis
- RN 4 (*guān yuán*): To tonify the original qi, nourish kidney, supplement deficiencies and treat general weakness
- DU 4 (*mìng mén*): To tonify kidney, regulate *du mai*, strengthen lumbar region, treat sexual dysfunction, secure essence and benefit lower limbs
- BL 23 (*shèn shù*): Back-*shu* point of the kidney to benefit the original qi and kidney yin

Supporting Points:

- SP 4 (*gōng sūn*): To harmonize the middle *jiao*, regulate the *chong* and *ren* vessels, regulate the qi and invigorate the spleen
- ST 25 (*tiān shū*): Front-*mu* point of the large intestine to regulate the intestines and invigorate the spleen

Recommended Formula: *Jīn Guì Shèn Qì Wán* (金匮肾气丸, Golden Cabinet's Kidney Qi Pill) from the *Essentials from the Golden Cabinet* (*Jīn Guì Yào Lüè*, 金匮要略)

Substitute Formula: *Yòu Guī Yǐn* (右归饮, Right-Restoring Drink)

Patent Formula: *Suō Quán Wán* (缩泉丸, Stream-Reducing Pill)

Summary Chart for *Xiāo Kě*

Patterns	Main Points	Supporting Points	Formulae
Dry Heat in the Lung	RN 12, LU 5, ST 36 PC 6, LU11, SP 6 LI 11	LU 7 for unbinding the chest and treating heart pain HT 7 for clearing heart heat	*Xiāo Kě Fāng* or *Yù Yè Tāng*
Severe Heat in the Stomach	BL 21, SP 6, ST 36 ST 34, KI 6, PC 6 SP 4	HT 9 for clearing heart heat and treat unconsciousness LI 11 for clearing heat in the large intestine	*Yù Nǚ Jiān* or *Bái Hǔ Jiā Rén Shēn Tāng* or *Zēng Yè Chéng Qì Tāng*
Deficiency Both Qi and Yin	BL 13, BL 20, BL 21, BL 23, ST 44, RN 6 RN 12, ST 36, KI 3, SP 6	SP 4 for fortifying spleen qi RN 4 for strengthening original qi	*Shēng Mài Yǐn* or *Shēn Líng Bái Zhú Sǎn* or *Liù Wèi Dì Huáng Wán*
Kidney Yin Deficiency	KI 3, HT 7, LV 3 BL 23, SP 6, LI 3	PC 7 for clearing heart heat and treating insomnia HT 5 for clearing heart heat and treating insomnia	*Liù Wèi Dì Huáng Wán* or *Dì Huáng Yǐn Zǐ*
Kidney Yin and Yang Deficiency	BL 20, RN 12, ST 36 KI 3, RN 4, DU 4 BL 23	SP 4 for fortifying spleen qi ST 25 for regulating the intestinal qi and moving stools	*Jīn Guì Shèn Qì Wán* or *Yòu Guī Yǐn*

CASE STUDY: Diabetes

Mr. Zhang, 53 years old.

Main Complaint: Thirst with excessive drinking and eating, profuse urine and weakness for over 3 years.

Medical History: The patient experienced severe thirst that could not be quenched by excessive drinking for 2 months, urgent hunger, frequent and profuse urination and weakness. His symptoms were slightly relieved by taking some Chinese medicinals. The patient took blood pressure medication for over 8 years. Three days ago, he drank a large amount of fluid which aggravated his symptoms. He had no history of externally-contracted febrile disease, diarrhea, vomiting and other internal diseases.

Presenting Symptoms: Severe thirst, excessive drinking, dry mouth, profuse urine, rapid digestion, mental fatigue, lack of strength, a red tongue tip and edges with a thin and yellow coating and thin and rapid pulse. He lost 6 kg in the past 2 months and had no lumbar and knee weakness, vertigo, tinnitus, aversion to cold or cold limbs.

Physical Examination: The patient was conscious and had red facial complexion, without abnormal findings in the heart and lung, the abdomen was flat and soft without tenderness and masses, and the liver and spleen could not be palpated below the ribs. There was an open and pus filled abscess on his back the size of 1 cm × 2 cm, which had not healed for a long time.

Laboratory Test: FBG 8.6 mmol/L, PBG 15.5 mmol/L (2 h after meals), Urine Glucose (+++), Urine Ketone (–).

Pattern Differentiation

These symptoms of thirst and excessive drinking with dry mouth, profuse urine, rapid digestion, red tongue tip and edges, thin and yellow coating, and rapid pulse belong to stomach heat impairing the body fluid demonstrating as *xiāo kě* syndrome of the upper and middle *jiao*. The lung governs qi and is the upper source of water, which distributes fluids though out the body. Due to the impairment of the lung by pathogenic dryness and heat, it fails to distribute the body fluid properly manifesting in the symptoms of severe thirst with excessive drinking. Since there is distribution disorder, the liquid moves downwards quickly and manifests as profuse urine. The *xiāo kě* syndrome of the middle *jiao* manifests as rapid digestion with urgent hunger and dry stool. This case does not demonstrate any *xiāo kě* of the lower *jiao*, since there is no lumbar and knee weakness, vertigo, and tinnitus.

This case is a combination of root yin deficiency with a pathogenic dry heat excess affecting both the upper and middle *jiao*. The pathogenic dry heat has entered the blood level causing blood heat and stasis binding with phlegm heat manifesting as the pus filled boil. In addition, since the qi and yin are impaired, the healthy qi fails to drain toxins and regenerate tissues, leading to delay in the healing.

Diagnosis

TCM Diagnosis: *Xiāo kě* of the upper and middle *jiao* due to lung and stomach dry and heat with qi deficiency and blood stasis

Western Medicine Diagnosis: Diabetes

Treatment

This is a case of *xiāo kě* of the upper and middle *jiao* affected with pathogenic dry and heat in the lung and stomach with qi deficiency and blood stasis.

Principles:

- Clear heat and resolve toxins
- Tonify qi and nourish yin
- Invigorate blood and unblock collaterals

Formula: Modified *Xiāo Kě Fāng* (Wasting-Thirst Formula), *Bái Hŭ Jiā Rén Shēn Tāng* (White Tiger Decoction plus Ginseng) combined with *Wŭ Wèi Xiāo Dú Yĭn* (Five Ingredients Toxin-Removing Beverage).

Ingredients:

天花粉	*tiān huā fěn*	15 g	Radix Trichosanthis
生地	*shēng dì*	15 g	Radix Rehmanniae
黄连	*huáng lián*	5 g	Rhizoma Coptidis
生石膏	*shí gāo*	15 g	Raw Gypsum Fibrosum
知母	*zhī mŭ*	10 g	Rhizoma Anemarrhenae
人参	*rén shēn*	5 g	Radix et Rhizoma Ginseng
桃仁	*táo rén*	10 g	Semen Persicae
金银花	*jīn yín huā*	10 g	Flos Lonicerae Japonicae
野菊花	*yě jú huā*	6 g	Flos Chrysanthemi Indici
紫花地丁	*zĭ huā dì dīng*	10 g	Herba Violae
玄参	*xuán shēn*	10 g	Radix Scrophulariae
天冬	*tiān dōng*	12 g	Radix Asparagi
麦冬	*mài dōng*	12 g	Radix Ophiopogonis
葛根	*gé gēn*	5 g	Radix Puerariae Lobatae
炙甘草	*zhì gān căo*	3 g	Radix et Rhizoma Glycyrrhizae Praeparata cum Melle

Formula Analysis

In this combined formula, *Xiāo Kě Fāng* (Wasting-Thirst Formula) can clear heat and promote body fluid, moisten the lung and quench thirst. *Bái Hŭ Jiā Rén Shēn Tāng* (White Tiger Decoction Plus Ginseng) combined with *gé gēn, mài dōng* and *xuán shēn* can boost qi, promote body fluid and quench thirst. *Wŭ Wèi Xiāo Dú Yĭn* (Five

Ingredients Toxin-Removing Beverage) can clear heat and resolve toxins, as well as dissipate abscess. *Táo rén* invigorates blood and resolves stasis. At the recovery stage of the abscess, it is important to drain toxin and regenerate tissues. Avoid overusing bitter and cold medicinals. As for boosting qi, avoid applying medicinals which are too warm and dry, such as *gān jiāng, bàn xià, guì zhī, xì xīn, má huáng,* and so on. This is to prevent further impairment of body fluid and worsening of the symptom.

Chinese Patent Medicines: *Xiāo Kě Wán* (Wasting-Thirst Pill), 10 pills were also given to the patient, half an hour before breakfast and dinner.

Follow-up Consultations

After taking 10 doses of the formula, the thirst reduced as well as the excessive drinking and eating and the urine also reduced. The blood glucose lowered to reach normal levels: FBG 6.5 mmol/L, PBG 11.3 mmol/L (2 h after meals).

KEY CLINICAL POINTS

1. *Xiāo Kě* syndrome is a severe condition which is commonly seen in clinic and normally affects middle aged and elderly people. The symptoms of excessive eating, drinking, profuse urine and emaciation are key symptoms to determine the severity of this disease. The prognosis will be favorable if the patient can begin appropriate treatment at an early stage, in addition to living a regular life style and diet. When children are affected by this syndrome, it usually stems from a congenital deficiency and proves to be more severe. Complications are very common in the syndrome since the healthy qi is very weak and other diseases are easily contracted and there is no defence mechanism of the body to counteract with the pathogenic factors.

2. A regular diet and controlling the amount of food and water intake can have a positive affect on this syndrome. Chinese medicine and acupuncture treatment can be used to supplement the healthy qi and reduce the pathogenic heat, stasis, dryness and phlegm.

3. Chronic cases of *xiāo kě* syndrome, such as diabetic retinopathy, cerebrovascular diseases, cardiovascular diseases, and renal diseases demonstrate blood stagnation and stasis. In these cases, it is important to promote blood circulation and remove blood stasis. The treatment must also take into account and protect the deficient root with medicinals, such as *dān shēn* (Radix et Rhizoma Salviae Miltiorrhizae), *chuān xiōng* (Rhizoma Chuanxiong), *yù jīn* (Radix Curcumae), *hóng huā* (Flos Carthami), *zé lán* (Herba Lycopi), *guǐ jiàn yǔ* (Ramulus Euonymi), and *shān zhā* (Fructus Crataegi).

BRIEF SUMMARY

The root of this case of *xiāo kě* syndrome is yin deficiency and its branch is pathogenic dryness and heat. At the initial stage, the pathogenic dryness and heat caused the symptoms of thirst and excessive hunger.

COMPREHENSION QUESTIONS

1. What is the etiology and pathomechanism of *xiāo kě*?
2. Multiple choice questions:

1) Which of the following symptoms is not a characteristic of *xiāo kě*?
A. Excessive drinking
B. Excessive eating
C. Profuse urine output
D. Profuse sweating
E. Emaciation

2) *Xiāo kě* mainly lies in following organs:
A. Lung, spleen and kidney
B. Lung, stomach and kidney
C. Heart, spleen and kidney
D. Liver, spleen and kidney
E. Heart, liver and kidney

3) The prominent symptoms of *xiāo kě* of the upper *jiao* are:
A. Lumbar and knee weakness
B. Rapid digestion with urgent hunger
C. Vexation, thirst and excessive drinking
D. Frequent and profuse urination
E. Turbid urine that is greasy

Answers

1. *Xiāo kě* is a disease with yin deficiency in chief and pathogenic dryness and heat as the branch. Manifestations of excessive thirst, hunger, profuse of yin deficiency and dryness-heat are often different in predominance due to the different disease course and disease severity. Generally, pathogenic dryness and heat retention is the main pathomechanism at the initial stage, while yin deficiency and blood stasis occur in the late stage. At later stage, there is yin and yang deficiency.

2. 1) D, 2) B, 3) C.

Part II
Heart Conditions

2.1 Chest *Bì* with Heart Pain

Chest *bì* with heart pain is a disease mainly manifesting as paroxysmal stuffiness, oppression and dull pain in the centre or the left side of the chest. In mild cases, these symptoms happen occasionally and last temporarily. In severe cases, the symptom of acute stabbing chest pain radiating down the left arm lasts for a long period of time sometimes accompanied by panting, restlessness, pale complexion, bluish lips, sweating, cold limbs, and extremely feeble pulse. These symptoms can be triggered by fatigue, cold weather and mental or emotional stress. However, in other cases, these symptoms arise at rest or during sleep especially in deficiency or elderly patients.

Chest pain is a symptom commonly seen in various coronary heart diseases. In Chinese medicine, we classified this symptom according to its accompanied signs and symptoms. When the chest pain presents in an acute situation there are signs of an excessive pattern which can be due to severe qi stagnation, cold retention, phlegm turbidity in the channels or blood stasis. However, in most cases of lingering chest pain, there is always an underlining deficiency of either the heart, liver, spleen and/or kidney. Other life habits and environmental stress can also increase the symptoms such as poor diet, excessive emotions and stress, internal invasion of excessive cold, overwork, trauma and excessive behaviour. All of these patterns and factors will obstruct the natural flow of chest yang qi and this stagnation causes local spasms and obstruction of the heart organ and channel.

The full etiopathology of chest *bì* is mainly due to a deficiency in the root with the presence of pathogenic excess in the branch, or simply said it is a combination of deficiency and excess. The presence of deficiency in the root causes the depletion of natural functions of the body due to deficiency of qi, yang, yin, blood causing the flow of qi to stagnate in the chest causing excessive chest pain and oppression and shortness of breath perceived as the excessive patterns.

The appropriate treatment protocol for one case will vary according to the stage of the disease. In acute stage, we will need to subdue the pathogenic factor and activate circulation of qi and move blood stasis. In the remission stage, we will need to nourish the deficiencies. Here is a summary list of the various patterns associated to chest *bì*, the most common pattern being heart qi deficiency.

CLINICAL PATTERNS DIFFERENTIATION AND TREATMENTS

1. Heart Blood Stasis

Symptoms: Chest and heart pain, stabbing pain often occurring at night with a fixed location, chest tightness, palpitations, restlessness, bluish lips, symptoms aggravated by anger and fatigue, a dark purple tongue with ecchymosis and a deep and choppy or knotted and intermittent pulse.

Treatment Principle:

- Activate blood and resolve stasis
- Dredge collaterals and stop chest pain

Main Acupuncture Points:

- HT 6 (*yīn xī*), PC 4 (*xī mén*): Both *xi*-cleft points to treat heart pain
- BL 15 (*xīn shù*): Back-*shu* point of the heart to treat heart pain and unbind the chest
- RN 14 (*jù què*): To treat chest and heart pain
- BL 17 (*gé shù*): Influential point of the blood to move blood to treat heart pain and palpitations
- RN 17 (*dàn zhōng*): Front-*mu* point of the pericardium to unbind the chest, treat palpitations and heart pain

Auricular Acupuncture Points: Heart, kidney, small intestine, sympathetic, *shen men*, subcortex, adrenal gland

Recommended Formula: *Táo Hóng Sì Wù Tāng* (桃红四物汤, Peach Kernel and Carthamus Four Substances Decoction) from the *Golden Mirror of the Medical Tradition* (*Yī Zōng Jīn Jiàn*, 医宗金鉴)

Substitute Formula:

- *Tōng Qiào Huó Xuè Tāng* (通窍活血汤, Orifice-Soothing and Blood-Activating Decoction)
- *Xuè Fǔ Zhú Yū Tāng* (血府逐瘀汤, Blood Stasis Expelling Decoction)

Patent Formula:

- *Fù Fāng Dān Shēn Dī Wán* (复方丹参滴丸, Compound Danshen Dropping Pills)
- *Sù Xiào Jiù Xīn Wán* (速效救心丸, Quick-Acting Pill for Heart Disease)
- *Tōng Xīn Luò Jiāo Náng* (通心络胶囊, Heart Collateral Unblocking Capsule)
- *Fù Fāng Dān Shēn Zhù Shè Yè* (复方丹参注射液, Compound Salvia Injection)
- *Chuān Xiōng Qín Zhù Shè Yè* (川芎嗪注射液, Ligustrazine Injection)

2. Cold Stagnation in the Chest

Symptoms: Sudden and sharp heart pain, chest pain radiating to the back, symptoms aggravated by exposure to cold, palpitations, shortness of breath, cold sensation of the body and limbs, spontaneous cold sweat, pale and white complexion, pale tongue with thin and white coating and a deep and tight or deep and thin pulse.

Treatment Principle:

- Warm yang and dissipate cold
- Promote free flow of heart yang

Main Acupuncture Points:

- BL 15 (*xīn shù*): Back-*shu* point of the heart to treat heart pain and unbind the chest
- BL 14 (*jué yīn shù*): Back-*shu* point of the pericardium to unbind the chest and treat heart pain
- PC 6 (*nèi guān*): *Luo*-connecting point of the pericardium to regulate the heart, unbind the chest and treat palpitations
- HT 5 (*tōng lǐ*): *Luo*-connecting point of the heart to treat heart pain
- RN 6 (*qì hǎi*): To fortify yang
- RN 4 (*guān yuán*): Front-*mu* point of the small intestine to regulate heart via small intestine

Recommended Formula: *Zhǐ Shí Xiè Bái Guì Zhī Tāng* (枳实薤白桂枝汤, Immature Bitter Orange, Chinese Chive and Cinnamon Twig Decoction) from the *Essentials from the Golden Cabinet* (*Jīn Guì Yào Lüè*, 金匮要略)

Substitute Formula:

- *Guā Lóu Xiè Bái Bái Jiǔ Tāng* (瓜蒌薤白白酒汤, Trichosanthes, Chinese Chive and White Wine Decoction)
- *Dāng Guī Sì Nì Tāng* (当归四逆汤, Chinese Angelica Frigid Extremities Decoction)

Patent Formula:

- *Guàn Xīn Sū Hé Wán* (冠心苏合丸, Storax Pill for Treating Coronary Heat Disease)
- *Sū Hé Xiāng Wán* (苏合香丸, Storax Pill)

3. Damp Phlegm Retention in the Chest

Symptoms: Chest tightness and suffocating heart pain, excessive phlegm, shortness of breath, heaviness of body and limbs, loss of appetite, nausea, obesity, fatigue, abdominal distention, loose stools, phlegm and sputum expectoration, pale and enlarged tongue with teeth marks and a greasy or white and slippery coating with a slippery pulse.

Treatment Principle:

- Activate and strengthen yang to expel dampness
- Resolve phlegm and unblock the channels
- Open the chest and stop pain

Main Acupuncture Points:

- RN 14 (*jù quē*): To treat chest and heart pain
- RN 17 (*dàn zhōng*): Influential point of the blood to treat heart pain
- PC 4 (*xī mén*): *Xi*-cleft point of the pericardium to treat heart pain

- ST 40 (*fēng lóng*): Main point for expelling phlegm and dampness from the lung, heart and chest
- LU 9 (*tài yuān*): *Yuan*-source point of the lung to nourish the lung qi and expel phlegm

Recommended Formula: Combine *Guā Lóu Xiè Bái Bàn Xià Tāng* (瓜蒌薤白半夏汤, Trichosanthes, Chinese Chive and Pinellia Decoction) from the *Essentials from the Golden Cabinet* (*Jīn Guì Yào Lüè*, 金匮要略) with *Dí Tán Tāng* (涤痰汤, Phlegm-Flushing Decoction) from the *Formulas to Aid the Living* (*Jì Shēng Fāng*, 济生方)

Substitute Formula: *Wēn Dǎn Tāng* (温胆汤, Gallbladder-Warming Decoction)

4. Qi and Blood Deficiency

Symptoms: Dull burning sensation in the chest and heart or sporadic chest stuffiness with convulsive palpitations, restlessness, insomnia, shortness of breath, symptoms aggravate with exertion, fatigue, dizziness, extremely pale complexion, spontaneous sweating, dry lips and mouth, red tongue with a thin dry coating with a choppy, empty and thin or thin and rapid pulse.

Treatment Principle:

- Tonify qi and nourish blood
- Invigorate qi and move blood
- Dredge collaterals and stop pain

Main Acupuncture Points:

- BL 15 (*xīn shù*): Back-*shu* point of the heart to treat heart pain and unbind the chest
- BL 17 (*gé shù*): Influential point of the blood to treat heart pain with palpitation
- BL 23 (*shèn shù*): Back-*shu* point of the kidney to benefit the original qi and kidney yin
- HT 6 (*yīn xì*): *Xi*-cleft point of the pericardium to treat heart pain
- HT 7 (*shén mén*): *Yuan*-source point of the heart to regulate and tonify the heart qi, stop heart pain and palpitation
- KI 3 (*tài xī*): *Yuan*-source point of the kidney to nourish kidney yin and yang
- SP 6 (*sān yīn jiāo*): To nourish the yin
- PC 6 (*nèi guān*): *Luo*-connecting point of the pericardium to regulate the heart, unbind the chest and treat palpitation and heart pain
- RN 17 (*dàn zhōng*): Front-*mu* point of the pericardium to unbind the chest and regulate qi, treat palpitation, irritability and heart pain

Recommended Formula: *Shēng Mài Sǎn* (生脉散, Pulse-Engendering Powder) from the *Origins of Medicine* (*Yī Xué Qǐ Yuán*, 医学启源)

Substitute Formula:

- *Rén Shēn Yǎng Yíng Tāng* (人参养营汤, Radix et Rhizoma Ginseng Tonify Decoction)
- *Tiān Wáng Bǔ Xīn Dān* (天王补心丹, Celestial Emperor Heart-Supplementing

Elixir)

Patent Formula: *Shēng Mài Yǐn* (生脉饮, Pulse-Engendering Beverage)

Summary Chart for Chest *Bì* with Heart Pain

Patterns	Main Points	Auricular Points	Formulae
Heart Blood Stasis	HT 6, PC 4, BL 15, RN 14, BL 17, RN 17	Heart, kidney, small intestine, sympathetic, *shen men*, subcortex, adrenal gland	*Táo Hóng Sì Wù Tāng*, *Tōng Qiào Huó Xuè Tāng* or *Xuè Fǔ Zhú Yū Tāng*
Cold Stagnation in the Chest	BL 15, BL 14, PC 6, HT 5, RN 6, RN 4	Heart, kidney, small intestine, sympathetic, *shen men*, subcortex, adrenal gland	*Zhǐ Shí Xiè Bái Guì Zhī Tāng*, *Guā Lóu Xiè Bái Bái Jiǔ Tāng* or *Dāng Guī Sì Nì Tāng*
Damp Phlegm Retention in the Chest	RN 14, RN 17, PC4, ST 40, LU 9	Heart, kidney, small intestine, sympathetic, *shen men*, subcortex, adrenal gland	Combine *Guā Lóu Xiè Bái Bàn Xià Tāng* with *Dí Tán Tāng* or *Wēn Dǎn Tāng*
Qi and Blood Deficiency	BL 15, BL 17, BL 23, HT6, HT 7, KI 3, PC 6, SP 6, RN 17	Heart, kidney, small intestine, sympathetic, *shen men*, subcortex, adrenal gland	*Shēng Mài Sǎn*, *Rén Shēn Yǎng Yíng Tāng* or *Tiān Wáng Bǔ Xīn Dān*

CASE STUDY 1: Angina Pectoris

Ms. Zhao, 65 years old.

Main Complaint: Repeated stabbing pain in the left aspect of the chest for 3 months with aggravated symptoms in the last 2 months.

Medical History: The patient has a history of hyperlipidemia. Three months ago, the patient suffered of left sided stabbing pain in the chest for 2 minutes induced by fatigue. The symptoms resolved themselves with rest and the patient did not receive treatments for her symptoms. The pain on the left aspect of the chest occurred 2 to 3 times each day in the past 2 months. She was hospitalized in an AAA hospital and was given various western medication (Isosorbide Dinitrate, Betaloc, Aspirin, Simvastatin, and Perindopril) which relieved the symptoms. Two days prior, she did a lot of housework and lifted heavy objects which triggered severe chest pain later diagnosed as angina pectoris.

Presenting Symptoms: Fixed stabbing pain in the left aspect of the chest that occurs after heavy physical labor lasting from 2 to 3 minutes accompanied by chest oppression, palpitations, feverish feeling in the palms and soles and dizziness.

Tongue and Pulse: Purple darkish tongue body with thin and white coating and a deep and wiry pulse.

Physical Examination: Temperature: 36.8℃, pulse: 78 bpm, respiration: 18 bpm, blood pressure: 130/76 mmHg.

The patient is mentally active and cooperative. The skin and sclera are non-icteric. No hemorrhagic spots, macules and papules. No lip cyanosis and no distended jugular veins. No enlarged lymph nodes are found. Clear breath sounds are heard bilaterally. There is no projection at the precordium, the cardiac exam is normal and grade 2-3/6 systolic murmur without conduction is present. No abnormal findings of the liver and spleen. No percussion tenderness over the renal region. Flat abdomen without mass or bloating. No pitting edema in the lower limbs.

Other Medical Test Results:

ECG: V1 - V5 ST segment depresses at least 0.05 mv, low and flat T wave shows myocardial ischemia.

Echo: artherosclerosis of the aorta caused a decreased function of the left ventricle.

Coronary Angiography: stenotic left anterior descending coronary artery at 65%.

Blood Fat: TRIG 2.3mmol/L, TC 5.67mmol/L, LDL 3.8mmol/L.

Pattern Differentiation

The patient is elderly with a weak constitution and *zang-fu* organs as well as a deficient heart qi. Therefore, the heart is too weak to promote blood flow leading to blood stasis obstructing the heart vessels. This blockage causes severe fixed stabbing pain in the chest. When the patient performs physical labor, she depletes her qi which further damages and weakens the heart qi triggering the acute chest pain. The blood stasis in the heart accompanied by the lack of nourishment is seen in the chest oppression and palpitation. If the blood stagnates for a long period of time new blood can not be produced resulting in blood depletion. The symptoms of feverish sensation in palms and soles, dizziness, purple darkish tongue, and deep and wiry pulse are all signs of internal retention of blood stasis and qi stagnation.

Diagnosis

TCM Diagnosis: Chest *bì* due to blood stasis in the heart and heart qi depletion

Western Medicine Diagnosis: Angina pectoris

Treatment

The main pathomechanism of this case is blood stasis and qi stagnation in the heart vessels causing the chest pain.

Principles:

- Invigorate blood and dissolve stasis
- Disperse obstruction and arrest pain
- Tonify qi and strengthen the heart

Formula: Modified *Xuè Fŭ Zhú Yū Tāng* (血府逐瘀汤, Blood Mansion Stasis-Expelling Decoction)

Ingredients:

当归	*dāng guī*	15 g	Radix Angelicae Sinensis
赤芍	*chì sháo*	10 g	Radix Paeoniae Rubra
川芎	*chuān xiōng*	15 g	Rhizoma Chuanxiong
桃仁	*táo rén*	5 g	Semen Persicae
红花	*hóng huā*	5 g	Flos Carthami
柴胡	*chái hú*	5 g	Radix Bupleuri
枳壳	*zhǐ qiào*	10 g	Fructus Aurantii
三七	*sān qī*	5 g	Radix et Rhizoma Notoginseng (powder)
生地	*shēng dì*	15 g	Radix Rehmanniae
川牛膝	*chuān niú xī*	15 g	Radix Cyathulae
蒲黄	*pú huáng*	15 g	Pollen Typhae

Formula Analysis

In the formula, *dāng guī, chì sháo, chuān xiōng, táo rén*, and *hóng huā* are used to unblock the heart vessels by invigorating blood and dispelling stasis. The combination of *chái hú, zhǐ qiào* and *chuān niú xī* can regulate the movement of qi and activates blood. *Tián qī* and *pú huáng* serve to dispel stasis and stop pain. *Shēng dì* cools blood and clears heat and, when combined with *dāng guī*, can dispel stasis without impairing blood. All ingredients combined can dissolve blood stasis, unblock heart vessels and nourish blood to treat chest oppression and heart pain.

Follow-up Consultations

After taking the formula for 14 days, the symptoms of chest oppression and heart pain were considerably reduced and there was no more insomnia. However, there were symptoms of abdominal distention and dry mouth showing signs of qi stagnation and internal fluid depletion so *chuān xiōng* was removed from the formula, while *yù zhú* (Rhizoma Polygonati Odorati) 15 g and *mù xiāng* (Radix Aucklandiae) 10 g were added. After another 14 doses of the modified formula, the symptoms of chest oppression and heart pain were completely resolved.

CASE STUDY 2: Chest Oppression

Mr. Zhang, 75 years old.

Main Complaint: Repeated left chest oppression and pain for 3 years with increased severity for 1 day.

Medical History: The patient began to experience left sided chest oppression and localized pain 3 years ago which lasted for about 1 minute and was relieved with rest. Later, the attacks became more severe and more frequent and could only be relieved by administrating sublingual nitroglycerin, or nifedipine. Coronary angiography demonstrated the patient had angina pectoris. At present, the patient is mainly treated with Elantan and Betaloc. He experienced left sided chest oppression and pain twice on the day of the consultation with accompanied dizziness and back distention. The patient particularly enjoys fatty, sweet, and heavy flavored food.

Presenting Symptoms: Left sided chest oppression and pain radiating to the back, nausea, dizziness, body heaviness, palpitations, shortness of breath, fatigue, lack of strength, sputum, numbness of the hands, obesity, pale tongue with thick and greasy coating and a slippery pulse.

Physical Examination: Temperature: 36.8 ℃, pulse: 82 bpm, respiration: 18 bpm, blood pressure: 138/86 mmHg, body weight: 75 kg.

The patient was mentally active and cooperative. The skin and sclera are non-icteric. No hemorrhagic spots, macules and papules. No lip cyanosis and no distended jugular veins. No enlarged lymph nodes are found. Clear breath sounds are heard bilaterally. There is no projection at the precordium, the cardiac exam is normal, regular rhythm, $A_2 > P_2$, and grade 3/6 systolic murmur can be heard at the apex region. The fourth heart sound conducting to the left armpit is present. No abnormal findings in the liver and spleen. No percussion tenderness over the renal region. Flat abdomen without shifting. No pitting edema in the lower limbs.

Other Medical Text Results:

ECG: V1 - V3 ST segment depresses 0.1 mv, low and flat T wave shows myocardial ischemia.

24h ECG: ST-T change indicates myocardial ischemia. There are altogether 862 times of ventricular premature beat. The fastest heart rate is 132 beats/min and the slowest 48 beats/min.

Echo: Sclerosis of the aorta, enlarged left atrium, and decreased function of the left ventricle.

Coronary Angiography: Stenotic left circumflex coronary artery at the centre for 75%.

Blood Fat: TRIG 2.3 mmol/L, TC 5.67 mmol/L, LDL 3.8 mmol/L.

Blood Sugar: 5.6 mmol/L.

Pattern Differentiation

The patient flavors having a diet composed of fatty, sweet and heavy flavored food which causes the failure of the spleen to transport the fluids and food while engendering phlegm-damp retention in the interior causing obesity. Phlegm is classified as a yin pathogen since it is heavy and sticky which obstructs the heart vessels and inhibits the movement of qi demonstrated in this patient as left sided chest oppression and pain. The collaterals of the heart are distributed on both shoulders and connect to the back-*shu* points. As the heart collaterals are blocked by phlegm turbidity, the pain radiates to the shoulders and upper back where the channels reach. If the phlegm turbidity affects the spleen, the stomach fails to harmonize and direct the qi downward, while the clear yang fails to ascend, resulting in body heaviness, nausea, dizziness, and excessive sputum. Qi deficiency of the heart and spleen accompanied by depletion of the heart vessels leads to symptoms of palpitations, shortness of breath, fatigue and lack of strength. The retention of phlegm obstructing the channels inhibits the natural flow of blood and manifest as numbness of the limbs. Pale tongue with a thick and greasy coating, and a slippery pulse confirming the internal obstruction of pathogenic phlegm.

Diagnosis

TCM Diagnosis: Chest *bì* due to internal obstruction of pathogenic phlegm

Western Medicine Diagnosis: Angina pectoris

Treatment

The main pathomechanism of this case is pathogenic phlegm obstructing the heart vessels accompanied by qi and blood stagnation.

Principles:

- Unblock yang and purge pathogen
- Dissolve phlegm and unblock collaterals
- Nourish heart and stop pain

Formula: Modified *Guā Lóu Xiè Bái Bàn Xià Tāng* (Trichosanthes, Chinese Chive and Pinellia Decoction).

Ingredients:

瓜蒌	*guā lóu*	15 g	Fructus Trichosanthis
薤白	*xiè bái*	10 g	Bulbus Allii Macrostemi
法半夏	*fǎ bàn xià*	10 g	Rhizoma Pinelliae Praeparatum
陈皮	*chén pí*	10 g	Pericarpium Citri Reticulatae
茯苓	*fú líng*	15 g	Poria
白术	*bái zhú*	15 g	dry-fried Rhizoma Atractylodis Macrocephalae
石菖蒲	*shí chāng pú*	15 g	Rhizoma Acori Tatarinowii
郁金	*yù jīn*	15 g	Radix Curcumae
丹参	*dān shēn*	15 g	Radix et Rhizoma Salviae Miltiorrhizae
川芎	*chuān xiōng*	15 g	Rhizoma Chuanxiong
枳壳	*zhǐ qiào*	10 g	Fructus Aurantii

Formula Analysis

In this formula, *guā lóu* is used to open the chest, dissipate masses and dissolve phlegm. *Xiè bái* is acrid and warm and it is used to unblock yang, dissipate masses, eliminate phlegm, and descend qi. *Bàn xià, chén pí* and *zhǐ qiào* are combined to dissolve phlegm and rectify qi. *Bái zhú* and *fú líng* strengthen the effect of fortifying spleen and dissolving phlegm. *Yù jīn, dān shēn* and *chuān xiōng* are added to invigorate blood, dissolve stasis and unblock collaterals. All the ingredients act together to unblock yang in the chest area and dissolve phlegm, dissipate masses and stop chest pain.

Follow-up Consultations

On the 2nd consultation, after taking 7 doses of the formula, the symptoms of chest oppression and pain occurred once or twice a week, the expectoration and nausea disappeared, but there were still signs of phlegm obstruction transforming into heat, such as dry mouth, bitter taste in the mouth, and yellow tongue coating. According to the changes in symptoms, *huáng qín* (Radix Scutellariae) 10 g and *zhú rú* (Caulis Bambusae in Taenia) 10 g were added to the previous formula to dissolve phlegm heat.

On the 3rd consultation, after taking 14 doses of the above formula, the symptoms of chest oppression and pain were completely resolved.

Clinical Analysis

In this case, as the patient is elderly, we would expect a deficiency pattern. The signs and symptoms of excessive sputum, thick greasy tongue coating illustrate severe pathogenic phlegm in the chest area. The formula *Guā Lóu Xiè Bái Bàn Xià Tāng* (Trichosanthes, Chinese Chive and Pinellia Decoction) was first recorded in the *Essentials from the Golden Cabinet* (*Jīn Guì Yào Lüè*) in the Chapter of *Chest Bì, Heart Pain and Shortness of Breath*, Line 4 which states: "For chest *bì* manifesting with the inability to lie down, and heart pain pulling to the back, *Guā Lóu Xiè Bái Bàn Xià Tāng* is indicated." Originally, this formula is composed of three medicinals *guā lóu, xiè bái* and *bàn xià* which are prepared in wine to increase the blood flow and remove pain. This formula is used to treat excessive retention of pathogenic phlegm upsurging and affecting the chest causing chest oppression and pain with the inability of lying down. *Guā lóu* and *xiè bái* unblock the yang qi in the chest and open the chest while *bàn xià* warms the centre and increases the function of expelling phlegm of the other two medicinals. This formula pattern is commonly used for a *taiyin* syndrome pattern affecting the upper and chest area with excessive sputum. It can be combined with other phlegm relieving formulas such as *Èr Chén Tāng* (二陈汤, Two Matured Substances Decoction) or *Dí Tán Tāng* (涤痰汤, Phlegm-Flushing Decoction) when there is presence of excessive phlegm to dredge the pathogenic phlegm and fortify the spleen.

CLINICAL KEY POINTS

The pattern differentiation of chest *bì* is primary characterized by the nature of pain in the chest. Chest *bì* due to excessive pattern can be seen as stabbing chest pain caused by blood stasis, colic chest pain due to yang deficiency and cold retention, oppressive chest and rib-side pain with frequent sighing resulting from qi stagnation, chest pain presenting with excessive sputum and a greasy tongue coating belonging to pathogenic phlegm retention in the chest. Chest *bì* due to a deficiency pattern can be seen as dull pain with shortness of breath and malar flush caused by qi and blood deficiency. As mentioned before the disease pattern usually presents with a combination of deficiency in the root and excess in the branch.

Furthermore, the acute and severe cases of chest *bì* need to be addressed appropriately. If the chest pain does not relieve or aggravates with the treatment, or if it is a very severe case, we need to seek emergency care by taking sublingual nitroglycerin or similar treatment immediately. However, if the pain gradually decreases and the tongue coating changes from thick to thin then we can continue the treatment and expect a positive prognosis. In some cases, we need to consider taking both western and Chinese medication at the same time.

CASE STUDY 3: Chronic Chest Oppression and Pain

Mr. Chen, 43 years old. Hospitalized on December 5th, 2000.

Main Complaint: Repeated chest oppression and pain for 3 months, increasing during the last day.

Medical History: The patient experienced chest oppression and pain 3 months ago which was diagnosed as coronary heart disease and given an angioplasty to add a stent. All symptoms relieved after the surgery. Yesterday, the patient suffered from chest oppression and lack of strength. As there was no efficacy from taking Isosorbide Mononitrate, he was hospitalized.

The patient was suffering from mental fatigue, shortness of breath, oppressive pain in the chest, mental confusion, easily woken up and was diagnosed with qi and yin depletion. The patient was given Chinese medicinals to tonify qi and nourish yin, and Western medicine was used to dilate coronary vessels, reduce coagulation and control the symptoms. However, after more than 10 days of these treatments, there was no improvement. The patient refused to have a coronal artery angiography. Therefore, he was asked to consult Dr. Deng Tie-tao.

Presenting Symptoms: Mental fatigue, shortness of breath, oppressive pain in the chest, mental confusion, restless sleep, poor appetite, pale red tongue with thin and white coating and a deficient pulse which is floating in the *guān* position.

Diagnosis

TCM Diagnosis: chest *bì* due to deficiency of both qi and yin with phlegm obstructing the collaterals

Western Medicine Diagnosis: Angina pectoris, type 2 diabetes and hyperlipemia.

Treatment

The main pathomechanism of this case is deficiency of both qi and yin which fails to nourish the heart as well as retention of pathogenic phlegm that obstructs the collaterals and inhibits heart vessels.

Principles:

- Tonify qi and nourish yin
- Invigorate blood and dredge channel
- Nourish spleen and resolve phlegm

Ingredients:

党参	*dǎng shēn*	24 g	Radix Codonopsis
黄芪	*huáng qí*	30 g	Radix Astragali
玉米须	*yù mǐ xū*	30 g	Stigma Maydis
桑寄生	*sāng jì shēng*	30 g	Herba Taxilli
山药	*shān yào*	30 g	Rhizoma Dioscoreae
茯苓	*fú líng*	15 g	Poria
白术	*bái zhú*	15 g	Rhizoma Atractylodis Macrocephalae
三七	*sān qī*	3 g	Radix et Rhizoma Notoginseng (powder infused)
炙甘草	*zhì gān cǎo*	3 g	Radix et Rhizoma Glycyrrhizae Praeparata cum Melle
枳壳	*zhǐ qiào*	6 g	Fructus Aurantii
化橘红	*huà jú hóng*	6 g	Exocarpium Citri Grandis

Follow-up Consultations

2nd consultation, on December 30th.

After taking 7 days of this formula, the chest oppression and pain were slightly alleviated and there was improvement in the mental state. The tongue was tender and light red with a thin and slightly yellow coating and the pulse was deficient. These signs demonstrated qi deficiency of both the heart and spleen leading to the retention of turbid phlegm, so it should be treated by fortifying the heart and spleen and dissolving the phlegm by adding 50 g of *wǔ zhuǎ lóng* (Herba Iponoeae) and 10 g of *zhú rú* (Caulis Bambusae in Taenia).

3rd consultation, on January 6th.

All symptoms were completely relieved and the patient was discharged from the hospital. He continued to take prescribed medication from Dr. Deng Tie-tao and there were no relapse of the chest oppression and pain.

BRIEF SUMMARY

Clearly identifying the pathological causes of chest *bì* is primordial to be able to decide on an effective treatment approach whether we are providing acupuncture or Chinese medicinals. Since the heart is often involved in chest *bì*, we need to make a clear judgement on the severity of the acute cases and bring necessary emergency care. Often, in acute cases we will need to sedate the heart and move blood stasis while raising the yang and relieving the pain. In chronic cases, we need to pay attention to the heart qi, blood, yin and yang deficiency. The syndrome will also include some blood stasis in chronic cases obstructing and preventing appropriate nourishment to come to the heart. We can also nourish other organs which might also be affected such as the liver, spleen, and kidney.

COMPREHENSION QUESTIONS

1. What are the syndrome patterns and appropriate formulas for chest *bì*?
2. How do we differentiate chest *bì* with heart pain from stomachache and rib-side pain?
3. What are the key prevention methods for chest *bì*?
4. Multiple choice questions:

1) Mr. Li, 49 years old. The patient presented with sudden chest colic pain radiating to the back which were often triggered and aggravated in cold weather, aversion to cold, cold extremities, cold sweating, palpitations, shortness of breath with a pale red tongue and a white coating, and a deep and tight pulse. The recommended formula is:

A. *Wū Tóu Chì Shí Zhī Wán* (Monkshood and Halloysite Pill)
B. *Sū Hé Xiāng Wán* (Storax Pill)
C. *Zhǐ Shí Xiè Bái Guì Zhī Tāng* (Immature Bitter Orange, Chinese Chive and Cinnamon Twig Decoction) plus *Dāng Guī Sì Nì Tāng* (Chinese Angelica Frigid Extremities Decoction)
D. *Zhǐ Shí Xiè Bái Bái Jiǔ Tāng* (Immature Bitter Orange, Chinese Chive and Wine Decoction)
E. *Dāng Guī Sì Nì Tāng* (Chinese Angelica Frigid Extremities Decoction)

2) Ms. Zhang, 68 years old. The patient presented with dull chest pain which aggravated sometimes and were triggered after exertion, lethargy, lack of strength, shortness of breath, reluctance to speak, palpitations, spontaneous sweating, pale darkish tongue with teeth marks, thin and white coating, and a moderate and weak pulse. The treatment method is to:

A. Tonify qi and invigorate blood, unblock vessels and stop pain
B. Tonify qi and nourish yin, invigorate blood and stop pain
C. Tonify qi and blood, invigorate blood and stop pain
D. Tonify qi and resolve phlegm, diffuse *bi* and stop pain

3) Mr. Zhou, 73 years old. The patient presented with intermittent dull chest oppression, palpitations, shortness of breath, fatigue, reluctance to speak, vertigo, dizziness, vexation, somnolence, hot sensation in the palms and soles, reddish tongue with no coat, and a thin and weak pulse. The recommended formula is:

A. *Shēng Mài Săn* (Pulse-Engendering Powder) plus *Zhì Gān Căo Tāng* (Honey-Fried Licorice Decoction)
B. *Bā Zhēn Tāng* (Eight-Gem Decoction)
C. *Zuŏ Guī Wán* (Left-Restoring Pill)
D. *Shēn Fù Tāng* (Ginseng and Aconite Decoction)
E. *Shēn Qí Dì Huáng Tāng* (Ginseng Astragali Rehmannia Decoction)

4) Ms. Hu, 67 years old. The patient presented with chest oppression and pain, palpitations, vexation, insomnia, night sweats, weakness of the lumbar and knees, tinnitus, vertigo, dizziness, hot sensation of the face, profuse sweating, crimson tongue with scanty coating, and a thin and rapid pulse. The treatment method is to:

A. Tonify the heart and kidney, invigorate blood and calm the mind
B. Tonify the kidney and nourish yin
C. Tonify heart qi, invigorate blood and dissolve stasis
D. Tonify qi and nourish yin, invigorate blood and stop pain
E. Nourish the yin and tonify the kidney, supplement the heart and calm the mind

5) Mr. Chen, 49 years old. The patient presented with chest pain sometimes radiating to the shoulder, shortness of breath, symptoms that aggravate in cold weather, palpitations, sweating, aversion to cold, cold limbs, edema of the lower limbs, lumbar weakness, pale complexion, pale white lips and nails, pale white tongue, and a deep and thin pulse. The recommended formula is:

A. *Shēn Fù Tāng* (Ginseng and Aconite Decoction) plus *Yòu Guī Wán* (Right-Restoring Pill)
B. *Bŭ Yáng Huán Wŭ Tāng* (Yang-Supplementing and Five-Returning Decoction)
C. *Guā Lóu Xiè Bái Guì Zhī Tāng* (Trichosanthis, Chinese Chive and Cinnamon Twig Decoction) plus *Dāng Guī Sì Nì Tāng* (Chinese Angelica Frigid Extremities Decoction)
D. *Shēng Mài Săn* (Pulse-Engendering Powder) plus *Zhì Gān Căo Tāng* (Honey-Fried Licorice Decoction)
E. *Guā Lóu Xiè Bái Bàn Xià Tāng* (Trichosanthes, Chinese Chive and Pinellia Decoction)

6) Mr. Tian, 68 years old. The patient presented with chest oppression, frequent heart pain, cold limbs, excessive sweating, pale complexion, cyanotic lips, deficient vexation, restlessness, blue purplish tongue, and an extremely thin pulse. The recommended formula is:

A. *Bā Zhēn Tāng* (Eight-Gem Decoction)
B. *Shēn Fù Lóng Mŭ Tāng* (Ginseng, Aconite, Keel and Oyster Shell Decoction)
C. *Shēn Fù Tāng* (Ginseng and Aconite Decoction) plus R*òu Guì Wán* (Cinnamon Pill)
D. *Shēng Mài Săn* (Pulse-Engendering Powder) plus *Zuŏ Guī Yĭn* (Left-Restoring Beverage)
E. *Bŭ Yáng Huán Wŭ Tāng* (Yang-Supplementing and Five-Returning Decoction)

7) Ms. Wang, 69 years old. The patient presented with chest pain and oppression, panting, palpitations, shortness of breath, lack of strength, aversion to cold, cold limbs, edema of the lower limbs, pale complexion and lips, pale and enlarged tongue with a slippery, deep and thin pulse. The treatment method is to:
A. Restore yang and tonify qi to rescue from depletion
B. Tonify the heart and kidney, invigorate blood and calm the mind
C. Tonify heart qi, invigorate blood and dissolve stasis
D. Tonify qi and nourish yin, invigorate blood and stop pain
E. Warm yang and promote urination, unblock channels and stop pain

Answers

1. A. For heart blood stasis pattern, we use *Táo Hóng Sì Wù Tāng* (Peach Kernel and Carthamus Four Substances Decoction);

B. For cold retention in the chest pattern, we use *Zhĭ Shí Xiè Bái Guì Zhī Tāng* (Immature Bitter Orange, Chinese Chive and Cinnamon Twig Decoction) plus *Dāng Guī Sì Nì Tāng* (Chinese Angelica Frigid Extremities Decoction);

C. For damp phlegm retention in the chest, we combine *Guā Lóu Xiè Bái Bàn Xià Tāng* (Trichosanthes, Chinese Chive and Pinellia Decoction) with *Dí Tán Tāng* (Phlegm-Flushing Decoction);

D. For the deficiency of both qi and yin, we use *Shēng Mài Săn* (Pulse-Engendering Powder) plus *Zhì Gān Căo Tāng* (Honey-Fried Licorice Decoction);

E. For the yin deficiency of heart and kidney, we use *Zuŏ Guī Wán* (Left-Restoring Pill);

F. For the heart yang deficiency, we use *Shēn Fù Tāng* (Ginseng and Aconite Decoction) plus *Yòu Guī Wán* (Right-Restoring Pill).

2. To recognize a stomachache and differentiate it from chest pain we can observe the location of the pain lies in the upper abdomen area and there is a local tenderness. The pain is mainly distending and lasts for a long time. In addition, there are some accompanied symptoms related to the digestive system, such as poor appetite and slow digestion, nausea, and vomiting. In addition, various medical tests can confirm a disorder of the stomach rather than a problem from the chest or heart such as an ultrasound, gastroenterography, gastroscope, and amylase test.

To differentiation rib-side pain from the chest pain, we can observe that the affected area relates to the side of the body and is usually at the right rib-side. There will be tenderness below the edge of the lower ribs. There are also some accompanied symptoms, such as no desire for greasy food, jaundice and fever. In addition, various medical tests such as gastroenterography, cholecystography, gastroscope, test of liver function, and amylase test can be helpful to make the differentiation.

3. To prevent chest pain or to accelerate the healing process from chest pain, the patient can follow these life style changes:

A. Maintain a proper and regular diet. Light flavored food should be taken instead of fatty and greasy food. Have small meals more frequently and have a very light dinner;

B. Dress according to the weather and avoid contracting cold. Pay special attention during the changes of seasons or during drastic weather;

C. Maintain a healthy attitude and avoid mental stress or excessive emotion such as anger, joy and grief;

D. Avoid overwork, excessive fatigue and physical labor;

E. When experiencing sudden heart pain immediately administer sublingual nitroglycerin or similar medicine and stay calm;

F. When the heart pain is severe and lasts for a long time, the patient should be rushed to the hospital and, after the situation is stabilized, rest in bed for the following 1 to 2 days. The diet during the rest should consist of mainly fluids. Confirm that the patient has regular bowel movements and prevent from bedsore;

G. Limit the intake of sugar and salt and avoid smoking and alcohol;

H. Pay close attention to the blood pressure, pulse, heart and respiration rate to identify abnormalities in the early stage.

4. 1) C, 2) A, 3) A, 4) E, 5) A, 6) B, 7) E.

2.2 Palpitation

Palpitation refers to an abnormal heart beat that ranges from unnoticed skipped heart beats or accelerated heart rate to very strong and noticeable heart beats causing chest tightness and pain. Palpitation can happen in healthy individuals; however, in severe cases can be accompanied with symptoms such as tightness and pain in the chest, dizziness, and difficult breathing or cough. Palpitations can be a symptom of various different heart conditions such as anxiety, phobias, hyperthyroidism, myocarditis, tachycardia, bradycardia, rheumatic fever, coronary heart diseases, asthma, emphysema, fever, drug abuse and other diseases.

In Chinese medicine, we understand palpitation to have two different main root causes; one of which is a physical root referred to as *"zheng chong"* (怔忡) in Chinese and the other has a psychological root referred to as *"jing ji"* (惊悸). These two causes have different pathomechanisms; the former is due to a weakness of the heart usually with a chronic history and the latter is due to an emotional excess more often seen in acute cases and is triggered by excessive emotions. There is a clear overlap of the symptoms of palpitation, chest tightness and shortness of breath. Furthermore, a chronic manifestation of one of the root causes can influence the other to arise temporarily.

There are six commonly known patterns associated to heart palpitations. We review them with some of their commonly seen acupuncture and Chinese medical treatment principles and prescriptions.

CLINICAL PATTERNS DIFFERENTIATION AND TREATMENTS

1. Heart and Gall Bladder Qi Deficiency

Symptoms: Palpitations which aggravate with anxiety or paranoia, easily frightened and timid personality, insomnia, dream disturbed sleep, fatigue, normal or pale tongue body with a thin white coating, in chronic cases or congenital deficient constitutions, a deep and thin crack that might reach the tip, a slightly weak, thready and rapid or thready and wiry pulse.

Treatment Principle:

- Pacify the mind and soothe the spirit
- Nourish and calm the heart

Main Acupuncture Points:

- BL 15 (*xīn shù*): Back-*shu* point of the heart to treat heart pain and unbind the chest

- BL 19 (*dān shù*): Back-*shu* point of the gallbladder to harmonize the qi and relieve fright
- PC 5 (*jiān shǐ*): To unbind the chest and transform phlegm, calm the spirit and descend qi
- PC 6 (*nèi guān*): To regulate the heart pain and stop palpitation, unbind the chest and calm the spirit
- PC 7 (*dà líng*): *Yuan*-source point of the pericardium to unbind the chest, regulate qi and calm the spirit
- HT 7 (*shén mén*): *Yuan*-source point of the heart to tonify the original qi of the heart and stop palpitation
- RN 14 (*jù quē*): To regulate and tonify the original qi of the heart, stop heart pain and palpitation
- DU 20 (*bǎi huì*): To raise the qi, regulate liver yang, benefit the heart and calm the spirit
- GB 40 (*qiū xū*): *Yuan*-source point of the gallbladder to fortify the gallbladder
- HT 9 (*shào chōng*): To treat palpitations, calm the spirit and resolve acute heart conditions

Supporting Points:

- HT 5 (*tōng lǐ*): *Luo*-connecting point of the heart to treat heart pain
- ST 36 (*zú sān lǐ*): To support the middle qi and support the healthy qi

Recommended Formula: *Ān Shén Dìng Zhì Wán* (安神定志丸, Mind-Tranquilizing Pill) from the *Medical Revelations* (*Yī Xué Xīn Wù*, 医学心悟)

Substitute Formula: *Tiān Wáng Bǔ Xīn Dān* (天王补心丹, Celestial Emperor Heart-Supplementing Elixir)

Patent Formula: *Hǔ Pò Ān Shén Wán* (琥珀安神丸, Chrysophoron Spirit-Calming Pill)

2. Heart Blood Deficiency

Symptoms: Palpitations with or without anxiety, generally worsening at night, insomnia with difficulty falling asleep, dream disturbed sleep, anxiety with panic attacks, forgetfulness, low concentration, dizziness, blurry vision, fatigue, poor appetite, abdominal distention, spontaneous sweating, pale complexion, pale tongue body with a thin white coating and a wiry and weak pulse.

Treatment Principle:

- Tonify heart qi and blood
- Calm the spirit and stop palpitations

Main Acupuncture Points:

- SP 6 (*sān yīn jiāo*): To nourish the yin and invigorate blood
- RN 14 (*jù quē*): To regulate and tonify the original qi of the heart, stop heart pain and palpitations

- ST 36 (*zú sān lǐ*): To nourish blood and support the middle qi
- HT 5 (*tōng lǐ*): *Luo*-connecting point of the heart to treat heart pain
- BL 20 (*pí shù*): Back-*shu* point of the spleen to produce and contain the blood
- EX-HN 3 (*yìn táng*): To calm the mind and treat insomnia
- HT 7 (*shén mén*): *Yuan*-source point of the heart to regulate and tonify the original qi of the heart, stop heart pain and palpitations
- BL 15 (*xīn shù*): Back-*shu* point of the heart to treat heart pain and unbind the chest
- BL 17 (*gé shù*): Influential point of the blood to activate the blood circulation, dispel stasis, unbind the chest and treat heart pain and palpitations

Supporting Points:

- DU 20 (*bǎi huì*) and BL 52 (*zhì shì*): To treat forgetfulness
- BL 42 (*pò hù*): To treat profuse dreaming
- DU 10 (*líng tái*) and DU 24 (*shén tíng*): To resolve anxiety

Recommended Formula: *Guī Pí Tāng* (归脾汤, Spleen-Restoring Decoction) from the *Formulas to Aid the Living* (*Jì Shēng Fāng*, 济生方)

Substitute Formula: *Tiān Wáng Bǔ Xīn Dān* (天王补心丹, Celestial Emperor Heart-Supplementing Elixir) plus *Sì Wù Tāng* (四物汤, Four Substances Decoction)

Patent Formula: *Rén Shēn Yǎng Róng Wán* (人参养荣丸, Gineseng Supporting and Nourishing Decoction Pill)

3. Heart Yang Deficiency

Symptoms: Palpitations which are either initiated or aggravated by movement and alleviate with rest, shortness of breath with exertion, chest tightness, fatigue, aversion to cold, cold extremities, spontaneous sweating, pale complexion with dark circles under the eyes, blue lips, edema with scanty urination, nocturia or frequent urination, swollen and purple tongue body with a white or greasy coating and a deficient, wiry, weak, slow, or knotted pulse.

Treatment Principle:

- Warm and tonify heart yang
- Calm the spirit and stop palpitations

Main Acupuncture Points:

- BL 15 (*xīn shù*): Back-*shu* point of the heart to treat heart pain and unbind the chest
- BL 14 (*jué yīn shù*): Back-*shu* point of the pericardium to unbind the chest, treat heart pain and palpitations
- PC 6 (*nèi guān*): *Luo*-connecting point of the pericardium to regulate the heart, unbind the chest and treat palpitations, insomnia and heart pain
- PC 7 (*dà líng*): *Yuan*-source point of the pericardium to tonify heart qi and blood, promote circulation, unbind the chest and treat palpitations
- HT 5 (*tōng lǐ*): *Luo*-connecting point of the heart to calm the spirit and stop heart

pain

- HT 7 (*shén mén*): *Yuan*-source point of the heart to regulate and tonify the original qi of the heart, stop heart pain and palpitations
- RN 4 (*guān yuán*): To tonify the original qi, benefit essence and regulate *chong mai* and *ren mai*
- RN 14 (*jù quē*): To regulate and tonify the original qi of the heart, stop heart pain and palpitations
- ST 36 (*zú sān lǐ*): To support the middle qi and support the healthy qi

Supporting Points:

- DU 20 (*bǎi huì*): To raise the yang
- BL 18 (*gān shù*): Back-*shu* point of the liver to regulate the qi flow and harmonize the liver

Recommended Formula: *Guì Zhī Gān Cǎo Lóng Gǔ Mǔ Lì Tāng* (桂枝甘草龙骨牡蛎汤, Cinnamomi, Licorice, Keel and Oyster Decoction) from the *Treatise on Cold Damage* (*Shāng Hán Lùn*, 伤寒论) plus *Shēn Fù Tāng* (参附汤, Ginseng and Aconite Decoction) from the *Corrections and Annotations to Fine Formulas for Women* (*Jiào Zhù Fù Rén Liáng Fāng*, 校注妇人良方)

Substitute Formula: *Sì Nì Tāng* (四逆汤, Frigid Extremities Decoction)

4. Heart and Kidney Disharmony

Symptoms: Palpitations, restlessness, poor sleep, dizziness, blurred vision, fever, vexing heat in the five centers, tinnitus, lumbago, pale tongue body with a thin white coating and a thready and rapid pulse.

Treatment Principle:

- Nourish yin and purge fire
- Nourish the heart and calm the mind

Main Acupuncture Points:

- BL 23 (*shèn shù*): Back-*shu* point of the kidney to benefit the original qi and kidney yin
- KI 3 (*tài xī*): *Yuan*-source point of the kidney to nourish kidney yin and yang and strengthen the lumbus
- HT 6 (*yīn xì*): *Xi*-cleft point of the heart to clear heat and calm the spirit, alleviate night sweats, stop heart pain and irritability
- HT 7 (*shén mén*): *Yuan*-source point of the heart to regulate and tonify the original qi of the heart, stop heart pain and palpitations
- PC 7 (*dà líng*): *Yuan*-source point of the pericardium to tonify heart qi and blood, promote circulation, unbind the chest and treat palpitations

Supporting Points:

- BL 52 (*zhì shì*): To tonify the kidney essence
- KI 4 (*dà zhōng*): *Luo*-connecting point of the kidney to tonify kidney, clear heat and calm the spirit

Recommended Formula: *Tiān Wáng Bŭ Xīn Dān* (天王补心丹, Celestial Emperor Heart-Supplementing Elixir) from the *Corrections and Annotations to Fine Formulas for Women* (*Jiào Zhù Fù Rén Liáng Fāng*, 校注妇人良方)

Substitute Formula: *Huáng Lián Ē Jiāo Tāng* (黄连阿胶汤, Coptis and Donkey-Hide Gelatin Decotion)

5. Water Retention Affecting the Heart

Symptoms: Palpitations, dizziness, vertigo, chest and epigastric distention, scanty urination, edema mainly on lower limbs, aversion to cold, cold extremities, thirst without a desire for drinking, nausea, vomiting clear phlegm and excessive salivation or drooling, white and slippery tongue coating and a slippery and wiry pulse.

Treatment Principle:

- Warm heart yang to expel congealed cold rheum
- Tonify qi and promote urination

Main Acupuncture Points:

- BL 15 (*xīn shù*): Back-*shu* point of the heart to treat heart pain and unbind the chest
- BL 23 (*shèn shù*): Back-*shu* point of the kidney to benefit the original qi and kidney yin
- KI 5 (*shuĭ quán*): *Xi*-cleft point of the kidney to regulate *chong* and *ren mai* and treat dysuria
- RN 14 (*jù quē*): To regulate and tonify the original qi of the heart, stop heart pain and palpitations
- RN 4 (*guān yuán*): To tonify the original qi and benefit essence, regulate *chong* and *ren mai* and alleviate enuresis
- RN 8 (*shén què*): Warm with salt moxa to warm yang, regulate fluid metabolism and treat edema
- RN 9 (*shuĭ fēn*): To regulate fluid metabolism and treat edema
- HT 7 (*shén mén*): *Yuan*-source point of the heart to regulate and tonify the original qi of the heart, stop heart pain and palpitations
- PC 6 (*nèi guān*): *Luo*-connecting point of the pericardium to regulate the heart, unbind the chest and treat palpitations and heart pain
- SP 9 (*yīn líng quán*): *He*-sea point of the spleen to regulate fluid passages, benefit the lower *jiao*, resolve dampness and treat edema, incontinence and enuresis

Supporting points:

- KI 7 (*fù liū*): To tonify kidney yang and clear deficient fire, regulate fluid passages and resolve edema
- KI 9 (*zhù bīn*): To clear the heart and resolve phlegm

Recommended Formula: *Líng Guì Zhú Gān Tāng* (苓桂术甘汤, Poria, Cinnamon Twig, Atractylodes Macrocephala and Licorice Decoction) from the *Essentials from the Golden Cabinet* (*Jīn Guì Yào Lüè*, 金匮要略)

Substitute Formula: *Zhēn Wǔ Tāng* (真武汤, True Warrior Decoction)

6. Heart Blood Stasis

Symptoms: Palpitations and sporadic chest pain which are worse during the night, chest stuffiness or stabbing pain, a tendency toward emotional outbursts, purple lips, varicose veins on chest and face, sometimes accompanied by liver qi stagnation symptoms, dark or crimson tongue body with ecchymosis and a thin white coating, enlarged and dark colored sublingual veins with a deep and choppy or wiry or intermittent pulse.

Treatment Principle:

- Promote blood circulation and resolve blood stasis
- Regulate qi and unblock the channels
- Unbind the chest and stop chest pain

Main Acupuncture Points:

- BL 15 (*xīn shù*): Back-*shu* point of the heart to treat heart pain and unbind the chest
- BL 17 (*gé shù*): Influential point of the blood to activate the blood circulation, dispel stasis, unbind the chest, treat heart pain and palpitations
- BL 14 (*jué yīn shù*): Back-*shu* point of the pericardium to unbind the chest and treat heart pain
- RN 17 (*dàn zhōng*): Front-*mu* point of the pericardium and influential point of qi to unbind the chest, activate qi and treat palpitations, irritability and heart pain
- RN 6 (*qì hǎi*): To harmonize blood, regulate qi and treat stroke
- PC 4 (*xì mén*): *Xi*-cleft point of the pericardium to activate blood circulation, dispel stasis, cool blood, stop bleeding, calm the spirit and treat palpitations and heart pain
- PC 5 (*jiān shǐ*): To unbind the chest, transform phlegm, calm the spirit and descend qi
- PC 6 (*nèi guān*): *Luo*-connecting point of the pericardium to regulate the heart, unbind the chest and treat palpitations and heart pain
- SP 6 (*sān yīn jiāo*): To nourish the yin, invigorate blood and treat insomnia
- HT 5 (*tōng lǐ*): *Luo*-connecting point of the heart to treat heart pain
- SP 10 (*xuè hǎi*): To promote blood flow, dispel blood stasis and calm the spirit

Supporting Points:

- PC 3 (*qū zé*): *He*-sea point of the pericardium to tonify heart qi, treat palpitations and irritability
- HT 3 (*shào hǎi*): *He*-sea point of the heart to clear heat, calm the spirit and treat heart pain
- RN 6 (*qì hǎi*): To harmonize blood, regulate qi and treat stroke

Recommended Formula: *Táo Rén Hóng Huā Jiān* (桃仁红花煎, Fried Peach Kernel Safflower Decoction) from the *[Chen] Su-An Medical Record* (*Sù Ān Yī Àn*, 素庵医案)

Substitute Formula: *Xuè Fŭ Zhú Yū Tāng* (血府逐瘀汤, Blood Stasis Expelling Decoction)

Patent Formula: *Xīn Shū Băo Jiāo Náng* (心舒宝胶囊, Heart Comforting Capsules)

Summary Chart for Palpitation

Patterns	Main Points	Supporting Points	Formulae
Heart and Gall Bladder qi Deficiency	BL 15, BL 19, PC 5, PC 6, PC 7, HT 7, RN 14, DU 20, GB 40, HT 9	HT 5 for heart pain ST 36 for healthy qi insufficiency	*Ān Shén Dìng Zhì Wán* or *Tiān Wáng Bŭ Xīn Dān*
Heart Blood Deficiency	SP 6, RN 14, ST 36, HT 5, BL 20, EX-HN 3, HT 7, BL 15, BL 17	DU 20 and BL 52 for forgetfulness BL 42 for profuse dreaming DU 10 and DU 24 for anxiety	*Guī Pí Tāng* or *Tiān Wáng Bŭ Xīn Dān* plus *Sì Wù Tāng*
Heart Yang Deficiency	BL 15, BL 14, PC 6, PC 7, HT 5, HT 7, RN 4, RN 14, ST 36	DU 20 for yang collapse BL 18 for liver disharmony	*Guì Zhī Gān Căo Lóng Gŭ Mŭ Lì Tāng* plus *Shēn Fù Tāng*
Heart and Kidney Disharmony	BL 23, KI 3, HT 6, HT 7, PC 7	BL 52 for kidney-essence insufficiency KI 4 for heat and irritability	*Tiān Wáng Bŭ Xīn Dān* or *Huáng Lián Ē Jiāo Tāng*
Water Retention affecting the Heart	BL 15, BL 23, KI 5, RN 14, RN 4, RN 8, RN 9, HT 7, PC 6, SP 9	KI 7 for edema KI 9 for heart-phlegm	*Líng Guì Zhú Gān Tāng* or *Zhēn Wŭ Tāng*
Heart Blood Stasis	BL 15, BL 17, BL 14, RN 17, RN 6, PC 4, PC 5, PC 6, SP 6, HT 5, SP 10	PC 3 for heart qi depletion HT 3 for irritability and pain RN 6 for qi and blood disorders and stroke	*Táo Rén Hóng Huā Jiān* or *Xuè Fŭ Zhú Yū Tāng*

CASE STUDY : Chronic Palpitation

Ms. Peng, 58 years old.

Main Complaint: Aggravated palpitations and shortness of breath after exertion for 8 years accompanied by edema of lower limbs for 3 days.

Medical History: The patient had suffered from left sided chest stuffiness and pain accompanied by flustered complexion and panting for 8 years after walking up the stairs. She was diagnosed with coronary heart disease with a cardiac function grade II. She was then administered Su Xiao Jiu Xin Pills which is a combination of Chinese medicinals and nitroglycerin. Other medication included aspirin, Isosorbide Mononitrate and Enalapril which controlled the symptoms for 6 years. Two years ago, the patient started to experience palpitations and shortness of breath due to exhaustion. Concurrently, she also suffered abdominal distension and productive cough with bloody sputum. She was treated with diuretics, cardiotonics, vasodilators, and anti-neurohumoral therapies which again relieved her symptoms. Three days ago, she went mountain climbing and then she felt chest oppression, palpitations and shortness of breath with an inability to lie down. In addition, the patient's occupation is to perform manual labor which leaves her exhausted every night. Within the family medical history, the father also suffers from coronary heart disease.

Presenting Symptoms: Palpitations and panting aggravated after exertion, unable to lie down, productive cough with frothy sputum, edema of the face and lower extremities, aversion to cold, cold limbs, cyanotic lips, scanty urine, poor appetite, abdominal distension, listlessness complexion, spontaneous sweating, pale tongue with a slippery coating and a deep, intermittent and slow pulse.

Physical Examination: Temperature: 36.7 ℃, pulse: 106 bpm, respiration: 26 bpm, blood pressure: 126/75 mmHg. The patient was mentally clear and aware but she looked obviously exhausted. The skin and sclera were non-icteric. There was no enlarged lymph nodes. Edema was obvious on her face with cyanotic lips and distended jugular veins. Hepatojugular reflux was positive. Moist rales were heard in the lower lung lobes. Cardiac dullness enlarged, heart rate was irregular. Premature beat was heard for 1-3/min. At cardiac apex, a 3/6 blowing systolic murmur that conducted to the left armpit was heard. In the tricuspid region, a 3/6 blowing systolic murmur and a prominent pulmonary second sound were heard. Her abdomen was flat with no shifting dullness. There was no percussion tenderness over both kidney regions. There was significant pitting edema over the lower limbs.

Other Medical Test Results:

ECG: Atrial premature beat, left ventricular hypertrophy and strain

Color Echocardiography: Enlarged left atrium, enlarged left and right ventricles, mild mitral and tricuspid regurgitation, decreased systolic function of the left ventricle

Chest X-ray: Increased hilar vascular shadows and enlarged heart shadow to the left

Urine Routine Test: Protein +

Blood Fat: TRIG 1.9 mmol/L, CHOL 4.3 mmol/L, LDL 3.16 mmol/L

Blood Sugar: 5.1 mmol/L

Renal Functions: BUN 9.2 umol/L, SCr 126 μmol/L

Pattern Differentiation

When observing this case study, we see that the combination of chronic heart disease, constitutional deficiency and overwork has created a severe heart yang qi depletion. This chronic condition combined with overwork has also caused the kidney yang to become depleted as well. This insufficiency of both heart and kidney yang causes blood stagnation which leads to palpitations, shortness of breath, and orthopnea, which are aggravated by exertion. Failure of kidney qi to expel fluids through the bladder causes internal retention of water dampness, manifesting as scanty urine, and edema of the face and lower limbs. If the retention of water qi adversely flows upward and affects the heart and lung, it causes symptoms of cough with frothy sputum. Kidney yang deficiency fails to nourish the spleen yang which in turn fails in its function of transportation and transformation causing more internal rheum to accumulate. This internal retention of rheum causes symptoms of poor appetite, abdominal distension, aversion to cold and cold limbs. The symptoms of listlessness and spontaneous sweating are symptoms of heart qi deficiency. The severe yang deficiency also contributes to lack of circulation and blood stasis in the heart and vessels causing the cyanotic lips. The pale tongue with a slippery coating and the deep and slow pulse are signs of water retention attacking the heart and vessels due to yang deficiency.

Diagnosis

TCM Diagnosis: Heart failure due to yang deficiency with rheum retention
Western Medicine Diagnosis: Coronary heart failure

Treatment

The pathomechanism of this case is mainly caused by insufficiency of heart and kidney yang qi, blood stasis, internal retention of water-rheum under the skin and internally aggressing the heart and lung.

Principles:

- Warm and tonify the heart and kidney yang
- Unblock yang and remove stasis
- Remove internal water-rheum and promote urination

Formula: Combined a modified *Zhēn Wǔ Tāng* (True Warrior Decoction) with *Wǔ Líng Sǎn* (Five Substances Powder with Poria).

Ingredients:

附片	*fù piàn*	5 g	Radix Aconiti Lateralis Praeparata
白参	*bái shēn*	10 g	Radix Ginseng Alba
黄芪	*huáng qí*	15 g	Radix Astragali
桂枝	*guì zhī*	10 g	Ramulus Cinnamomi
茯苓	*fú líng*	15 g	Poria
泽泻	*zé xiè*	15 g	Rhizoma Alismatis
猪苓	*zhū líng*	15 g	Polyporus
白术	*bái zhú*	15 g	Rhizoma Atractylodis Macrocephalae
车前子	*chē qián zǐ*	15 g	Semen Plantaginis
丹参	*dān shēn*	15 g	Radix et Rhizoma Salviae Miltiorrhizae
川芎	*chuān xiōng*	10 g	Rhizoma Chuanxiong
葶苈子	*tíng lì zǐ*	6 g	Semen Lepidii

Formula Analysis

In this formula, *fù piàn* and *guì zhī* act to warm and boost the heart and kidney yang. *Bái shēn* and *huáng qí* strengthen qi and nourish heart for supporting the heart and vessels. *Bái zhú* and *fú líng* fortify the spleen for transforming qi and promote urination. *Zé xiè, zhū líng* and *chē qián zǐ* promote urination. *Dān shēn* and *chuān xiōng* invigorate blood and remove stasis. *Tíng lì zǐ* acts to diffuse the lung and transform water retention.

Chinese Patent Medicine: The patient was also administered a patent formula of *Qí Lì Qiáng Xīn Jiāo Náng* (Astragalus and Lepidium Heart-Boosting Capsules) at 2-3 capsules, 3 times a day.

Follow-up Consultations

On the 2nd consultation, after taking 7 days of the formula, the urine output increased, the palpitations and shortness of breath were alleviated, and the patient was able to lie down with a heart rate of 88 bpm. 14 packages of the same formula were prescribed.

On the 3rd consultation, the symptoms of palpitations, shortness of breath, and edema were completely relieved and there was no pitting edema of the lower limbs. The heart rate was 76 bpm. However, there was still poor appetite and aversion to cold in the abdomen. The former formula was modified by removing *zé xiè* and *zhū líng* and adding *gān jiāng* 5 g and *shā rén* 5 g to warm yang and fortify the spleen.

The patient continued taking this formula for 2 months to consolidate the treatment and there were no more symptoms.

Clinical Analysis

In the *Treatise on Cold Damage* (*Shāng Hán Lùn*, 伤寒论) Clause 316, it states: "*Shaoyin* disease, if not finished on the second and third day, and by the fourth or fifth day, there is abdominal pain, the urination is not free, the four limbs are heavy and aching, and there is spontaneous diarrhea, this is because of water qi. If the person either has a cough, or urination is free, or there is diarrhea, or vomiting, *Zhēn Wǔ Tāng* governs." In this case, the patient has scant urination which is causing the lower abdominal cold sensation and the edema of the lower extremities. The accumulated water rheum moves upward aggressing the heart and causing palpitation and chest tightness as well as the cough with frothy sputum. In this case, there is still an external yin pattern of *shaoyin* and there is still signs of facial edema which can be treated with *Zhēn Wǔ Tāng*. Since this case is very severe and has a long history, the formula *Wǔ Líng Sǎn* was added to promote the urination and remove internal rheum. Clause 71 states: "*Taiyang* syndrome, after sweat promotion, profuse sweating starts, so there are stomach dryness, and irritability which leads to insomnia. If there is a desire for drinking water, drink moderately. This will help to harmonize the stomach and heal. If the pulse is floating and urination is inhibited, with a slight fever and incessant thirst, *Wǔ Líng Sǎn* governs." This clause describes that in external syndrome with inhibited urination we can prescribe *Wǔ Líng Sǎn* to disinhibit urination and relieve the upward moving of the water rheum causing irritability. On the third consultation, the chief complaint of the patient was mainly relieved, however the symptoms of aversion to cold, cold sensation in the lower abdomen and aversion to cold were still present. This was a sign that the retention of cold in the lower abdomen was more severe, the medicinals *zé xiè* and *zhū líng* were removed because they are in cold nature and the edema was already resolved. The medicinals *gān jiāng* 5 g and *shā rén* 5 g were added for their warm nature and their ability to warm the middle and fortify the spleen to restore appetite.

CLINICAL KEY POINTS

Generally speaking, the diagnosis of heart failure is primarily identified by the principal symptoms of palpitations, shortness of breath or panting and general weakness. Depending on the severity, it is usually accompanied by abdominal distension, poor appetite, scanty urine, edema, cyanotic complexion, lips and nails, jugular vein distension, masses below the rib side, or orthopnea, perspiration, cold limbs, pale complexion, productive cough with bloody and frothy sputum, and occasional dizziness and fainting.

The disease location of heart failure mainly lies in the heart, but it also involves the lung, spleen, liver and kidney depending on the severity and medical history. The treatment of heart failure at the early stage is mainly to fortify the heart and lung, invigorate blood and resolve stasis, nourish yin and blood. At the middle and late stages, the treatment is to warm and supplement the heart and kidney, unblock yang and promote urination. At the critical stage, the treatment is mainly to rescue yang and nourish yin to rescue from desertion.

In addition, for herbs prescribed in the formula, it is suggested the use of some heart-strengthening Chinese medicinals such as *tíng lì zǐ, wǔ jiā pí* (from the northern areas of China), *huáng qí* and *rén shēn*.

BRIEF SUMMARY

The occurrence of heart failure is usually related to the long standing weakness of the constitution, emotional excesses, extreme fatigue, or prolonged perspiration. The main location of this disease lies in the heart but attention also needs to be given to the kidney, spleen, lung and liver depending on the case. When the heart lacks nourishment or when there is an obstruction in the heart, we need to provide immediate attention to restore the function of the heart and avoid death. In less severe cases and chronic cases which are not in need of immediate emergency care, acupuncture and Chinese medicinal treatments can be given according to the pattern differentiation to nourish the heart, unblock the yang, calm the mind, and relieve palpitations.

COMPREHENSION QUESTIONS

1. What are the commonly used formulas for all patterns of palpitation?
2. How to differentiate heart failure from wheezing and thoracic rheum retention?
3. What are the key healthcare habits for heart conditions?
4. Multiple choice questions:

1) Mr. Ling, 66 years old. The patient suffers from flustered complexion and shortness of breath which aggravated after exertion, fatigue, weakness, listlessness, reluctance to speak, dry cough with scant sputum, pale complexion, pale red tongue with teeth marks and a whitish tongue coating and a deep and thin pulse. The treatment principle is to:

A. Tonify the heart and lung
B. Nourish yin and heart
C. Tonify qi and nourish yin
D. Tonify qi and invigorate blood
E. Warm the kidney and promote urination

2) Ms. Yang, 73 years old. The patient has suffered from coronary heart disease for 5 years. Her clinical manifestations are palpitations, panting after exertion, fatigue, weakness, reluctance to speak, spontaneous sweating, night sweating, dry throat and mouth, dizziness, vexation, red tongue with a scanty coating and a thin and rapid pulse. The recommended formula is:

A. *Shēn Qí Dì Huáng Tāng* (Ginseng Astragalus Rehmannia Decoction)
B. *Shēng Mài Săn* (Pulse-Engendering Powder)
C. *Sì Jūn Zĭ Tāng* (Four Gentlemen Decoction)
D. *Zhēn Wŭ Tāng* (True Warrior Decoction)
E. *Liù Wèi Dì Huáng Tāng* (Six-Ingredient Rehmannia Decoction)

3) Ms. Shen, 49 years old. The patient suffered from palpitations and panting aggravated after exertion, unable to lie down, aversion to cold, cold limbs, spontaneous sweating, listlessness, scanty urine, mild edema of the lower limbs, pale and enlarged tongue and a deep and slow pulse. The recommended formula is:

A. *Yòu Guī Wán* (Right-Restoring Pill)
B. *Yòu Guī Yĭn* (Right-Restoring Beverage)
C. *Jīn Guì Shèn Qì Wán* (Golden Cabinet's Kidney Qi Pill)
D. *Shēn Fù Lóng Mŭ Tāng* (Ginseng, Aconite, Keel and Oyster Shell Decoction)
E. Combination of *Guì Zhī Gān Căo Lóng Gŭ Mŭ Lì Tāng* (Cinnamon Twig, Licorice, Keel and Oyster Shell Decoction) and *Jīn Guì Shèn Qì Wán* (Golden Cabinet's Kidney Qi Pill)

4) Mr. Shu, 58 years old. The patient suffered from palpitations, shortness of breath, fatigue, lack of strength, panting aggravated after exertion, jugular vein distension, masses below the rib side, mild edema of the feet, cyanotic lips, tongue with teeth marks and a deep and choppy pulse. The treatment principle is:

A. Tonify qi and warm yang
B. Tonify qi and invigorate blood
C. Tonify qi and nourish yin
D. Tonify yang and promote urination
E. Tonify the heart and lung

5) Ms. Shen, 69 years old. The patient suffered from palpitations and panting, productive cough with whitish and frothy sputum, unable to lie down, distress in the chest and gastric region, scanty urine, edema of the lower limbs, pale and greasy tongue coating with a wiry and slippery pulse. The recommended formula is:

A. *Zhēn Wŭ Tāng* (True Warrior Decoction)
B. *Wŭ Líng Săn* (Five Substances Powder with Poria)
C. *Èr Chén Tāng* (Two Matured Substances Decoction)
D. *Tíng Lì Dà Zăo Xiè Fèi Tāng* (Lepidium and Jujube Lung-Draining Decoction)
E. *Qīng Jīn Huà Tán Tāng* (Metal-Clearing and Phlegm-Transforming)

6) Ms. Jin, 81 years old. The patient suffered from hypertension for 30 years accompanied by continuous flustered complexion and panting with more exhalation than inhalation, aggravation after exertion, tight shoulders and sagging abdomen, oily sweat, dry mouth and throat, constipation, edema of the whole body, scanty urine, red tongue without coating and an extremely feeble pulse. The recommended formula is:

A. *Rén Shēn Yăng Róng Tāng* (Ginseng Supporting and Nourishing Decoction)
B. *Shēn Fù Lóng Mŭ Tāng* (Ginseng, Aconite, Keel and Oyster Shell Decoction)
C. *Zhēn Wŭ Tāng* (True Warrior Decoction)
D. Combination of *Shēn Fù Lóng Mŭ Tāng* (Ginseng, Aconite, Keel and Oyster Shell Decoction) and *Shēng Mài Săn* (Pulse-Engendering Powder)
E. *Zuŏ Guī Yĭn* (Left-Restoring Beverage)

Answers

1. A. For heart and gallbladder qi deficiency, use *Ān Shén Dìng Zhì Wán* (Mind-Tranquilizing Pill) or *Tiān Wáng Bŭ Xīn Dān* (Celestial Emperor Heart-Supplementing Elixir)

B. For heart blood deficiency, use *Guī Pí Tāng* (Spleen-Restoring Decoction) or *Tiān Wáng Bŭ Xīn Dān* (Celestial Emperor Heart-Supplementing Elixir) plus *Sì Wù Tāng* (Four Substances Decoction)

C. For heart and kidney yang deficiency, use *Guì Zhī Gān Căo Lóng Gŭ Mŭ Lì Tāng*

(Cinnamomi, Licorice, Keel and Oyster Decoction) plus *Shēn Fù Tāng* (Ginseng and Aconite Decoction)

D. For heart and kidney disharmony, use *Tiān Wáng Bǔ Xīn Dān* (Celestial Emperor Heart-Supplementing Elixir)

E. For water retention affecting the heart, use *Líng Guì Zhú Gān Tāng* (Poria, Cinnamon Twig, Atractylodes Macrocephala and Licorice Decoction), *Zhēn Wǔ Tāng* (True Warrior Decoction) or *Tíng Lì Dà Zǎo Xiè Fèi Tāng* (Lepidium and Jujube Lung-Draining Decoction)

F. For heart blood stasis, use *Táo Rén Hóng Huā Jiān* (Fried Peach Kernel Safflower Decoction) or *Xuè Fǔ Zhú Yū Tāng* (Blood Stasis Expelling Decoction)

2. Wheezing is clinically characterized as sudden shortness of breath with stifling sound in the throat. When the wheezing begins, the patient may also have signs of orthopnea or cyanotic lips. These patients have no history of heart disease or related symptoms such as palpitations, edema, masses below the rib side, and so on. The onset of wheezing is usually triggered by allergenic substances such as pollen, chemicals or some kinds of food.

The thoracic rheum also presents with the symptoms of palpitations and shortness of breath, but it is combined with the signs and symptoms of pericardial effusion, such as interrupted pulse, low blood pressure, and distant heart sound. It is diagnosed by X-ray and ultrasound.

3. The key healthcare points that patients can perform in case of heart diseases are the following:

A. Stay aware to maintain a stable heart rate, heart rhythm, respiration, blood pressure by monitoring the heart on a daily basis and with regular ECG. If there are sudden severe signs of a heart pain, seek immediate medical emergency care.

B. Maintain a healthy schedule between rest and work that is suitable for your ability. Perform mild daily exercise such as walking or single limb motion.

C. Maintain a healthy positive attitude and a quiet lifestyle with low stress and reduce physical and emotional burden.

D. Maintain a healthy and appropriate diet. The food chosen should be easy to digest and nutritious. Do not choose fatty, greasy and food which are difficult to digest. Take smaller meals more often during the day with a low sodium intake.

4. 1) A, 2) B, 3) E, 4) B, 5) D, 6) D.

2.3 Insomnia

Insomnia is a disease characterized by various types of sleeping disorders often due to the inability of the mind to rest. The inability to sleep well is characterized by the inability to fall asleep, frequently waking up during the night, having dreamful sleep, having very superficial sleep and waking up exhausted. All of these conditions fall under sleeping disorders of insomnia. These conditions are very often seen and almost everyone has suffered various degrees of insomnia which lasted either for a short period of time or for many years. Insomnia can be a primary symptom or it can also be a secondary symptom to other diseases.

In Chinese medicine, the disease of primary insomnia is located in the heart and results from the lack of nourishment of the heart blood not anchoring the spirit and not letting the mind rest. This condition is also caused by disorders of other organs such as of the liver, gallbladder, spleen, stomach and kidney. There are excessive and deficiency patterns of the listed organs which affect the heart and inhibit the spirit to fully rest at night. The patterns listed below describe the various differentiations according to the presenting symptoms. Once we have identified the correct pattern causing insomnia, we can restore balance and health with the appropriate treatment principles.

CLINICAL PATTERNS DIFFERENTIATION AND TREATMENTS

1. Liver Qi Stagnation

Symptoms: Difficulty falling asleep and dream disturbed sleep, aggravated with stress, depression, irritability with emotional outbursts, headaches (mostly frontal or temporal), tense shoulders and neck, hypochondrium tension or discomfort, frequent sighing, dizziness, irregular menstrual cycle, poor appetite, normal or dark tongue body, a thin white or yellow coating. In some cases, the long standing qi stagnation causes internal heat which can be seen in symptoms such as thirst, bitter taste in the mouth, red eye, redness of the edges of the tongue and a thick yellow coating, a rapid and wiry pulse.

Treatment Principle:

- Soothe liver qi and drain liver fire
- Calm the spirit and nourish the heart

Main Acupuncture Points:

- LV 3 (*tài chōng*): *Yuan*-source point of the liver to clear liver damp heat and fire, spread liver qi, nourish blood and yin and regulate menstruation
- PC 6 (*nèi guān*): *Luo*-connecting point of the pericardium to unbind the chest and calm the spirit
- BL 18 (*gān shù*): Back-*shu* point of the liver to clear liver and gall bladder fire, regulate and smoothen the qi flow, resolve depression and harmonize liver
- BL 19 (*dǎn shù*): Back-*shu* point of the gallbladder to harmonize the qi, resolve emotional outbursts, clear liver and gallbladder damp heat and nourish yin
- BL 15 (*xīn shù*): Back-*shu* point of the heart to clear fire, unbind the chest and resolve insomnia
- GB 20 (*fēng chí*): To clear heat, treat headache and resolve insomnia
- HT 7 (*shén mén*): *Yuan*-source point of the heart to regulate and tonify the original of the heart, stop heart pain and resolve insomnia
- EX-HN 24 (*ān mián*): To calm the mind, pacify the liver and resolve insomnia
- EX-HN 3 (*yìn táng*): To calm the mind

Supporting Points:

- SJ 5 (*wài guān*) and GB 39 (*xuán zhōng*): To treat lateral headaches
- SP 6 (*sān yīn jiāo*): To alleviate poor digestion
- LV 2 (*xíng jiān*) and GB 44 (*zú qiào yīn*): To clear liver and gallbladder fire

Recommended Formula: *Lóng Dǎn Xiè Gān Tāng* (龙胆泻肝汤, Gentian Liver-Draining Decoction) from the *Secrets from the Orchid Chamber* (*Lán Shì Mì Cáng*, 兰室秘藏)

Substitute Formula: *Dāng Guī Lóng Huì Wán* (当归龙荟丸, Chinese Angelica, Gentian, and Aloe Pill)

Patent Formula: *Shū Mián Jiāo Náng* (舒眠胶囊, Sleep-Soothing Capsule)

2. Internal Stagnation of Phlegm Heat

Symptoms: Insomnia which is characterized by excessive dreaming or waking up early with difficulty falling back asleep, palpitations which are aggravated by anxiety, profuse yellow sputum, irritability and restlessness, dizziness and vertigo, heavy sensation of the head, chest fullness, poor appetite, belching, bitter taste in the mouth, nausea, vomiting, red tongue body and tip with a greasy yellow coating and a wiry or slippery and rapid pulse.

Treatment Principle:

- Clear heat and transform phlegm
- Harmonize the middle *jiao* and calm the spirit
- Calm the heart and treat insomnia

Main Acupuncture Points:

- DU 20 (*bǎi huì*): To supplement and raise the qi, regulate liver yang, benefit the heart and calm the spirit

- RN 12 (*zhōng wǎn*): To invigorate the spleen and harmonize the stomach
- LU 5 (*chǐ zé*): *He*-sea point of the lung to clear heat and regulate fluids
- ST 25 (*tiān shū*):Front-*mu* point of the large intestine to regulate the intestines, resolve damp heat, rectify qi and eliminate accumulations
- ST 40 (*fēng lóng*): To expel phlegm and dampness from the lungs, heart and chest
- ST 36 (*zú sān lǐ*): To tonify the spleen and nourish the healthy qi
- PC 6 (*nèi guān*): *Luo*-connecting point of the pericardium to regulate the heart, unbind the chest and treat heart pain
- ST 34 (*liáng qiū*): *Xi*-cleft point of the stomach to harmonize the stomach and regulate the qi
- ST 45 (*lì duì*): To clear stomach heat, calm the spirit, dredge the channel and resolve insomnia with profuse dreaming

Supporting Points:

- GB 43 (*xiá xī*): To clear damp heat from the gallbladder channel and reduce swelling
- DU 19 (*hòu dǐng*) and DU 24 (*shén tíng*): To treat anxiety

Recommended Formula: *Huáng Lián Wēn Dǎn Tāng* (黄连温胆汤, Coptis Gallbladder-Warming Decoction) from the *Important Formulas Worth a Thousand Gold Pieces for Emergency* (*Bèi Jí Qiān Jīn Yào Fāng*, 备急千金要方)

Substitute Formula:

- *Dí Tán Tāng* (涤痰汤, Phlegm-Flushing Decoction)
- *Shēng Tiě Luò Yǐn* (生铁落饮, Iron Flakes Beverage)

3. Severe Heat in the Heart

Symptoms: Insomnia characterized by waking up frequently and nightmares, irritability and anxiety, palpitations, thirst with a desire for cold drinks, bitter taste in the mouth, mouth and tongue ulcers, red and hot complexion, dark urine or painful urination, red tongue body especially at the tip with a yellow coating and rapid and surging pulse.

Treatment Principle:

- Clear heart fire and calm the spirit
- Nourish the heart yin and treat insomnia

Main Acupuncture Points:

- HT 8 (*shào fǔ*): Fire point to clear heart heat, calm the spirit and stop pain
- PC 8 (*láo gōng*): To clear heart heat, cool blood, calm spirit and alleviate irritability
- HT 7 (*shén mén*): *Yuan*-source point of the heart to regulate and tonify the original qi of the heart, stop heart pain and palpitations
- BL 15 (*xīn shù*): Back-*shu* point of the heart to clear heart fire, calm the spirit, unbind the chest and regulate qi

- SP 6 (*sān yīn jiāo*): To nourish yin, invigorate blood, treat hypertension, insomnia and various gynaecological disorders
- KI 6 (*zhào hǎi*): To clear deficient fire and regulate the *yin qiao mai*
- EX-HN 24 (*ān mián*): To calm the mind and treat insomnia
- EX-HN 3 (*yìn táng*): To calm the mind and improve sleep

Supporting Points:

- HT 9 (*shào chōng*): To clear heart heat, calm the spirit, stop heart pain, treat fever, stroke and loss of consciousness
- PC 7 (*dà líng*): To clear heart heat, cool blood, unbind the chest, calm spirit and alleviate irritability

Recommended Formula: *Zhū Shā Ān Shén Wán* (朱砂安神丸, Cinnabar Spirit-Calming Pill) from the *Elucidation of Medicine* (*Yī Xué Fā Míng*, 医学发明)

Substitute Formula: *Cí Zhū Wán* (磁朱丸, Loadstones and Cinnabar Pill)

Patent Formula: *Zhū Shā Ān Shén Wán* (朱砂安神丸, Cinnabar Spirit-Calming Pill)

4. Heart and Gall Bladder qi Deficiency

Symptoms: Insomnia and frequently waking up at night with the inability to fall back asleep, anxiety and palpitations, various phobias, paranoia, shortness of breath, fatigue, depression, spontaneous sweating, a normal or pale tongue body with a thin white coating and a wiry and thready pulse.

Treatment Principle:

- Tonify gall bladder qi and alleviate phobias
- Calm the spirit and mind
- Nourish the heart and treat insomnia

Main Acupuncture Points:

- DU 20 (*bǎi huì*): To supplement and raise the qi, regulate liver yang, benefit the heart and calm the spirit
- PC 7 (*dà líng*): *Yuan*-source point of the pericardium to tonify heart qi and blood, promote circulation, unbind the chest and treat palpitations
- HT 7 (*shén mén*): *Yuan*-source point of the heart to regulate and tonify the original qi of the heart, stop heart pain and palpitations
- GB 40 (*qiū xū*): *Yuan*-source point of the gallbladder to clear heat and activate the channel
- ST 36 (*zú sān lǐ*): To support the middle and nourish the healthy qi
- BL 23 (*shèn shù*): Back-*shu* point of the kidney to benefit the original qi and kidney yin
- BL 52 (*zhì shì*): To tonify the kidney essence
- BL 47 (*hún mén*): To spread liver qi
- EX-HN 24 (*ān mián*): To calm the mind and treat insomnia
- EX-HN 3 (*yìn táng*): To calm the mind and improve sleep

Supporting Points:
- HT 5 (*tōng lǐ*): *Luo*-connecting point of the heart to treat heart pain
- BL 7 (*tōng tiān*): To clear heat
- EX-HN 16 (*fà jì xué*): To treat insomnia and calm the spirit

Recommended Formula: *Ān Shén Dìng Zhì Wán* (安神定志丸, Mind-Tranquilizing Pill) from the *Medical Revelations* (*Yī Xué Xīn Wù*, 医学心悟)

Substitute Formula: *Suān Zǎo Rén Tāng* (酸枣仁汤, Sour Jujube Decoction)

5. Heart and Kidney Disharmony

Symptoms: Insomnia with frequently waking up covered in hot sweat, restlessness, irritability, palpitations, vexing heat in the five centers (chest, palms and soles), night sweats, dry mouth and throat, dizziness, tinnitus, forgetfulness, lumbago, nocturnal seminal emission, red tongue body with scant or no coating and a wiry and rapid pulse.

Treatment Principle:
- Nourish the heart and kidney yin
- Clear fire and calm the spirit to treat insomnia

Main Acupuncture Points:
- PC 8 (*láo gōng*): To clear heart heat, cool blood, calm spirit and alleviate irritability
- PC 7 (*dà líng*): *Yuan* point of the pericardium to tonify heart qi and blood, promote circulation, unbind the chest and treat palpitations
- KI 3 (*tài xī*): *Yuan*-source point of the kidney to nourish kidney yin and yang
- HT 7 (*shén mén*): *Yuan*-source point of the heart to regulate and tonify the heart, stop heart pain and palpitations
- LV 3 (*tài chōng*): To relieve chest congestion and irritability
- BL 15 (*xīn shù*): Back-*shu* point of the heart to treat heart pain and unbind the chest
- BL 14 (*jué yīn shù*): Back-*shu* point of the pericardium to unbind the chest and treat heart pain
- BL 23 (*shèn shù*): Back-*shu* point of the kidney to benefit the original qi and kidney yin
- EX-HN 16 (*fà jì xué*): To treat forgetfulness, insomnia and calm the spirit
- EX-HN 24 (*ān mián*): To calm the mind and treat insomnia
- EX-HN 3 (*yìn táng*): To calm the mind and improve sleep
- SP 6 (*sān yīn jiāo*): To nourish the yin, invigorate blood, treat hypertension, insomnia and various gynaecological disorders

Supporting Points:
- SI 19 (*tīng gōng*) and SJ 3 (*zhōng zhǔ*): To treat dizziness
- HT 5 (*tōng lǐ*): To treat heart pain with arrhythmia

Recommended Formula: Combine *Jiāo Tài Wán* (交泰丸, Peaceful Interaction) from the *Han's Clear View of Medicine* (*Hán Shì Yī Tōng*, 韩氏医通) with *Liù Wèi Dì Huáng Wán* (六味地黄丸, Six Ingredients Rehmannia Pill) from the *Qian's Key to Diagnosis and Treatment of Children's Diseases* (*Qián Shì Xiǎo Ér Yào Zhèng Zhí Jué*, 钱氏小儿药证直诀)

Substitute Formula:

- *Huáng Lián Ē Jiāo Tāng* (黄连阿胶汤, Coptis and Donkey-Hide Gelatin Decoction)
- *Tiān Wáng Bǔ Xīn Dān* (天王补心丹, Celestial Emperor Heart-Supplementing Elixir)

Patent Formula: *Bǔ Nǎo Ān Shén Piàn* (补脑安神片, Brain-Tonifying and Mind-Calming Tablet)

6. Deficiency of Spleen qi and Heart Blood

Symptoms: Palpitations generally worse at night, insomnia with difficulty falling asleep, dream disturbed sleep, anxiety with panic attacks, forgetfulness, low concentration, dizziness, blurry vision with "floaters", fatigue, poor appetite with abdominal distention after meals, spontaneous sweating, pale complexion, a tendency to bruise easily, pale tongue body with a thin white coating and a wiry and weak pulse.

Treatment Principle:

- Tonify spleen qi and nourish heart blood
- Calm the mind and treat insomnia

Main Acupuncture Points:

- BL 21 (*wèi shù*): Back-*shu* point of the stomach to regulate digestion and harmonize the middle qi
- RN 12 (*zhōng wǎn*): To regulate qi and invigorate spleen
- ST 25 (*tiān shū*): Front-*mu* point of the large intestine to regulate the intestines and invigorate the spleen
- ST 36 (*zú sān lǐ*): To tonify the spleen, nourish the healthy qi, nourish blood and resolve insomnia
- ST 40 (*fēng lóng*): To nourish the spleen, clear phlegm, calm the spirit, treat dizziness and alleviate pain
- ST 44 (*nèi tíng*): To resolve insomnia, clear fire and treat irritability
- ST 45 (*lì duì*): To calm the spirit, dredge the channel and resolve insomnia

Supporting Points:

- SP 4 (*gōng sūn*): To harmonize the middle *jiao*, regulate the *chong mai* and *ren mai*, regulate the qi and invigorate the spleen
- HT 2 (*qīng líng*): To regulate qi and blood, activate the channel and stop pain

Recommended Formula: *Guī Pí Tāng* (归脾汤, Spleen-Restoring Decoction) from the *Formulas to Aid the Living* (*Jì Shēng Fāng*, 济生方)

Substitute Formula: *Yǎng Xīn Tāng* (养心汤, Heart-Tonifying Decoction)

Patent Formula:

- *Zǎo Rén Ān Shén Jiāo Náng* (枣仁安神胶囊, Jujube Spirit-Calming Capsule)

- *Guī Pí Wán* (归脾丸, Spleen-Restoring pills)

Summary Chart for Insomnia

Patterns	Main Points	Supporting Points	Formulae
Liver Qi Stagation	LV 3, PC 6, BL 18, BL 19, BL 15, GB 20, HT 7, EX-HN 24, EX-HN 3	SJ 5 and GB 39 for lateral headaches SP 6 for poor digestion LV 2 and GB 44 for liver and gallbladder fire	*Lóng Dăn Xiè Gān Tāng* or *Dāng Guī Lóng Huì Wán*
Internal Stagnation of Phlegm Heat	DU 20, RN 12, LU 5, ST 25, ST 40, ST 36, PC 6, ST 34, ST 45	GB 43 for damp-heat in the gallbladder and swelling DU 19 and DU 24 for anxiety	*Huáng Lián Wēn Dăn Tāng, Dí Tán Tāng* or *Shēng Tiě Luò Yĭn*
Severe Heat in the Heart	HT 8, PC 8, HT 7, BL 15, SP 6, KI 6, EX-HN 24, EX-HN 3	HT 9 for fever, stroke and loss of consciousness PC 7 for blood heat and irritability	*Zhū Shā Ān Shén Wán* or *Cí Zhū Wán*
Heart and Gall Bladder Qi Deficiency	DU 20, PC 7, HT 7, GB 40, ST 36, BL 23, BL 52, BL 47, EX-HN 24, EX-HN 3	HT 5 for heart pain BL 7 for internal heat EX-HN 16 for insomnia and irritability	*Ān Shén Dìng Zhì Wán* or *Suān Zăo Rén Tāng*
Heart and Kidney Disharmony	PC 8, PC 7, KI 3, HT 7, LV 3, BL 15, BL 14, BL 23, EX-HN 16, EX-HN 24, EX-HN 3, SP 6	SI 19 and SJ 3 for dizziness HT 5 for heart pain with arrhythmia	*Jiāo Tài Wán* plus *Liù Wèi Dì Huáng Wán, Huáng Lián Ē Jiāo Tāng* or *Tiān Wáng Bŭ Xīn Dān*
Deficiency of Spleen qi and Heart Blood	BL 21, RN 12, ST 25, ST 36, ST 40, ST 44, ST 45	SP 4 for middle *jiao* insufficiency HT 2 for qi and blood disharmony	*Guī Pí Tāng* or *Yăng Xīn Tāng*

CASE STUDY 1: Chronic Insomnia

Mr. Zhang, 53 years old, retired. 1st consultation on 21st June, 2004

Main Complaint: Insomnia with excessive dreams for over 10 years.

Medical History: Ten years ago, due to severe pressure at work, the patient experienced difficulty in falling asleep and was easily waken with difficulty in falling asleep again. He also experienced vivid and excessive dreams and could only sleep at most from 3 to 4 hours a night. In the morning, he felt tired and was unable to concentrate which greatly affected his work and daily life. He consulted many doctors and was given various oral prescription of sleeping pills such as Estazolam. The medication was effective at first but symptoms relapsed after he stopped taking them. Presently, the patient refused to take these medications because of their severe side effects. Therefore, he sought help from Chinese medicine. In addition, the patient has also been taking high blood pressure medication for the last 10 years which stabilized his blood pressure. The patient was also diagnosed with chronic gastritis five years prior to consultation which he was successfully treated with Sunflower Stomach-Recovering Pill (*Kuí Huā Wèi Kāng Líng*).

Presenting Symptoms: Insomnia with poor appetite, scanty stool, normal urination, lethargy, a thin red tongue with little coating and a thready and rapid pulse.

Physical Examination: Temperature: 36.3 ℃, pulse: 86 bpm, respiration: 19 bpm, blood pressure: 135/80 mmHg. The patient was thin, aware, cooperative but reacted slowly and showed a poor spirit. He spoke clearly and slowly. The patient could only extract his tongue outward half of the way, normal strength and muscle tone, with upper and lower extremity strength of grade 5. There were no abnormal findings in the CT scan of the brain.

Pattern Differentiation

The elderly patient showed a severe lack of nourishment which lasted a long time with severe stress at work which impaired the liver and kidney yin leading to relatively exuberant liver yang. The exuberance liver fire disturbed the spirit and instigated a disharmony between the heart and kidney of over active heart fire with kidney yin deficiency manifesting in the red tongue with scanty coating as well as the thready and rapid pulse. In this case the symptom of insomnia mainly lies in the pathogenic heart fire inhibiting the spirit and mind to rest deeply while it is also affected with the yin depletion of the liver and kidney. Generally speaking, this case of insomnia pertains to a deficiency in the root yin with an excess of empty fire in the branch.

Diagnosis

TCM Diagnosis: Insomnia due to yin deficiency with internal heat harassing the heart spirit

Western Medicine Diagnosis: Chronic Insomnia

Treatment

The main pathomechanism of this case is liver and kidney yin deficiency which fails to control the uprising empty fire harassing the heart which can also be seen as a disharmony of the heart and kidney.

Principles:

- Nourish liver and kidney
- Subdue pathogenic heart heat
- Nourish blood and calm the mind

Formula: Modified *Liù Wèi Dì Huáng Wán* (Six-Ingredient Rehmannia Pill) combined with modified *Suān Zǎo Rén Tāng* (Sour Jujube Decoction)

Ingredients:

熟地黄	*shú dì huáng*	15 g	Radix Rehmanniae Praeparata
山药	*shān yào*	15 g	Rhizoma Dioscoreae
山茱萸	*shān zhū yú*	10 g	Fructus Corni
泽泻	*zé xiè*	10 g	Rhizoma Alismatis
茯苓	*fú líng*	15 g	Poria
牡丹皮	*mŭ dān pí*	15 g	Cortex Moutan
酸枣仁	*suān zăo rén*	15 g	Semen Ziziphi Spinosae
茯神	*fú shén*	15 g	Sclerotium Poriae Pararadicis
知母	*zhī mŭ*	10 g	Rhizoma Anemarrhenae
川芎	*chuān xiōng*	10 g	Rhizoma Chuanxiong
合欢花	*hé huān huā*	15 g	Flos Albiziae
柏子仁	*băi zĭ rén*	15 g	Semen Platycladi
夜交藤	*yè jiāo téng*	15 g	Caulis Polygoni Multiflori
炙甘草	*zhì gān căo*	5 g	Radix et Rhizoma Glycyrrhizae Praeparata cum Melle

Formula Analysis

In this clinical case, the insomnia pertains to the pattern of yin deficiency with uprising pathogenic empty heat harassing the heart spirit. *Liù Wèi Dì Huáng Wán* (Six-Ingredient Rehmannia Pill) was chosen to nourish yin and supplement the kidney essence. *Suān Zăo Rén Tāng* (Sour Jujube Decoction) serves to clear heart heat, remove vexation, nourish blood and calm the mind. *Hé huān huā, băi zĭ rén* and *yè jiāo téng* are combined to nourish the heart and calm the mind. All these medicinals are combined to enrich yin, clear empty heat, nourish blood and calm the mind.

Chinese Patent Medicine: *Băi Zĭ Yăng Xīn Wán* (柏子养心丸, Arborvitae Seed Heart-Nourishing Pill) was also taken orally to nourish the heart blood and calm the mind to treat insomnia. The patient was instructed to take 8 pills three times a day and avoid taking raw, cold, fatty, and greasy food.

Follow-up Consultations

2nd consultation: After taking 10 doses of the medication, the sleep quality improved and he could sleep for about five to six hours a night. However, there was still some difficulty to fall asleep and it took the patient about 30 minutes to an hour in the bed before falling asleep. The prior formula was given with the addition of 20 g of both raw *lóng gŭ* and *mŭ lì* to calm the mind.

3rd consultation: After having another 15 doses of the medication, the patient reported that he could sleep a total of 8 hours every night with good quality and all the other symptoms also subsided. A follow-up visit 3 months later confirmed that the patient had no relapse and continued having a good quality of sleep.

CASE STUDY 2: Acute Insomnia

Mr. Tian Zhen-ping, 63 years old. 1st consultation on February 12th, 2012.

Main Complaint: Severe insomnia with weakness and tingling of the limbs for two months with aggravation for a week.

Medical History: The patient had severe insomnia and self administered 2 mg of Estazolam to be able to get some sleep. Two months ago, his lower limbs, especially of the right side, became numb without any known cause. The numbness developed from his foot moving up the leg slowly while the symptoms increased within the last week. In addition, there was an obvious lack of strength in the foot and a heavy sensation of the lower extremities while walking. The patient did not suffer from any headache, poor appetite, nausea or vomiting but shown symptoms of dizziness, flustered complexion, chest oppression, shortness of breath and occasional pain in epigastric area. All symptoms aggravated after exertion. His urine and stool were normal and there was no sign of over salivation. The tongue was dark red with white and thick coating and the pulse was deep and thin.

Physical Examination: Temperature: 36 ℃, pulse: 74 bpm, respiration: 19 bpm, blood pressure: 130/80 mmHg. The patient showed normal facial muscles and strength of the upper limbs. The right leg strength was normal (4+), however the left leg had a slight weakness (4–). Muscle tone was normal with symmetrical tendon reflex. There was decrease in the shallow sensation of the wrist and knee joints.

Pattern Differentiation

The pathomechanism of this case of insomnia is a combination of deficiency and excess causing the combination of his symptoms. The patient has a long history of liver yin and kidney essence deficiency. The liver yin is closely related to the blood causing a blood deficiency increased by the kidney essence depletion. This blood depletion first caused the insomnia inhibiting the spirit to rest and the body to fully recuperate at night. The blood depletion also caused the lack of nourishment to the muscles and tendons causing the numbness and weakness in the lower limbs. The lack of nourishment caused a qi depletion of the spleen and stomach, inhibiting the spleen natural function of transforming and transporting the food nutrients. The weak spleen also causes an accumulation of phlegm in the channel causing the symptoms of dizziness and thick greasy tongue coating. This retention of phlegm blocking the channels is inhibiting the blood circulation causing the numbness of the extremities as well as the weakness of the lower limbs.

Diagnosis

TCM Diagnosis: Insomnia due to phlegm stasis obstructing the collaterals with liver and kidney yin deficiency causing depletion of the sea of marrow

Western Medicine Diagnosis: Acute insomnia

Treatment

Principles:

- Supplement liver blood and kidney yin
- Supplement the essence and nourish the sea of marrow
- Nourish spleen qi and transform phlegm
- Calm the mind to improve sleep

Acupuncture Point Combination:

Acupuncture treatments were given in the afternoon once a day, retaining the needles 30 minutes each time.

- DU 20 (*băi huì*) and EX-HN 1 (*sì shén cōng*): To bring the healthy yang to the head and nourish the sea of marrow
- EX-HN 3 (*yìn táng*) and HT 7 (*shén mén*): To clear heart heat and calm the mind
- SP 6 (*sān yīn jiāo*): To nourish the three yin channels and promote blood circulation in the lower limbs
- BL 62 (*shēn mài*), KI 6 (*zhào hăi*) and LV 3 (*tài chōng*): To nourish the root and kidney essence
- ST 36 (*zú sān lĭ*) and ST 40 (*fēng lóng*): To nourish the stomach, drain phlegm and promote the circulation in the lower limbs

Follow-up Consultations

The patient recovered fully after 20 days (2 courses of treatment).

KEY CLINICAL POINTS

There are 3 important clinical points we need to keep in mind when we treat patients suffering from either acute or chronic insomnia. We must remember to recreate a deeper level of internal balance in the qi, blood, yin and yang of every *zang-fu* organ. Any excess need to be subdued and deficient organs need to be nourished. Second, we need to tend to the main complaint and add medicinals to calm the mind and treat insomnia. Sleep is an important aspect of our body mind connection. When insomnia becomes the primary complaint it is detrimental to reinstate a balance in the daily life in our physical, mental and emotional conditions. Avoiding any physical, mental or emotional stress and overstrain is important for a quick recovery. In some cases, insomnia might cause some unstable emotional state as well as some psychological disorder or depression. Suggesting or offering some psychological assistance is also part of the treatment of insomnia.

Additionally, it is important to remember to tend to the blood stasis which is commonly present in cases of stubborn or chronic insomnia with vexation, dark or bruised tongue. We will need to remove blood stasis and activate blood circulation. In case of blood stasis with chronic insomnia, we can consider the formula *Xuè Fŭ Zhú Yū Tāng* (Blood Mansion Stasis-Expelling Decoction) to invigorate blood and dissolve stasis, soothe the liver and rectify qi. It can also activate the collaterals and calm the mind, nourish yin and clear heart heat.

BRIEF SUMMARY

Many patients suffer from insomnia as a primary or a secondary symptom. When the body is deficient or infected with a pathogen the mind is unable to rest fully and deeply causing various levels of insomnia. We must first identify if the insomnia is a primary or a secondary symptom. When it is a primary symptom we identify the pattern differentiation and treat it accordingly. If the insomnia is a secondary symptom, we must identify the primary cause of disease and treat it accordingly, then the insomnia will resolve itself. Chronic cases of insomnia might also need some counselling to fully restore the mental and emotional balance.

COMPREHENSION QUSTIONS

1. What are the clinical manifestations of insomnia?
2. What are the different patterns and recommended formulas for insomnia?
3. What main changes in life style can patients undertake to support their treatment when suffering from insomnia?
4. Multiple choice questions:

1) Ms. Chen, 55 years old. Main complaint is insomnia for over 5 years with frequent signing. The patient suffers from restless sleep with frequent indigestion and bloating especially when she is irritated or angry. The pulse is tight and wiry and the tongue is red with a thin white coating. What is the recommended formula?

A. *Lóng Dăn Xiè Gān Tāng* (Gentian Liver-Draining Decoction)
B. *Dí Tán Tāng* (Phlegm-Flushing Decoction)
C. *Zhū Shā Ān Shén Wán* (Cinnabar Spirit-Calming Pill)
D. *Huáng Lián Wēn Dăn Tāng* (Coptis Gallbladder-Warming Decoction)
E. *Cí Zhū Wán* (Loadstones and Cinnabar Pill)

2) The main pathomechanism of insomnia is closely related to disorder of which main organs:

A. The heart, the spleen, the liver and the kidney
B. The heart, the spleen, the liver, the kidney and the stomach
C. The heart, the gallbladder, the liver, the spleen and the kidney
D. The heart, the lung, the spleen and the kidney
E. The heart, the lung, the stomach and the kidney

3) The disease location of insomnia is mainly located which organ?
A. The brain
B. The spleen
C. The kidney
D. The heart
E. The liver

4) If the insomnia pertains to the pattern of heart and kidney disharmony, the recommended formula is?
A. *Ān Shén Dìng Zhì Tāng* (Spirit and Mind Calming Pill)
B. *Jiāo Tài Wán* (Heart and Kidney Interacting Pill)
C. *Liù Wèi Dì Huáng Wán* (Six-Ingredient Rehmannia Pill) plus *Jiāo Tài Wán* (Peaceful Interaction)
D. *Zhū Shā Ān Shén Wán* (Cinnabar Spirit-Calming Pill)
E. *Suān Zǎo Rén Tāng* (Sour Jujube Decoction)

Answers

1. In mild cases, patients have either difficulty to fall asleep, restless sleep or are easily woken up with the inability to fall asleep again for a continuous 3 weeks. While in severe cases, patients can not sleep all night due to various causes such as overthinking, anxiety and so on. In severe cases, the insomnia is often accompanied by headache, dizziness, palpitations, forgetfulness, lethargy, weakness, restlessness and excessive dreaming. Often these patients have a history of improper diet, emotional stress, mental or physical overstrain, anxiety and physical weakness. Also these patients will not demonstrate any organic disorders that may hinder sleep.

2. There are various causes identified in Chinese medicine that may cause insomnia. Here is a list of the most common ones with the recommended formulas:

A. Liver qi stagnation: The recommended formula is *Lóng Dǎn Xiè Gān Tāng* (Gentian Liver-Draining Decoction) or *Dāng Guī Lóng Huì Wán* (Chinese Angelica, Gentian, and Aloe Pill).

B. Stagnation of phlegm heat: The recommended formula is *Huáng Lián Wēn Dǎn Tāng* (Coptis Gallbladder-Warming Decoction) or *Dí Tán Tāng* (Phlegm-Flushing Decoction).

C. Severe heat attacking the heart: The recommended formula is *Zhū Shā Ān Shén Wán* (Cinnabar Spirit-Calming Pill) or *Cí Zhū Wán* (Loadstones and Cinnabar Pill).

D. Heart and gall bladder qi deficiency: The recommended formulas is *Ān Shén Dìng Zhì Wán* (Mind-Tranquilizing Pill) or *Suān Zǎo Rén Tāng* (Sour Jujube Decoction).

E. Heart and kidney disharmony: The recommended formula is *Jiāo Tài Wán* (Peaceful Interaction), *Liù Wèi Dì Huáng Wán* (Six Ingredients Rehmannia Pill) or *Tiān Wáng Bǔ Xīn Dān* (Celestial Emperor Heart-Supplementing Elixir).

F. Spleen qi and heart blood deficiency: The recommended formula is *Guī Pí Tāng*

(Spleen-Restoring Decoction) or *Yǎng Xīn Tāng* (Heart Tonifying Decoction).

3. Patients suffering from insomnia have an interest of reducing their daily emotional, mental and physical stress so that their mind can rest at night. Normally, the body and mind have a natural response to slow down and rest in the evening. However, when the body is diseased, the spirit is unable to fully let go of the stress of the day and it remains over stimulated at night causing the mind and body unable to rest. In this sense it is important for insomnia patients to restore a healthy and balanced physical state during the day and to be able to rest at night. This balance includes restoring a regular diet that is taken at regular times without any overly spicy, greasy, sweet and salty food, going to bed at regular times, and avoiding excessive physical exercises like running or jogging right before sleep.

4. 1) A, 2) A, 3) D, 4) C.

2.4 Forgetfulness

Forgetfulness is defined as decreased long-term and/or short-term memory. In Chinese medicine, it is believed that poor memory is related to deficiency of heart blood, spleen qi and kidney essence. In some cases, it is also due to a combination of the various syndromes with stagnation of qi and blood or retention of turbid phlegm harassing the upper part of the body.

While the deficiency patterns of forgetfulness are more common, the excessive patterns are commonly seen in acute cases of trauma or during periods of excessive mental or emotional stress. For example, the forgetfulness can be caused by excessive anxiety damaging the heart and spleen qi consuming the blood causing a lack of nourishment to the brain. However, in most cases forgetfulness is due to deficient patterns such as a prolonged illness impairing essence and blood, qi and blood deficiency due to old age, or excessive loss of blood due to trauma or surgery causing a lack of nourishment to the brain. The excess patterns of forgetfulness are often a result of internal damage of seven excessive emotions causing internal fire or retention of turbid phlegm clouding the upper. Below are the common patterns of forgetfulness with their acupuncture and medicinal treatment approaches.

CLINICAL PATTERNS DIFFERENTIATION AND TREATMENTS

1. Spleen Qi and Heart Blood Deficiency

Symptoms: Poor memory, absent-mindedness, poor concentration, insomnia with difficulty falling asleep and dreamful sleep, palpitations, anxiety, phobias, dizziness, blurry vision, fatigue, poor appetite, abdominal fullness, pale complexion, menorrhagia, pale tongue with a thin white coating and a wiry and weak pulse.

Treatment Principle:

- Nourish spleen and heart
- Tonify qi and blood
- Calm the spirit and nourish essence

Main Acupuncture Points:

- DU 20 (*bǎi huì*): To supplement the qi and raise the yang
- HT 7 (*shén mén*): *Yuan* point of the heart to treat forgetfulness, tonify the original qi of the heart and calm the spirit
- BL 15 (*xīn shù*): Back-*shu* point of the heart to nourish the original qi of the heart

- BL 17 (*gé shù*): Influential point of the blood to activate the blood circulation and dispel stasis
- BL 20 (*pí shù*): Back-*shu* point of the spleen to nourish the spleen and control the blood
- EX-HN 3 (*yìn táng*): To calm the mind and treat insomnia

Supporting Points:

- BL 42 (*pò hù*): To resolve profuse dreaming
- EX-HN 16 (*fā jì xué*): To treat vertigo and headaches

Recommended Formula: *Guī Pí Tāng* (归脾汤, Spleen-Restoring Decoction) from the *Formulas to Aid the Living* (*Jì Shēng Fāng*, 济生方)

Substitute Formula: *Rén Shēn Yǎng Róng Tāng* (人参养荣汤, Ginseng Supporting and Nourishing Decoction)

Patent Formula:

- *Guī Pí Wán* (归脾丸, Spleen-Restoring Pill)
- *Rén Shēn Yǎng Róng Wán* (人参养荣丸, Ginseng Supporting and Nourishing Pill)

2. Heart and Kidney Yin Deficiency

Symptoms: Poor memory, insomnia with frequent waking up with heat sensations and hot sweats, restlessness, palpitation, anxiety, vexing heat in the five centers, night sweating, mouth and throat dryness, dizziness and tinnitus, lumbago, red tongue with scanty or no coating and a wiry and rapid pulse.

Treatment Principle:

- Nourish heart and kidney yin
- Clear heat and calm the spirit

Main Acupuncture Points:

- KI 3 (*tài xī*): *Yuan*-source point of the kidney to nourish yin and resolve insomnia
- HT 7 (*shén mén*): *Yuan*-source point of the heart to treat forgetfulness, tonify the original qi of the heart and calm the spirit
- DU 20 (*bǎi huì*): To benefit the heart, calm the spirit and regulate the mind
- BL 15 (*xīn shù*): Back-*shu* point of the heart to nourish the original qi of the heart and calm the spirit
- BL 23 (*shèn shù*): Back-*shu* point of the kidney to tonify kidney yin
- EX-HN 3 (*yìn táng*): To calm the spirit and treat insomnia

Supporting points:

- HT 5 (*tōng lǐ*): *Luo*-connecting point of the heart to treat heart pain with arrhythmia
- BL 43 (*gāo huāng*): To nourish yin and resolve asthmatic cough

Recommended Formula: *Tiān Wáng Bǔ Xīn Dān* (天王补心丹, Celestial Emperor Heart-Supplementing Elixir) from the *Corrections and Annotations to Fine Formulas for Women* (*Jiào Zhù Fù Rén Liáng Fāng*, 校注妇人良方)

Substitute Formula: *Huáng Lián Ē Jiāo Tāng* (黄连阿胶汤,Coptis and Donkey-Hide

Gelatin Decoction)

Patent Formula:

- *Tiān Wáng Bŭ Xīn Dān* (天王补心丹, Celestial Emperor Heart-Supplementing Elixir)
- *Jiàn Năo Wán* (健脑丸, Healthy Brain Pill)

3. Kidney Essence Deficiency

Symptoms: Poor memory, not recognizing relatives (more common in elderly patients) and disorientation, generalized malaise, emaciation, hair loss, lack of luster of hair or premature balding, weakness and soreness of lumbus and knees, decreased libido, impotence, infertility, frequent urination, nocturia, tinnitus, deafness, blindness, pale tongue with a thin coating and a wiry and weak pulse.

Treatment Principle:

- Nourish kidney essence
- Tonify spleen qi and nourish heart blood

Main Acupuncture Points:

- KI 3 (*tài xī*): *Yuan*-source point of the kidney to nourish yin and resolve insomnia
- ST 36 (*zú sān lĭ*): To tonify qi and nourish blood
- DU 20 (*băi huì*): To raise the yang and nourish the sea of marrow
- RN 4 (*guān yuán*): To tonify original qi and benefit essence
- RN 6 (*qì hăi*): To tonify original qi and blood, benefit essence and fortify yang
- DU 4 (*mìng mén*): To regulate the *du mai* and benefit the *ming men*

Supporting Points:

- KI 10 (*yīn gŭ*): To tonify kidney yang and resolve impotence
- ST 27 (*dà jù*): To nourish essence and resolve sexual dysfunctions

Recommended Formula: *Zuŏ Guī Wán* (左归丸, Left-Restoring Pill) from *The Complete Works of [Zhang] Jing-yue* (*Jĭng Yuè Quán Shū*, 景岳全书)

Substitute Formula: *Jīn Guì Shèn Qì Wán* (金匮肾气丸, Golden Cabinet's Kidney Qi Pill)

Patent Formula:

- *Zuŏ Guī Wán* (左归丸, Left-Restoring Pill)
- *Jīn Guì Shèn Qì Wán* (金匮肾气丸, Golden Cabinet's Kidney Qi Pill)

4. Blood and Phlegm Stagnation

Symptoms: Poor memory, absent-mindedness, poor concentration, slow speech, dull expression, purple tongue with bruises and thick white coating, enlarged and dark sublingual veins, slippery or wiry and choppy pulse.

Treatment Principle:

- Strengthen the spleen to resolve phlegm
- Invigorate blood and expel stasis

Main Acupuncture Points:

- BL 17 (*gé shù*): Influential point of the blood to activate blood circulation and dispel stasis

- PC 4 (*xì mén*): *Xi*-cleft point of the pericardium to activate blood circulation, dispel stasis and calm the spirit
- SP 10 (*xuè hǎi*): To promote blood flow, dispel blood stasis and calm the spirit
- DU 20 (*bǎi huì*): To raise the yang and nourish the sea of marrow
- ST 40 (*fēng lóng*): To expel phlegm and dampness, nourish the spleen and calm the spirit
- SP 3 (*tài bái*): *Yuan* point of the spleen to invigorate the spleen and resolve dampness, raise the clear and direct the turbid downward

Supporting Points:

- GB 20 (*fēng chí*): To resolve blood stasis
- EX-HN 1 (*sì shén cōng*): To improve memory, resolve insomnia and awaken the mind

Recommended Formula: *Shòu Xīng Wán* (寿星丸, God of Longevity Pill) from the *Beneficial Formulas from the Taiping Imperial Pharmacy* (*Tài Píng Huì Mín Hé Jì Jú Fāng*, 太平惠民和剂局方)

Substitute Formula:

- Combine *Tōng Qiào Huó Xuè Tāng* (通窍活血汤, Orifice-Soothing Blood-Activating Decoction) and *Èr Chén Tāng* (二陈汤, Two Matured Substances Decoction)
- Combine *Xuè Fǔ Zhú Yū Tāng* (血府逐瘀汤, Blood Stasis Expelling Decoction) and *Èr Chén Tāng* (二陈汤, Two Matured Substances Decoction)

Patent Formula: *Xuè Fǔ Zhú Yū Wán* (血府逐瘀丸, Blood Stasis Expelling Pill)

Summary Chart for Forgetfulness

Patterns	Main Points	Supporting points	Formulae
Spleen Qi and Heart Blood Deficiency	DU 20, HT 7, BL 15, BL 17, BL 20, EX-HN 3	BL 42 for profuse dreaming EX-HN 16 for vertigo and headaches	*Guī Pí Tāng* or *Rén Shēn Yǎng Róng Tāng*
Heart and Kidney Yin Deficiency	KI 3, HT 7, DU 20, BL 15, BL 23, EX-HN 3	HT 5 for arrhythmia BL 43 for yin deficiency with cough	*Tiān Wáng Bǔ Xīn Dān* or *Huáng Lián Ē Jiāo Tāng*
Kidney Essence Deficiency	KI 3, ST 36, DU 20, RN 4, RN 6, DU 4	KI 10 for impotence ST 27 for essence deficiency and sexual dysfunctions	*Zuǒ Guī Wán* or *Jīn Guì Shèn Qì Wán*
Blood and Phlegm Stagnation	BL 17, PC 4, SP 10, DU 20, ST 40, SP 3	GB 20 for blood stasis EX-HN 1 for poor memory with insomnia	*Shòu Xīng Wán* or combined *Tōng Qiào Huó Xuè Tāng* and *Èr Chén Tāng*

CASE STUDY 1: Chronic Forgetfulness

Mr. Li, 58 years old.

Main Complaint: Vertigo, numbness of the head with a decrease in memory for seven years with aggravation for a year.

Medical History: The patient suffered from intermittent vertigo, numbness of the head, decreased memory, and slow reaction seven years ago with no known cause of onset. He has not received treatment for these symptoms. In the recent year, the symptoms worsened greatly especially when he was tired. The short term memory was greatly affecting his life. Medical testing showed grade 2 retinal arteriosclerosis for which he was hospitalized. In addition, the patient had a history of hypotension for over 10 years with a blood pressure of 90/60 mmHg.

Presenting Symptoms: Decreased memory, slow mental reaction, indifferent expression, lethargy, poor spirit, low appetite, poor sleep, loose stool, aversion to cold, frequent urination, a thin, red tongue with scanty coating, and thin and rapid pulse.

Physical Examination: Temperature: 36.2 ℃, pulse: 73 bpm, respiration: 19 bpm, blood pressure: 120/75 mmHg. The patient was alert and cooperative but had poor spirit and slow reaction and a clear and slow speech. He had poor strength of both hands, muscle strength of the upper and lower limbs were normal (grade 5) with normal muscle tone and symmetric tendon reflex.

Pattern Differentiation

Long standing poor nutrition had hindered the blood and essence of the patient which caused a severe weakness of the spleen and stomach leading to internal retention of turbid phlegm obstructing the brain and vessels while also creating a blood deficiency not nourishing the brain. This lack of nourishment led to the declining of the brain marrow causing the mind and spirit to demonstrate a slow mental reaction and poor memory. In this case, the pathogenesis location lies in the deficiency of the essence not nourishing the brain and it is closely related to the heart, liver, spleen and kidney.

Diagnosis

TCM Diagnosis: Forgetfulness due to blood and essence depletion and turbid phlegm obstructing the orifices

Western Medicine Diagnosis: Poor memory with grade 2 retinal arteriosclerosis

Treatment

The main pathomechanism is long standing postnatal malnutrition and spleen-stomach weakness leading to internal retention of turbid phlegm obstructing the brain and vessels with blood depletion.

Principles:

- Strengthen the spleen and resolve phlegm
- Remove obstruction and open the orifices
- Nourish blood and essence

Formula: Modification of *Bàn Xià Bái Zhú Tiān Má Tāng* (Pinellia, Atractylodes Macrocephala and Gastrodia Decoction)

Ingredients:

半夏	*bàn xià*	8 g	Rhizoma Pinelliae
白术	*bái zhú*	10 g	Rhizoma Atractylodis Macrocephalae
茯苓	*fú líng*	10 g	Poria
天麻	*tiān má*	12 g	Rhizoma Gastrodiae
陈皮	*chén pí*	10 g	Pericarpium Citri Reticulatae
竹茹	*zhú rú*	10 g	Caulis Bambusae in Taenia
远志	*yuǎn zhì*	10 g	Radix Polygalae
石菖蒲	*shí chāng pú*	10 g	Rhizoma Acori Tatarinowii
丹参	*dān shēn*	15 g	Radix et Rhizoma Salviae Miltiorrhizae
当归	*dāng guī*	10 g	Radix Angelicae Sinensis
川牛膝	*chuān niú xī*	10 g	Radix Cyathulae
地龙	*dì lóng*	10 g	Pheretima
炙甘草	*zhì gān cǎo*	6 g	Radix et Rhizoma Glycyrrhizae Praeparata cum Melle

Formula Analysis

In this case of chronic forgetfulness, the lack of nourishment to the brain is caused by a combination of deficiency and excess. The deficiency of the spleen qi creates an accumulation of turbid phlegm in the interior which obstructs the orifice of the brain causing slow mental reaction and poor memory. In this case, we need to supplement the spleen qi and transform the phlegm while removing obstruction and opening the orifice. The formula *Bàn Xià Bái Zhú Tiān Má Tāng* is applied to fortify and warm the spleen with and remove dampness with *bàn xià, bái zhú, fú líng and chén pí. Shí chāng pú* and *yuǎn zhì* are added to dissolve phlegm to open the orifices. *Dāng guī* and *dān shēn* are combined to nourish and activate blood and unblock the orifices. All the medicinals are combined to fortify the spleen and dissolve phlegm, dissolve obstruction to open the orifices.

Follow-up Consultations

After 20 doses, the short term memory of the patient improved greatly and his mental reaction was quicker. After another 20 doses, his memory and reaction were normal and he was able to care for himself again.

CASE STUDY 2: Chronic Vertigo

Ms. Cheng, 53 years old. 1st consultation on February 2nd, 2012.

Main Complaint: Vertigo and forgetfulness for eight years with aggravation for 2 years.

Medical History: The patient suffered from intermittent vertigo with unknown cause of onset for 8 years ago while each episode lasted for many hours to days. The patient thought it was due to poor sleep and did not seek medical attention at the time. Accompanied symptoms were headache and forgetfulness. Two years prior, the patient took a CT scan which confirmed atrophy of the brain while the vertigo worsened. At that time the patient sought medical help with no results. Soon after, her insomnia became very severe and she was hospitalized.

Presenting Symptoms: Vertigo, decreased memory, insomnia, difficulty in falling asleep, a pale red tongue with a white coating and a wiry and thin pulse.

Physical Examination: Showed normal muscle tone and strength of the extremities while the bilateral Babinski reflex (–). An ultrasound of the neck vascular showed a slight presence of atherosclerosis plaque superior to the right collar bone.

Diagnosis

TCM Diagnosis: Vertigo and forgetfulness due to turbid phlegm obstructing the upper

Western Medicine Diagnosis: Vertigo and insomnia

Treatment

Principles:

- Strengthen the spleen and drain dampness
- Dispel phlegm and remove obstruction
- Open orifice and treat vertigo

Acupuncture Point Combination:

Acupuncture was given every day.

- DU 20 (*bǎi huì*), *sì shén cōng* (EX-HN 1): To open the orifice and nourish the brain, treat vertigo and forgetfulness
- DU 24 (*shén tíng*), *yìn táng* (EX-HN 3): To calm the mind and treat vertigo and insomnia
- Scalp Acupuncture: Vertigo and auditory Scalp Line (an area in a length of 4 cm between two horizontal lines with a point 1.5 cm directly above the apex of ear as the midpoint): To treat vertigo
- ST 36 (*zú sān lǐ*), ST 40 (*fēng lóng*) and SP 9 (*yīn líng quán*): To nourish the spleen and stomach and transform phlegm
- KI 3 (*tài xī*) and SP 6 (*sān yīn jiāo*): To nourish spleen and kidney essence and support the root

Manipulations: First insert the needles into DU 20 and DU 24 transversely with the needle tip facing each other. Then insert the needles in the four *sì shén cōng* points towards DU 20 transversely. Apply the depleting technique on ST 40, the supplementing technique on KI 3 and SP 6, and the even technique on the other points. In addition, a modification of *Bàn Xià Bái Zhú Tiān Má Tāng* (Pinellia,

Atractylodes Macrocephala and Gastrodia Decoction) was given.

Follow-up Consultations

After 21 days of treatments, she felt her memory had improved that the long-term memory was fine and the short-term memory was improving. The dizziness also resolved. The patient was asked to continue acupuncture treatments and try to prevent from contracting wind-cold, have light diet and avoid emotional stress.

KEY CLINICAL POINTS

1. When treating forgetfulness we need to first identify if the syndrome is due to a deficiency or an excess pattern or if it includes both patterns. The deficiency patterns of forgetfulness mainly lie in the depletion of the qi, blood, yin and yang of the heart, spleen, kidney and liver. The excess pattern is usually due to internal obstruction of phlegm-damp retention and stagnation of qi and blood. They can be identified from each other by their corresponding symptoms and signs.
2. Since kidney essence deficiency is often the basic pathomechanism causing forgetfulness, remember to add medicinals to fortify kidney, supplement essence and boost marrow when applying other medicinals to dissolve phlegm and open the orifices, remove stasis and unblock the orifices, as well as awaken the spirit by aromatic medicinals according to different patterns.
3. Prevention of forgetfulness is more important than treatment. We should encourage elderly people to think a lot, keep a good mood, have regular physical exercises, cultivate favorable life habits, and ensure sleep quality.

BRIEF SUMMARY

Clinically, forgetfulness is more often seen in deficiency patterns than excess patterns. Excessive anxiety, over thinking and overstrain hinders the heart qi and blood and spleen qi causing a severe blood depletion and lack of nourishment to the brain. Sexual indulgence, prolonged illness and old age can also contribute to the impairment of qi, blood, yin, yang and essence. Since the brain is the sea of marrow, a severe deficiency of kidney essence also leads to a malnourishment of the brain and causes forgetfulness. On the other hand, the excess patterns of the forgetfulness resulting from the internal damage of excessive emotions and various pathogens entering the collaterals such as cold, heat, dampness and phlegm cause obstruction of the orifices and cause forgetfulness. We need to consider both the root and branch in the treatment approach and nourish the brain and blood while removing obstructions and pathogens.

COMPREHENSION QUESTIONS

1. What are the diagnostic factors of forgetfulness?
2. What are the differentiation points of forgetfulness and dementia?
3. Multiple choice questions:

1) The basic pathomechanism of forgetfulness is:

A. Qi and blood insufficiency
B. Phlegm-damp clouding the brain
C. Kidney qi deficiency
D. Stagnation of static blood
E. Insufficiency of center qi

2) The symptoms and signs of the patient include forgetfulness, vertigo, headache, body heaviness, chest oppression, gastric stuffiness, palpitations, dark tongue, greasy coating, deep and wiry pulse. This is a pattern of:

A. Qi and blood insufficiency
B. Phlegm-damp clouding the brain
C. Kidney qi deficiency
D. Stagnation of static blood
E. Insufficiency of center qi

3) The symptoms and signs of the patient include decreased memory, forgetfulness, mental fatigue, poor appetite, abdominal distention, palpitations, insomnia, light coloured tongue, and week pulse. The proper treatment principle is to:

A. Supplement qi and nourish the heart
B. Boost the kidney and replenish essence
C. Dissolve stasis and open the orifices
D. Resolve stasis and open the orifice
E. Open the orifices and awaken the spirit

Answers

1. Forgetfulness is mainly characterized by chronic or acute decreased memory and easily forgeting notions. Low spirit, depression and mental disorder are often the triggers. Diseases, such as dementia, apoplexy, insomnia, depression, and mania, can all cause memory disorder, so they should be excluded.

2. Dementia and forgetfulness are both common diseases among the elderly. The former is resulted from organic disease of the brain that causes hypofunction of the brain and decreased intelligence, and is characterized by silly, dull-witted, changes of personality and emotions, being unable to recognize family members, and easy to get lost outside. With the aggravation of disease, the patient gradually loses the ability

to look after themselves. Forgetfulness is due to recession of cerebral functions, which is mainly characterized by easily to forget recent events. It has no changes of personality.

3. 1) C, 2) B, 3) A.

Part III

Liver Conditions

3.1 Dizziness & Vertigo

The dizziness is characterized with symptoms ranging from lightheadedness and giddiness to severe loss of balance. It may last for several seconds, for days and weeks. It is usually accompanied by symptoms of vertigo, nausea, blurry vision, and fainting. For mild cases, dizziness can be relieved by closing eyes and sitting to rest, while for serious cases, patients feel like the room is spinning and are very unstable which inhibits them from being able to stand up. Dizziness and vertigo are common symptoms related to hypertension, heat stroke, fever, Ménière's Disease, cardiovascular disorders and similar diseases in the Western medicine.

In Chinese medicine, dizziness and vertigo are mainly due to either a deficient or excess pattern affecting the upper. A common pattern is yin deficiency of the liver and kidney causing the hyperactive yang harassing the upper body. The deficiency patterns include depletion of qi and blood and kidney essence depletion not nourishing the brain. Complex patterns include severe spleen and stomach depletion not transforming the fluids causing an accumulation of dampness and phlegm blocking the clear yang from nourishing the upper. Long standing obstruction of the collaterals and trauma can cause blood stasis which can inhibit the flow of qi and blood of the channels in the upper body causing vertigo. Below is a summary of the most commonly seen patterns and treatment approaches for dizziness and vertigo.

CLINICAL PATTERNS DIFFERENTIATION AND TREATMENTS

1. Hyperactivity of Liver Fire

Symptoms: Sudden episodes of dizziness or vertigo usually triggered by emotional outburst, tinnitus, distending headaches which are aggravated by fatigue or excessive emotions, flushed face, restlessness, irritability, dreamful sleep, bitter taste in the mouth, nausea, red tongue with a yellow coating and a wiry pulse.

Treatment Principle:

- Pacify liver and subdue liver yang
- Nourish the liver and kidney yin and essence

Main Acupuncture Points:

• BL 18 (*gān shù*): Back-*shu* point of the liver to clear liver and gall bladder fire to regulate and smooth the flow of qi

• LV 3 (*tài chōng*): *Yuan*-source point of the liver to clear liver damp heat and fire, spread liver qi, nourish blood and yin

• GB 20 (*fēng chí*): To clear heat, treat headaches and resolve insomnia

• KI 3 (*tài xī*): *Yuan*-source point of the kidney to nourish kidney yin and yang, resolve insomnia and tinnitus

• BL 23 (*shèn shù*): Back-*shu* point of the kidney to benefit the original qi and kidney yin

• LV 2 (*xíng jiān*): To clear liver fire and spread liver qi

Supporting Points:

• SJ 5 (*wài guān*) and GB 39 (*xuán zhōng*): To treat lateral headaches

• PC 5 (*jiān shǐ*): To treat plum-pit sensation

Recommended Formula: *Tiān Má Gōu Téng Yǐn* (天麻钩藤饮, Gastrodia and Uncaria Beverage) from the *New Discussion on the Patterns and Treatment of Miscellaneous Disease* (*Zá Bìng Zhèng Zhì Xīn Yì*, 杂病证治新义)

Substitute Formula: *Dà Dìng Fēng Zhū* (大定风珠, Major Wind-Stabilizing Pill)

Patent Formula: *Tiān Má Gōu Téng Yǐn* (天麻钩藤饮, Gastrodia and Uncaria Beverage)

2. Qi and Blood Deficiency

Symptoms: Dizziness or vertigo triggered by fatigue and aggravated by exertion, a pale complexion, lusterless lips, fingernails and hair, poor memory, palpitation, poor sleep, shortness of breath, mental exhaustion, reluctance to speak, poor appetite, a pale tongue and a thready and weak pulse.

Treatment Principle:

• Tonify qi and nourish blood

• Strengthen spleen and stomach

Main Acupuncture Points:

• BL 20 (*pí shù*): Back-*shu* point of the spleen to invigorate spleen and control the blood, regulate and harmonize the middle *jiao*.

• ST 36 (*zú sān lǐ*): To tonify spleen, nourish blood and support the middle qi

• RN 17 (*dàn zhōng*): Influential point of qi to regulate qi and unbind the chest, treat irritability and resolve palpitation

• RN 6 (*qì hǎi*): To tonify the original qi, invigorate spleen and harmonize blood

• DU 20 (*bǎi huì*): To supplement and raise the qi, resolve tinnitus and dizziness

• RN 4 (*guān yuán*): To tonify deficiency and regulate *chong* and *ren mai*

Supporting Points:

• EX-HN 24 (*ān mián*) and EX-HN 3 (*yìn táng*): To calm the spirit and resolve insomnia

- EX-HN 16 (*fà jì xué*): To treat poor memory

Recommended Formula: *Guī Pí Tāng* (归脾汤, Spleen-Restoring Decoction) from the *Formulas to Aid the Living* (*Jì Shēng Fāng*, 济生方)

Substitute Formula: *Bŭ Zhōng Yì Qì Tāng* (补中益气汤, Center-Supplementing and Qi-Boosting Decoction)

Patent Formula: *Guī Pí Wán* (归脾丸, Spleen-Restoring Pill)

3. Kidney Essence Deficiency

Symptoms: Chronic dizziness or vertigo, listlessness, insomnia, dreamful sleep, poor memory, lumbar soreness, and tinnitus.

If there is kidney yin deficiency there will also be night sweating, vexing heat in the five centers, nocturnal emission, irregular menstruation, red tongue and a wiry, thready and rapid pulse.

If there is kidney yang deficiency there will be an aversion to cold, cold limbs, impotence and uterine cold, pale tongue and a deep, weak and slow pulse.

Treatment Principle:

- Nourish yin and tonify kidney essence for kidney yin deficiency
- Warm yang and tonify kidney essence for kidney yang deficiency
- Nourish the brain and arrest vertigo

Main Acupuncture Points:

- DU 20 (*băi huì*): To supplement and raise the qi, nourish the sea of marrow
- ST 27 (*dà jù*): To benefit kidney, nourish essence and treat impotence
- RN 4 (*guān yuán*): To tonify original qi, benefit the essence and nourish kidney
- SP 6 (*sān yīn jiāo*): To tonify kidney and nourish yin, resolve poor appetite and insomnia
- BL 23 (*shèn shù*): Back-*shu* point of the kidney to tonify kidney yin
- KI 6 (*zhào hăi*): To nourish kidney and clear deficient fire

Supporting Points:

- BL 30 (*bái huán shù*): To warm the uterus, regulate seminal emission and resolve lower back and limbs pain
- KI 3 (*tài xī*): *Yuan*-source point of the kidney to nourish kidney yin and yang, strengthen the lumbar region

Recommended Formula: *Zuŏ Guī Wán* (左归丸, Left-Restoring Pill) from *The Complete Works of [Zhang] Jing-yue* (*Jĭng Yuè Quán Shū*, 景岳全书)

Substitute Formula: *Yòu Guī Wán* (右归丸, Right-Restoring Pill)

Patent Formula: *Zuŏ Guī Wán* (左归丸, Left-Restoring Pill)

4. Phlegm Obstructing the Mind

Symptoms: Dizziness or vertigo with heaviness of the head, lack of concentration, chest stuffiness, nausea, obesity, poor appetite, sleepiness, white tongue with greasy coating and a soft or slippery pulse.

Treatment Principle:

- Expel dampness and resolve phlegm
- Strengthen the spleen and harmonize the stomach
- Open the orifices and treat dizziness

Main Acupuncture Points:

- ST 40 (*fēng lóng*): Main point for expelling phlegm and dampness, nourishing the spleen and calming the spirit
- BL 20 (*pí shù*): Back-*shu* point of the spleen to invigorate spleen and resolve phlegm, regulate and harmonize the middle *jiao*
- ST 36 (*zú sān lǐ*): To tonify spleen, nourish blood and support the middle qi
- PC 6 (*nèi guān*): To regulate stomach, unbind the chest and alleviate nausea
- BL 43 (*gāo huāng*): To tonify organs and resolve phlegm

Supporting Points:

- EX-HN 1 (*sì shén cōng*): To improve poor memory, resolve insomnia and open the mind
- SP 8 (*dì jī*): *Xi*-cleft point of the spleen to harmonize spleen, resolve dampness and improve appetite

Recommended Formula: *Bàn Xià Bái Zhú Tiān Má Tāng* (半夏白术天麻汤, Pinellia, Atractylodes Macrocephala and Gastrodia Decoction) from the *Medical Revelations* (*Yī Xué Xīn Wù*, 医学心悟)

Substitute Formula: *Wēn Dǎn Tāng* (温胆汤, Gallbladder-Warming Decoction)

Patent Formula: *Bàn Xià Tiān Má Wán* (半夏天麻丸, Pinellia and Gastrodia Pill)

5. Blood Stasis Obstructing the Mind

Symptoms: Dizziness or vertigo with a fixed headache, dark complexion, dark purple lips and fingernails, palpitations, insomnia, tinnitus, deafness, dark purple tongue with ecchymosis and a wiry and choppy or thready and choppy pulse.

Treatment Principle:

- Invigorate blood and dissolve stasis
- Open the orifice and clear the mind

Main Acupuncture Points:

- BL 15 (*xīn shù*): Back-*shu* point of the heart to resolve blood stasis and calm the spirit, unbind the chest and regulate qi
- GB 20 (*fēng chí*): To clear heat, treat headaches and resolve insomnia
- DU 16 (*fēng fǔ*): To benefit the upper and resolve dizziness
- SP 10 (*xuè hǎi*): To promote blood flow, dispel blood stasis and calm the spirit
- LV 3 (*tài chōng*): *Yuan*-source point of the liver to benefit qi, nourish blood and yin and clear head and eyes

Supporting Points:

- RN 4 (*guān yuán*): To resolve dysmenorrhea, regulate *chong* and *ren mai* and benefit the uterus

• EX-HN 1 (*sì shén cōng*): To improve poor memory, resolve insomnia and awaken the mind

Recommended Formula: *Tōng Qiào Huó Xuè Tāng* (通窍活血汤, Orifice-Soothing Blood-Activating Decoction) from the *Correction of Errors in Medical Works* (*Yī Lín Gǎi Cuò*, 医林改错)

Substitute Formula: *Xuè Fǔ Zhú Yū Tāng* (血府逐瘀汤, Blood Stasis Expelling Decoction)

Patent Formula: *Xuè Fǔ Zhú Yū Wán* (血府逐瘀丸, Blood Stasis Expelling Pill)

Summary Chart for Dizziness

Patterns	Main Points	Supporting Points	Formulae
Hyperactivity of Liver Fire	BL 18, LV 3, GB 20, KI 3, BL 23, LV 2	SJ 5 and GB 39 for lateral headaches PC 5 for plum-stone qi (globus hystericus)	*Tiān Má Gōu Téng Yǐn* or *Dà Dìng Fēng Zhū*
Qi and Blood Deficiency	BL 20, ST 36, RN 17, RN 6, DU 20, RN 4	EX-HN 24 for irritability and insomnia EX-HN 3 to calm the mind EX-HN 16 for poor memory accompanied by vertigo	*Guī Pí Tāng* or *Bǔ Zhōng Yì Qì Tāng*
Kidney Essence Deficiency	DU 20, ST 27, RN 4, SP 6, BL 23, KI 6	BL 30 for uterine cold, seminal emission and lumbago KI 3 to nourish kidney	*Zuǒ Guī Wán* or *Yòu Guī Wán*
Phlegm Obstructing the Middle *Jiao*	ST 40, BL 20, ST 36, PC 6, BL 43	EX-HN 1 for poor memory and insomnia SP 8 for dampness and poor appetite	*Bàn Xià Bái Zhú Tiān Má Tāng* or *Wēn Dǎn Tāng*
Blood Stasis affecting the Upper	BL 15, GB 20, DU 16, SP 10, LV 3	RN 4 for dysmenorrhea EX-CA 1 for irregular menstruation and uterine disorders	*Tōng Qiào Huó Xuè Tāng* or *Xuè Fǔ Zhú Yū Tāng*

CASE STUDY: Chronic Dizziness

Mr. Jiang, 57 years old.

Main Complaint: Recurrent dizziness and blurry vision for 5 years with aggravation for a week.

Medical History: The patient suffered from dizziness and blurry vision following a stressful and exhausting period 5 years ago. The symptoms went away with rest; however, the patient self administered Dogbane to lower his blood pressure since it reached 176/98 mmHg at the time. Following that episode, symptoms of dizziness, blurry vision, and neck distension would return with a fluctuating blood pressure between 160/92 and 170/96 mmHg. The patient mainly took Acertil, Lacidipine and Aspirin as medication to control it. The patient was later diagnosed with grade 2 hypertension and he also had a family history of hypertension. The week prior to the consultation, he quarrelled with others and had a sudden feeling of dizziness and irritability with insomnia and dreamful sleep which affected his work. He suffered from peripheral arteriosclerosis obliteration and was often impatient.

Presenting Symptoms: Dizziness, blurry vision, tinnitus, headache, distension of the head, flushed face and ears, restlessness, irritability, poor sleep, dreamful sleep, dry mouth with a bitter taste, dry difficult stools, chest stuffiness and distension, a red tongue with a thin yellow and dry coating and wiry pulse.

Physical Examination: Temperature: 37 ℃, pulse: 72 bpm, respiration: 20 bpm, blood pressure 156/112 mmHg with an average of 158/96 mmHg during the day and 142/92 mmHg in the evening. The patient was active and aware with no abnormal findings on the lymph nodes, lungs, heart, abdomen, liver, spleen and kidney. An ECG and colour sonography showed left ventricular enlargement and damage. Urine test was protein (+), blood cholesterol was TRIG 2.3 mmol/L, CHOL 5.6 mmol/L, LDL 3.56 mmol/L, blood sugar was 4.8 mmol/L, and the renal functions were BUN 6.7 umol/L, SCr 98 umol/L.

Pattern Differentiation

This patient was usually impatient and often quarrelled. In this case, the emotional disorder caused liver qi constraint which transformed into fire leading to hyperactivity of liver yang moving upwards and harassing the brain resulting in dizziness and blurry vision. In addition, the flow of qi and blood rushed upward with the liver yang hyperactivity and caused headache, distension of the head, flushed face and eyes, and tinnitus. The liver governs the flow of qi and when the liver is constricted it caused chest stuffiness and distress, impatience and irritability causing internal heat. Internal heat consumed the body fluids and the intestines failed to be moistened which caused a dry mouth with bitter taste and dry difficult stools. When the excessive heat disturbs the spirit, there are signs of insomnia and dreamful sleep. The red tongue with a thin, yellow and dry tongue coating and the wiry pulse were signs of liver yang hyperactivity.

Diagnosis

TCM Diagnosis: Dizziness due to liver yang hyperactivity harassing the upper
Western Medicine Diagnosis: Chronic dizziness

Treatment

In this case, the pathomechanism mainly lies in the emotional disorder causing the liver qi constraint transforming into liver fire moving upwards harassing the brain.

Principles:

- Soothe the liver qi and subdue yang
- Clear pathogenic fire and open orifices
- Calm the mind and treat dizziness

Formula: Modified *Tiān Má Gōu Téng Yǐn* (Gastrodia and Uncaria Decoction)

Ingredients:

天麻	*tiān má*	10 g	Rhizoma Gastrodiae
钩藤	*gōu téng*	19 g	Ramulus Uncariae Cum Uncis
石决明	*shí jué míng*	30 g	Concha Haliotidis
黄芩	*huáng qín*	10 g	Radix Scutellariae
栀子	*zhī zǐ*	10 g	Fructus Gardeniae
夏枯草	*xià kū cǎo*	10 g	Spica Prunellae
郁金	*yù jīn*	15 g	Radix Curcumae
草决明	*cǎo jué míng*	15 g	Semen Cassiae
生地	*shēng dì*	15 g	Radix Rehmanniae
牛膝	*niú xī*	15 g	Radix Achyranthis Bidentatae
桑寄生	*sāng jì shēng*	15 g	Herba Taxilli
茯神	*fú shén*	15 g	Sclerotium Poriae Pararadicis
夜交藤	*yè jiāo téng*	15 g	Caulis Polygoni Multiflori

Formula Analysis

In this formula, *tiān má* acts to dispel wind and subdue yang, relieve headache and dizziness. *Gōu téng* clears heat, extinguishes wind and subdues internal fire. The combination of these two medicinals soothes the liver and subdues overacting liver yang. *Shí jué míng* tranquilizes the liver and extinguishes internal wind. *Huáng qín, zhī zǐ* and *xià kū cǎo* clear the liver and purge fire. *Yù jīn* resolves constraint qi and clears pathogenic fire. *Shēng dì* and *cǎo jué míng* nourish blood, moisten intestines and relax bowels. *Niú xī* and *sāng jì shēng* strengthen the liver and kidney. *Fú shén* and *yè jiāo téng* nourish the blood and calm the mind. The combination of all the medicinals calms the liver and subdues overacting liver yang, and clears pathogenic fire and extinguishes wind.

Chinese Patent Medicines: *Mài Jūn Ān Piàn* (Peaceful Pulse Tablets) was given to the patient at the dosage of 3 tablets, 3 times a day.

Follow-up Consultations

On the 2nd consultation, after 7 doses of the above formula and patent medicine, the blood pressure was 148/94 mmHg. His bowels were normal and the symptom of dry mouth subsided. He still had numbness of the upper limbs and distending pain in the nape. Based on the previous formula, 15 g of *dì lóng* (Pheretima) and 15 g of *dāng guī* (Radix Angelicae Sinensis) were added to invigorate blood and unblock collaterals. *Gé gēn* (Radix Puerariae Lobatae) 10 g was added to relax the sinews and relieve convulsion.

On the 3rd consultation, after another 14 doses of the formula and patent medicine, the blood pressure was 140/92 mmHg. The patient still had mild dizziness, dreamful sleep, distention of the eyes, a pale red tongue with thin yellow coating and a wiry pulse. The patient continued with the same formula for another 14 doses which relieved the symptoms completely.

KEY CLINICAL POINTS

Though the cause for the symptoms of dizziness is mainly located in the brain, the pathomechanism is closely related to the disorder of the liver, spleen and kidney. Understanding the full complexity of the patterns helps to target the treatment to the root of the symptoms as well as symptoms themselves. Analysis on the combination of symptoms and comparing them to the list of symptoms in the pattern differentiation section will guide us to the appropriate treatment approaches, acupuncture point combinations and recommended formulas.

It is important to remember when treating dizziness and vertigo, the patterns are usually a combination of deficiency and excess. For example, deficiency of yin and essence with hyperactive yang affecting the upper, or deficiency of qi and blood not nourishing the brain causing internal wind, spleen qi deficiency not transforming fluids creating phlegm blocking the upper and so on.

In addition, dizziness and vertigo are closely related to hypertension which may lead to stroke causing coma or death. In this sense, it is important for these patients to be able to control their blood pressure and avoid more severe diseases. This is taken into account when modifying the medicinals in the formula by adding some medicinals to target the symptoms of high blood pressure with medicinals such as *gōu téng, xià kū cǎo,* and *gé gēn* for hyperactivity of liver yang pattern; *dì lóng, yì mǔ cǎo,* and *chuān niú xī* for blood stasis obstructing the orifices pattern; *bái sháo* and *xuán shēn* for liver and kidney yin deficiency pattern; *dù zhòng* and *sāng jì shēng* for kidney yang deficiency pattern.

COMPREHENSION QUESTIONS

1. What are the pattern differentiations and formulas for dizziness?
2. How can we differentiate dizziness from wind-strike?
3. How can a patient suffering from dizziness and vertigo participate in their healing?
4. Multiple choice questions:

1) Mr. Hou, 46 years old. The patient suffered from hypertension for 3 years with symptoms of headache, dizziness, tinnitus, poor memory, dry eyes, blurry vision, rib-

side dull pain, lumbar and knee soreness, dry throat and mouth, poor sleep, dreamful sleep, a red tongue with a scanty coating and a thin pulse. The recommended treatment principles are to:

A. Tonify the liver and kidney, nourish yin and essence
B. Nourish yin, soothe the liver and subdue liver yang
C. Soothe the liver and subdue pathogenic fire
D. Nourish yin, soothe the liver and brighten the vision
E. Tonify the kidney and soothe the liver

2) Mr. Kuang, 43 years old. The patient suffered from hypertension for a year with the symptoms of headache, dizziness, bitter taste in the mouth, dry throat, irritability, a red tongue with a yellow and greasy tongue coating and a wiry and slippery pulse. The recommended formula is:

A. *Tiān Má Gōu Téng Tāng* (Gastrodia and Uncaria Decoction)
B. *Zhī Zǐ Qīng Gān Tāng* (Gardenia Liver-Calming Decoction)
C. *Lóng Dǎn Xiè Gān Tāng* (Gentian Liver-Draining Decoction)
D. *Huáng Lián Wēn Dǎn Tāng* (Coptis Gallbladder-Warming Decoction)
E. *Zhèn Gān Xī Fēng Tāng* (Liver-Sedating and Wind-Extinguishing Decoction)

3) Ms. Xie, 56 years old. The patient suffered from hypertension for six years with accompanied symptoms of headache, dizziness, blurry vision, heaviness of the head, chest stuffiness, nausea, vomiting with foam, epigastric *pǐ* and fullness, poor appetite, mental fatigue, an enlarged tongue with teeth marks and a white and greasy tongue coating. The recommended formula is:

A. *Huáng Lián Wēn Dǎn Tāng* (Coptis Gallbladder-Warming Decoction)
B. *Tiān Má Gōu Téng Tāng* (Gastrodia and Uncaria Decoction)
C. *Bàn Xià Bái Zhú Tiān Má Tāng* (Pinellia, Atractylodes Macrocephala and Gastrodia Decoction)
D. *Liù Jūn Zǐ Tāng* (Six Gentlemen Decoction)
E. *Zhǐ Mí Fú Líng Wán* (Puzzle Resolving Poria Pill)

4) Mr. Peng, 67 years old. The patient suffered from hypertension for nine years with the accompanied symptoms of headache and dizziness which aggravated by exertion and induced by fatigue, mental exhaustion, reluctant to speak, lusterless complexion, pale lips and nails, palpitation, poor sleep, a pale tongue with a thin and white coating and a thin and weak pulse. The recommended treatment principle is to:

A. Fortify the spleen and qi
B. Tonify qi and nourish blood, strengthen the spleen and stomach
C. Tonify qi and blood
D. Strengthen the spleen and nourish the heart
E. Strengthen the spleen, soothe the liver, and harmonize the stomach

5) Mr. Ye, 72 years old. The patient suffered from hypertension for eight years with accompanied symptoms of headache with stabbing pain, dizziness, darkish complexion, purple darkish lips, dry and scaly skin, poor memory, palpitation, insomnia, tinnitus, hearing loss, a purple darkish tongue with a thin and choppy pulse. The recommended formula is:

A. *Xuè Fŭ Zhú Yū Tāng* (Blood Mansion Stasis-Expelling Decoction)
B. *Táo Hóng Sì Wù Tāng* (Peach Kernel and Carthamus Four Substances Decoction)
C. *Tōng Qiào Huó Xuè Tāng* (Orifice-Unblocking and Blood-Moving Decoction)
D. *Bŭ Yáng Huán Wŭ Tāng* (Yang-Supplementing and Five-Returning Decoction)
E. *Dān Shēn Yĭn* (Salvia Beverage)

6) Ms. Liu, 73 years old. The patient suffered from hypertension for 28 years and clinical manifestations of headache, dizziness, tinnitus, cold sensation of the body and limbs, palpitation, shortness of breath, soreness of the waist and knee, seminal emission, impotence, frequent and excessive nocturia, loose stool, a pale and enlarged tongue with a thin and weak pulse. The recommended treatment principle is to:

A. Fortify the spleen and kidney
B. Warm and supplement the kidney yang
C. Tonify the kidney and supplement essence
D. Warm and supplement the spleen and stomach
E. Nourish the kidney yin

Answers

1. There are 5 main patterns related to the symptoms of dizziness. Here is a summary of the main patterns with their recommended formula:

• For hyperactive liver fire, use *Tiān Má Gōu Téng Yĭn* (Gastrodia and Uncaria Beverage) or *Dà Dìng Fēng Zhū* (Major Wind-Stabilizing Pill)

• For kidney essence deficiency, use *Zuŏ Guī Wán* (Left-Restoring Pill) for yin deficiency, *Jì Shēng Shèn Qì Wán* (Life-Saving Kidney Qi Pill) for yang deficiency or *Yòu Guī Wán* (Right-Restoring Pill) for both yin and yang deficiency;

• For qi and blood deficiency, use *Guī Pí Tāng* (Spleen-Restoring Decoction) or *Bŭ Zhōng Yì Qì Tāng* (Center-Supplementing and Qi-Boosting Decoction);

• For turbid phlegm obstructing the mind, use *Bàn Xià Bái Zhú Tiān Má Tāng* (Pinellia, Atractylodes Macrocephala and Gastrodia Decoction) or *Wēn Dăn Tāng* (Gallbladder-Warming Decoction);

• For stasis obstructing the brain, use *Tōng Qiào Huó Xuè Tāng* (Orifice-Unblocking and Blood-Moving Decoction) or *Xuè Fŭ Zhú Yū Tāng* (Blood Stasis Expelling Decoction);

2. Wind-strike is a disease chiefly characterized as suddenly falling into a coma due to either a blood clot or bleeding in the brain with sequelea of hemiplegia, facial palsy, aphasia and half-body numbness. In comparison, the symptoms of dizziness

are a combination of the sensation of being unstable like the room is spinning around you accompanied with vertigo, tinnitus and headache. There are no symptoms of coma or paralysis involved with dizziness. However, in some cases, the symptoms of dizziness and vertigo can be precursors of wind-strike.

3. Patients suffering from dizziness can do various changes in the daily life to support a healthier life. Patients can give importance to spending quality time in nature or in a quiet environment every day to rest and recuperate from the emotional and mental stress. Taking short walks in parks, or practicing Tai ji or an activity the patient enjoys is recommended to calm the emotions and relax the mind.

Dietary changes can also be made as to avoid smoking, drinking alcohol, or eating salty and spicy food. Adding more fruits and vegetable while reducing the intake of greasy and fatty foods are best for the circulatory system. Adding foods which have been proven to reduce blood pressure such as celery, spinach, laver, lily, shitake mushroom, black agaric, wild rice shoot or seaweed are good supplements.

In addition, keeping a daily blood pressure log to inform the doctor and monitor the blood pressure is recommended.

4. 1) A, 2) D, 3) C, 4) B, 5) C, 6) B.

3.2 Wind-strike

Wind-strike is a disease chiefly characterized by the symptoms of sudden attack of slurred speech, disorientation and fainting and/or coma, similar to stroke. There are often sequelae of hemiplegia, facial palsy, aphasia and numbness of the limbs. In mild cases, there are light symptoms of tingling or numbness without falling into a full coma or having paralysis. In Western medicine, stroke is understood to be the results of a sudden internal hemorrhage or blood thrombosis in the brain characterized in various diseases such as cerebral hemorrhage, cerebral thrombosis, cerebral embolism and subarachnoid hemorrhage.

In Chinese medicine, there are many pathological patterns related to the acute onset as well as the sequelae themselves. Firstly, understanding that wind-strike is often caused by the dysfunction of multiple organs causing a severe adverse flow of qi and blood in the brain leading to obstruction in the brain vessels. In mild cases, the wind-strike disorder affects the channels and collaterals; while in serious cases, it affects the viscera and bowels which involves excess and deficiency patterns. There are excessive patterns of pathogenic phlegm, fire, cold, and blood stasis which are sometimes combined with deficiency patterns of qi and blood depletion, deficiency of the liver yin and blood, spleen and stomach qi or kidney yin, yang and essence. In the acute stage, the wind-strike is often caused by phlegm-fire and liver wind uprising affecting the brain. Soon after the sudden attack, the pathogenic yin prevails and the healthy yang of the patient declines and there is an obvious qi deficiency. In the later stage, there is apparent kidney essence depletion not nourishing the brain. The treatment principles will vary according to the type of pathogenic factors, the pattern differentiation as well as the stage of the pathology.

CLINICAL PATTERNS DIFFERENTIATION AND TREATMENTS

1. Channel Disorder Patterns

A. Sudden Hyperactivity of Liver Yang

Symptoms: Sudden facial paralysis, slurred speech or aphasia, numbness and heaviness of the extremities, hemiplegia, dizziness, headaches, vertigo, tinnitus, dreamful sleep, lower back and knee pain, dryness of the throat, constipation, dark and scanty urination, red tongue with scanty or greasy coating and a wiry, thready and rapid or wiry and slippery pulse.

Treatment Principle:

- Nourish yin and subdue yang
- Expel wind and unblock the collaterals

Main Acupuncture Points:

- GB 20 (*fēng chí*): To expel wind and clear heat, treat headaches and resolve hearing and balancing disorders
- KI 3 (*tài xī*): *Yuan*-source point of the kidney to nourish yin and yang and clear deficient heat
- BL 18 (*gān shù*): Back-*shu* point of the liver to clear liver and gall bladder fire, spread liver qi, nourish blood, pacify wind and calm the spirit
- LV 3 (*tài chōng*): *Yuan*-source point of the liver to clear pathogenic fire and dampness, subdue yang and pacify wind, nourish blood and yin
- DU 20 (*băi huì*): To subdue liver yang, pacify wind, nourish the sea of marrow and treat stroke and aphasia
- DU 16 (*fēng fŭ*): To expel wind, nourish marrow and calm the spirit

Supporting Points:

- SP 6 (*sān yīn jiāo*): To tonify liver and kidney, nourish yin and resolve painful muscular contractions

Recommended Formula: *Tiān Má Gōu Téng Tāng* (天麻钩藤汤, Gastrodia and Uncaria Decoction) from the *New Discussion on the Patterns and Treatment of Miscellaneous Disease* (*Zá Bìng Zhèng Zhì Xīn Yì*, 杂病证治新义)

Substitute Formula: *Líng Jiăo Gōu Téng Tāng* (羚角钩藤汤, Antelope Horn and Uncaria Decoction)

Patent Formula: *Ān Gōng Niú Huáng Wán* (安宫牛黄丸, Peaceful Palace Bovine Bezoar Pill)

B. Wind Phlegm Obstructing the Channels

Symptoms: Skin numbness of palms and soles, sudden deviation of the mouth and eye, slurred speech, hemiplegia, dysphagia, excessive salivation which is difficult to expectorate, chills, fever, dizziness, headaches, loss of muscle motor coordination or numbness or limb hypertonicity, joint soreness or pain, a dark tongue with a thin and white or yellow coating and a floating and rapid or wiry and slippery pulse.

Treatment Principle:

- Fortify the qi to transform phlegm
- Nourish blood to extinguish internal wind
- Open the orifices and unblock the collaterals

Main Acupuncture Points:

- GB 20 (*fēng chí*): To expel wind and clear heat, treat headaches and resolve hearing loss and vertigo

- LI 4 (*hé gǔ*): To expel wind and phlegm, treat mouth and eye deviation and upper limb paralysis
- ST 40 (*fēng lóng*): To expel phlegm and dampness
- BL 40 (*wěi zhōng*): To treat hemiplegia due to stagnated dampness and benefit lower back and knees
- SP 6 (*sān yīn jiāo*): To resolve phlegm and lower limb pain and spasms
- EX-UE 9 (*bā xié*): To expel wind and treat finger and upper limb numbness and spasms

Supporting Points:

- EX-HN 1 (*sì shén cōng*): To open the orifices and awaken the mind
- ST 4 (*dì cāng*): To expel wind, stop salivation and resolve facial paralysis and pain

Recommended Formula: *Zhēn Fāng Bái Wán Zǐ* (真方白丸子, Effective White Pill) from the *Formulas from the Auspicious Bamboo Hall* (*Ruì Zhú Táng Fāng*, 瑞竹堂方)

Substitute Formula: *Bàn Xià Bái Zhú Tiān Má Tāng* (半夏白术天麻汤, Pinellia, Atractylodes Macrocephala and Gastrodia Decoction) plus *Qiān Zhèng Sǎn* (牵正散, Symmetry-Correcting Powder)

Patent Formula: *Zhòng Fēng Huí Chūn Wán* (中风回春丸, Stroke Recovery Pill)

C. Phlegm Heat in the *Fu*-Organs

Symptoms: Sudden loss of consciousness, locked jaw, clenched fists, muscle rigidity, stool and urine retention, flushed face, fever, rapid breathing, halitosis, excessive salivation, throat-rales, restlessness and irritability, hiccups, a red tongue with yellow and greasy coating and wiry, slippery and surging pulse.

Treatment Principle:

- Clear liver heat and subdue yang rising
- Expel wind and transform phlegm
- Unblock channels and open orifices

Main Acupuncture Points:

- LI 11 (*qū chí*): To clear heat and cool blood, expel wind and transform phlegm, resolve upper limb paralysis and benefit the throat
- ST 44 (*nèi tíng*): To clear fire, expel phlegm and resolve irritability
- ST 40 (*fēng lóng*): To expel phlegm and dampness
- ST 25 (*tiān shū*): Front-*mu* of the large intestine to resolve phlegm heat, harmonize stomach and regulate the intestines
- DU 26 (*shuǐ gōu*): To restore consciousness and clear fire
- GB 20 (*fēng chí*): To expel wind and clear heat, treat headaches and resolve hearing loss and vertigo

Supporting Points:

- HT 8 (*shào fǔ*): To clear heat from the heart and small intestine, calm the spirit and alleviate pain

- LI 4 (*hé gǔ*): To expel phlegm, treat upper limb paralysis and locked jaws

Recommended Formula: *Táo Hé Chéng Qì Tāng* (桃核承气汤, Peach Kernel Qi-Guiding Decoction) from the *Treatise on Cold Damage* (*Shāng Hán Lùn*, 伤寒论) plus *Dí Tán Tāng* (涤痰汤, Phlegm-Flushing Decoction) from the *Fine Formulas of Wonderful Efficacy* (*Qí Xiào Liáng Fāng*, 奇效良方)

Substitute Formula: *Xīng Lóu Chéng Qì Tāng* (星蒌承气汤, Arisaema and Trichosanthes Qi-Guiding Decoction)

Patent Formula:

- *Ān Gōng Niú Huáng Wán* (安宫牛黄丸, Peaceful Palace Bovine Bezoar Pill)
- *Niú Huáng Qīng Xīn Wán* (牛黄清心丸, Bovine Bezoar Heart-Clearing Pill)

D. Qi Deficiency and Blood Stasis

Symptoms: Unilateral body weakness, loss of motor and sensory coordination, fatigue, edema or numbness of limbs, facial paralysis, pale complexion, poor appetite, loose stools, slurred speech, dark purple tongue with petechiae and white coating and a thready, choppy and weak pulse.

Treatment Principle:

- Tonify qi and invigorate blood to remove blood stasis
- Unblock the collaterals and open orifices

Main Acupuncture Points:

- RN 6 (*qì hǎi*): To tonify original qi, invigorate spleen and harmonize blood
- SP 10 (*xuè hǎi*): To promote blood flow and dispel stasis, harmonize menstruation and calm the spirit
- ST 36 (*zú sān lǐ*): To tonify qi and invigorate blood, treat stroke and lower limb paralysis
- DU 20 (*bǎi huì*): To raise the qi, nourish the sea of marrow and treat stroke
- BL 17 (*gé shù*): Influential point of the blood to activate blood circulation and dispel stasis
- BL 20 (*pí shù*) plus BL 21 (*wèi shù*): Back-*shu* points of spleen and stomach to nourish qi, invigorate blood and harmonize the middle *jiao*

Supporting Points:

- EX-LE 6 (*dǎn náng xué*): To treat muscular atrophy and lower limb numbness
- ST 4 (*dì cāng*): To resolve facial paralysis and pain

Recommended Formula: *Bǔ Yáng Huán Wǔ Tāng* (补阳还五汤, Yang-Supplementing and Five-Returning Decoction) from the *Correction of Errors in Medical Works* (*Yī Lín Gǎi Cuò*, 医林改错)

Substitute Formula: *Táo Hóng Sì Wù Tāng* (桃红四物汤, Peach Kernel and Carthamus Four Substances Decoction)

Patent Formula: *Zhòng Fēng Huí Chūn Wán* (中风回春丸, Stroke Recovery Pill)

E. Wind-Stirring due to Yin Deficiency

Symptoms: Sudden facial paralysis, sudden deviation of the mouth and eyes, headache, tinnitus, blurry vision, dreamful sleep, tongue stiffness and slurred speech or aphasia, heavy sensations of the limbs or hemiplegia, lower back and knee pain, throat dryness, constipation, dark scanty urination, a red tongue with scanty or greasy coating and a wiry, thready and rapid or wiry and slippery pulse.

Treatment Principle:

- Nourish yin and subdue uprising yang
- Nourish blood and expel wind
- Open orifices and unblock the collaterals

Main Acupuncture Points:

- KI 3 (*tài xī*): *Yuan*-source point of the kidney to nourish yin and yang, strengthen the lower back and knees
- BL 23 (*shèn shù*): Back-*shu* point of the kidney to tonify kidney yin
- LV 3 (*tài chōng*): *Yuan*-source point of the liver to soothe liver, subdue yang and pacify wind, nourish blood and yin
- SP 6 (*sān yīn jiāo*): To tonify liver and kidney, nourish yin and resolve muscle pain and spasm
- LI 4 (*hé gǔ*): To expel wind, treat deviation of the mouth and eye and upper limb paralysis
- EX-UE 9 (*bā xié*): To expel wind and treat numbness and spasm of the finger and upper limbs

Supporting Points:

- DU 21 (*qián dǐng*): To subdue liver yang, clear eyes and calm spirit
- GB 20 (*fēng chí*): To expel wind, benefit eyes, treat headaches and resolve hearing loss and vertigo

Recommended Formula: *Zhèn Gān Xī Fēng Tāng* (镇肝息风汤, Liver-Sedating and Wind-Extinguishing Decoction) from the *Records of Chinese Medicine with Reference to Western Medicine* (*Yī Xué Zhōng Zhōng Cān Xī Lù*, 医学衷中参西录)

Substitute Formula: *Sì Wù Tāng* (四物汤, Four Substances Decoction) plus *Dà Dìng Fēng Zhū* (大定风珠, Major Wind-Stabilizing Pill)

Patent Formula:

- *Zhī Bǎi Dì Huáng Wán* (知柏地黄丸, Anemarrhena, Phellodendron and Rehmannia Pill)
- *Dà Bǔ Yīn Wán* (大补阴丸, Major Yin-Supplementing Pill)

Summary Chart for Wind-Strike: Channel Disorders

Channel Patterns	Main Points	Supporting Points	Formulae
Sudden Hyperactivity of Liver Yang	GB 20, KI 3, BL 18, LV 3, DU 20, DU 16	SP 6 for muscle contractions	*Tiān Má Gōu Téng Tāng* or *Líng Jiǎo Gōu Téng Tāng*

Continued

Channel Patterns	Main Points	Supporting Points	Formulae
Wind Phlegm Obstructing the Meridians	GB 20, LI 4, ST 40, BL 40, SP 6, EX-UE 9	EX-HN 1 to open the orifices ST 4 for excessive salivation and facial paralysis	*Zhēn Fāng Bái Wán Zǐ* or *Bàn Xià Bái Zhú Tiān Má Tāng* plus *Qiān Zhèng Sǎn*
Phlegm Heat in the *Fu* Organs	LI 11, ST 44, ST 40, ST 25, DU 26, GB 20	HT 8 for heart and small intestine heat LI 4 for upper limb paralysis and locked jaw	*Táo Hé Chéng Qì Tāng* plus *Dí Tán Tāng* or *Xīng Lóu Chéng Qì Tāng*
Qi Deficiency and Blood Stasis	RN 6, SP 10, ST 36, DU 20, BL 17, BL 20	EX-LE 6 for muscular atrophy and lower limb numbness ST 4 for facial paralysis	*Bǔ Yáng Huán Wǔ Tāng* or *Táo Hóng Sì Wù Tāng*
Wind Stirring due to Yin Deficiency	KI 3, BL 23, LV 3, SP 6, LI 4, EX-UE 9	DU 21 for liver yang rising GB 20 for hearing loss and vertigo	*Zhèn Gān Xī Fēng Tāng* or *Sì Wù Tāng* plus *Dà Dìng Fēng Zhū*

2. Organ Disorder Patterns

A. Wind Fire Obstructing the Heart

Symptoms: Sudden collapse with loss of consciousness, hemiplegia, contractions and rigidity of the limbs, deviation of the tongue and mouth, squinting and redness of the eyes, flushed face, locked jaw, neck stiffness, fist clenching, a dark red tongue with dry and yellow or black coating and a wiry pulse.

Treatment Principle:

- Clear pathogenic fire and expel wind
- Open the orifices and soothe the heart

Main Acupuncture Points:

- DU 16 (*fēng fǔ*): To expel wind and clear heat, nourish marrow and calm the spirit
- BL 62 (*shēn mài*): To treat stroke and unconsciousness, resolve head and eye disorders
- LV 2 (*xíng jiān*): To clear fire and spread liver qi, expel wind and clear head, calm spirit and treat mouth deviation
- LI 11 (*qū chí*): To clear heat and cool blood, expel wind and phlegm, resolve upper limb paralysis and benefit the throat
- DU 26 (*shuǐ gōu*): To restore consciousness and clear fire
- LU 7 (*liè quē*): To expel wind, benefit the head, loosen the neck and regulate the

ren vessel

Supporting Points:

- EX-HN 1 (*sì shén cōng*): To open the orifices and awaken the mind
- GB 20 (*fēng chí*): To expel wind and heat, benefit neck and eyes, treat headaches and resolve hearing and balancing disorders

Recommended Formula: *Tiān Má Gōu Téng Tāng* (天麻钩藤汤, Gastrodia and Uncaria Decoction) from the *New Discussion on the Patterns and Treatment of Miscellaneous Disease* (*Zá Bìng Zhèng Zhì Xīn Yì*, 杂病证治新义) plus *Zǐ Xuě Dān* (紫雪丹, Purple Snow Elixir)

Substitute Formula: *Líng Jiǎo Gōu Téng Tāng* (羚角钩藤汤, Antelope Horn and Uncaria Decoction)

Patent Formula: *Ān Gōng Niú Huáng Wán* (安宫牛黄丸, Peaceful Palace Bovine Bezoar Pill)

B. Phlegm Fire Obstructing the Heart

Symptoms: Sudden collapse with loss of consciousness, snoring and wheezing accompanied by phlegm expectoration, difficult movement and convulsions of affected limb, mouth and tongue deviation, flushed face, eye redness, hot sensations, restlessness, dark red tongue with yellow and greasy or dry coating, and wiry, slippery and rapid pulse.

Treatment Principle:

- Soothe liver and expel wind
- Resolve phlegm and subdue fire
- Open the orifices

Main Acupuncture Points:

- PC 6 (*nèi guān*): *Luo* point of the pericardium to clear heart heat and calm the spirit
- DU 26 (*shuǐ gōu*): To restore consciousness and clear fire, arrest convulsions
- ST 40 (*fēng lóng*): To transform phlegm and dampness and clear heart phlegm
- SI 3 (*hòu xī*): To clear wind and heat, resolve pain and rigidity of head and neck muscles, treat stroke
- DU 16 (*fēng fǔ*): To clear heat, nourish sea of marrow and treat disorders along *du* vessel
- LV 2 (*xíng jiān*): To clear liver fire, spread liver qi and relax sinews to benefit muscle rigidity

Supporting Points:

- 12 *jing*-well points: To treat post stroke hemiplegia and edema, clear heat and arrest convulsions
- SJ 3 (*zhōng zhǔ*): To expel wind and heat and treat finger rigidity

Recommended Formula: *Líng Yáng Jiǎo Tāng* (羚羊角汤, Antelope Horn Decoction) from *The Refined in Medicine Remembered* (*Yī Chún Shèng Yì*, 医醇賸义)

Substitute Formula: *Qīng Qì Huà Tán Wán* (清气化痰丸, Qi-Clearing and Phlegm-Transforming Pill)

Patent Formula: *Ān Gōng Niú Huáng Wán* (安宫牛黄丸, Peaceful Palace Bovine Bezoar Pill)

C. Phlegm and Dampness Obstructing the Heart

Symptoms: Sudden loss of consciousness, locked jaw, clenched fists, urine retention, constipation, limb rigidity or contractions, heaviness and numbness of the head, occasional aphasia, profuse phlegm expectoration, a pale enlarged tongue with thick and greasy white coating and a deep, slippery and slow pulse.

Treatment Principle:

- Dry dampness and resolve phlegm
- Invigorate spleen and stomach
- Open the orifices

Main Acupuncture Points:

- PC 6 (*nèi guān*): *Luo* point of the pericardium to regulate heart, unbind the chest and calm the spirit
- DU 26 (*shuǐ gōu*): To restore consciousness and arrest convulsions
- RN 12 (*zhōng wǎn*): Front-*mu* point of the stomach to harmonize spleen and stomach
- ST 8 (*tóu wéi*): To regulate stomach and clear the head
- ST 40 (*fēng lóng*): To transform phlegm and dampness, clear heart phlegm, harmonize stomach and nourish spleen
- SP 9 (*yīn líng quán*): To expel dampness and regulate spleen and stomach

Supporting Points:

- EX-HN 1 (*sì shén cōng*): To open the orifices and awaken the mind
- DU 20 (*bǎi huì*): To raise qi, open the orifices, awaken the mind, nourish the sea of marrow and treat stroke and aphasia

Recommended Formula: *Dí Tán Tāng* (涤痰汤, Phlegm-Flushing Decoction) from the *Fine Formulas of Wonderful Efficacy* (*Qí Xiào Liáng Fāng*, 奇效良方)

Substitute Formula: *Sū Hé Xiāng Wán* (苏合香丸, Storax Pill)

Patent Formula:

- *Ān Gōng Niú Huáng Wán* (安宫牛黄丸, Peaceful Palace Bovine Bezoar Pill)
- *Sū Hé Xiāng Wán* (苏合香丸, Storax Pill)

D. Depletion of Original Qi

Symptoms: Sudden collapse, loss of consciousness with an open mouth and closed eyes, shallow breathing, cold limbs, profuse sweating, urinary and fecal incontinence, limb flaccidity or paralysis, tongue flaccidity, slurred speech, lower back and knee pain, palpitations, dizziness, blurred vision, a thin and small tongue with scanty coating and a thready, weak or faint pulse.

Treatment Principle:

- Nourish yin and supplement qi
- Tonify kidney and nourish essence
- Open the orifices

Main Acupuncture Points:

- PC 6 (*nèi guān*): *Luo* point of the pericardium to regulate heart, treat palpitations and tongue disorders
- DU 26 (*shuǐ gōu*): To restore consciousness and arrest convulsions
- RN 4 (*guān yuán*): To tonify original qi and benefit kidney essence, regulate *chong* and *ren* vessels and treat stroke
- RN 8 (*shén què*): To warm yang and rescue collapse, regulate fluid passages and disinhibit urine retention
- RN 6 (*qì hǎi*): To tonify original qi and essence, treat stroke and diffused muscular weakness
- DU 20 (*bǎi huì*): To raise qi and yang, open the orifices and awaken the mind, nourish the sea of marrow and treat post stroke aphasia

Supporting Points:

- BL 38 (*fú xì*): To relax sinews and alleviate pain, soothe muscle contractions and treat lower back and limb painful paralysis
- EX-HN 22 (*shàng lián quán*): To benefit tongue and speech

Recommended Formula: *Shēn Fù Tāng* (参附汤, Ginseng and Aconite Decoction) from the *Revised Yan's Prescriptions for Rescuing Lives* (*Chóng Dìng Yán Shì Jì Shēng Fāng*, 重订严氏济生方)

Substitute Formula: *Huí Yáng Jiù Jí Tāng* (回阳救急汤, Yang-Returning Emergency Decoction)

Patent Formula: *Shēng Mài Yǐn* (生脉饮, Pulse-Engendering Beverage)

Summary Chart for Wind-strike: Organ Disorders

Organ Patterns	Main Points	Supporting Points	Formulae
Wind-Fire Obstructing the Heart	DU 16, BL 62, LV 2, LI 11, DU 26, LU 7	EX-HN 1 for opening the orifices GB 20 for hearing and balancing disorders	*Tiān Má Gōu Téng Tāng* plus *Zǐ Xuě Dān* or *Líng Jiǎo Gōu Téng Tāng*
Phlegm-Fire Obstructing the Heart	PC 6, DU 26, ST 40, SI 3, DU 16, LV 2	12 *jing*-well points for post stroke hemiplegia and edema SJ 3 for finger rigidity	*Líng Yáng Jiǎo Tāng* or *Qīng Qì Huà Tán Wán*
Phlegm and Dampness Obstructing the Heart	PC 6, DU 26, RN 12, ST 8, ST 40, SP 9	EX-HN 1 to open the orifices DU 20 for post stroke aphasia	*Dí Tán Tāng* or *Sū Hé Xiāng Wán*

Continued

Organ Patterns	Main Points	Supporting Points	Formulae
Depletion of Original Qi	PC 6, DU 26, RN 4, RN 8, RN 6, DU 20	BL 38 for lower back and limb paralysis and contractions EX-HN 22 for tongue and speech disorders	*Shēn Fù Tāng* or *Huí Yáng Jiù Jí Tāng*

3. Post Stroke Sequelae Treatment Approach

A. Hemiplegia

Symptoms: Hemiplegia, unilateral contracture, flaccidity or numbness of affected limb, edema of the hands and feet on affected side, slurred speech, mouth and eye deviation, pale and lusterless complexion, a pale-purple or deviated tongue with thin white coating, thready, choppy and weak pulse.

Treatment Principle:

- Tonify qi and invigorate blood
- Unblock the collaterals and activate limbs

Main Acupuncture Points:

- DU 20 (*băi huì*): To regulate qi, nourish the sea of marrow and treat stroke and speech disorders
- LI 15 (*jiān yú*): To treat hemiplegia, shoulder and arm pain and upper limb contractions
- LI 4 (*hé gŭ*): To treat pain and motor disorders of upper limbs and head
- GB 34 (*yáng líng quán*): To relax sinews, benefit joints and treat lower limb numbness and pain
- ST 36 (*zú sān lĭ*): To tonify qi and invigorate blood, treat stroke and lower limb paralysis
- SP 10 (*xuè hăi*): To promote blood flow, dispel stasis and invigorate spleen to resolve edema

Supporting Points:

- EX-HN 22 (*shàng lián quán*): To benefit tongue and speech
- ST 41 (*jiě xī*): To treat lower limb pain and weakness

Recommended Formula: *Bŭ Yáng Huán Wŭ Tāng* (补阳还五汤, Yang-Supplementing and Five-Returning Decoction) from the *Correction of Errors in Medical Works* (*Yī Lín Găi Cuò*, 医林改错)

Substitute Formula: *Táo Hóng Sì Wù Tāng* (桃红四物汤, Peach Kernel and Carthamus Four Substances Decoction)

Patent Formula: *Zhòng Fēng Huí Chūn Wán* (中风回春丸, Stroke Recovery Pill)

B. Slurred Speech

Symptoms: Tongue stiffness, slurred speech and unilateral skin numbness on the limbs, wiry and slippery pulse.

Treatment Principle:

- Dispel wind and resolve phlegm
- Open the orifices and unblock the collaterals

Main Acupuncture Points:

- RN 23 (*lián quán*): Local point to treat post stroke speech disorders
- DU 15 (*yǎ mén*): To benefit the tongue and speech disorders
- EX-HN 12 (*jīn jīn*): To treat aphasia and tongue stiffness
- SJ 1 (*guān chōng*): To benefit the throat and speech
- LI 12 (*zhǒu liáo*): To activate the channel and resolve skin numbness
- LI 11 (*qū chí*): To expel wind and resolve phlegm, treat skin disorders and benefit upper limbs

Recommended Formula: *Shén Xiān Jiě Yǔ Dān* (神仙解语丹, Immortal Pellets for Treating Aphasia) from the *Corrections and Annotations to Fine Formulas for Women* (*Jiào Zhù Fù Rén Liáng Fāng*, 校注妇人良方)

Substitute Formula: *Dí Tán Tāng* (涤痰汤, Phlegm-Flushing Decoction)

C. Deviation of the Eye and Mouth

Symptoms: Loss of motor and sensory co-ordination of facial muscles, drooling, difficult movement of affected eye and mouth.

Treatment Principle:

- Dispel wind and resolve phlegm
- Open the orifices and unblock the collaterals

Main Acupuncture Points:

- BL 2 (*cuán zhú*): Local point to expel wind and treat eye and mouth deviation
- ST 4 (*dì cāng*) plus ST 6 (*jiá chē*): Local point to treat facial paralysis and muscle contractions
- ST 42 (*chōng yáng*): *Yuan*-source point of the stomach to transform phlegm and treat eye and mouth deviation
- SJ 17 (*yì fēng*): To expel wind, treat eye and mouth deviation, resolve trismus
- LI 4 (*hé gǔ*) and LV 3 (*tài chōng*): To expel wind, spread qi and treat eye, mouth and tongue disorders
- GB 20 (*fēng chí*): To expel wind and treat eye disorders

Recommended Formula: *Qiān Zhèng Sǎn* (牵正散, Symmetry-Correcting Powder) from the *Secret Formulas of the Yang Family* (*Yáng Shì Jiā Cáng Fāng*, 杨氏家藏方)

Substitute Formula: *Yù Zhēn Sǎn* (玉真散, True Jade Powder)

Patent Formula: *Dà Huó Luò Wán* (大活络丸, Channel-Activating Bolus)

Summary Chart for Post-Stroke Sequelae

Post-Stroke Sequelae	Main Points	Supporting Points	Formulae
Hemiplegia	DU 20, LI 15, LI 4 GB 34, ST 36, SP 10	EX-HN 22 for benefiting tongue and speech ST 41 for treating lower limb pain and weakness	*Bŭ Yáng Huán Wŭ Tāng* or *Táo Hóng Sì Wù Tāng*
Slurred Speech	RN 23, DU 15, EX-HN 12, SJ 1, LI 12, LI 11		*Shén Xiān Jiě Yŭ Dān* or *Dí Tán Tāng*
Deviation of the Eye and Mouth	BL 2, ST 4, ST 42, SJ 17, LI 4, GB 20		*Qiān Zhèng Săn* or *Yù Zhēn Săn*

CASE STUDY 1: Left-sided Hemiplegia

Mr. Lu, 48 years old.

Main Complaint: Numbness and weakness of the left side of the body for 2 days.

Medical History: The patient had a history of alcohol drinking and smoking. He also suffered from 3 years of hypertension and took 1 tablet of *Zhenju* Hypotensor 2 times a day. The day prior to consultation, the patient suddenly felt numbness of the left side of his body with some lack of strength. He also suffered from a severe headache, vertigo, bitter taste in the mouth, dry throat and nausea which did not relieve after rest. The morning of the consultation, the weakness of the left side of the body worsened and his speech was distorted. A CT scan showed high density imaging in the right basal ganglia so he was admitted to the hospital for further treatment. There was no fainting prior to the symptoms; vomiting, convulsion of the limbs and fecal and urine incontinence did not occur all through the disease course.

Presenting Symptoms: Left half-body numbness and weakness, speech disorder, headache, vertigo, bitter taste in the mouth, dry throat, nausea, red tongue, yellow and greasy tongue coating, wiry and powerful pulse.

Physical Examination: Temperature: 37.0 ℃, pulse: 98 bpm, respiration: 20 bpm, blood pressure: 160/80 mmHg. The patient was aware and conscious. He showed some aphasia, shallow left nasolabial groove, left deviation of tongue, supple neck, hypomyotonia of the left half body, tendon reflex left (+)/right (++), muscle strength of the left upper extremity 0-1 degree, muscle strength of the quadriceps femoris 3 degree, muscle strength of the tibialis anterior and gastrocnemius 2 degree, no response to plantar reflex, normal pinprick sensation all over the body.

Pattern Differentiation

This patient is nearly at his fifties with clear signs of liver and kidney yin deficiency. The deficiency of the yin fails to control the hyperactive liver yang from moving upwards and affecting the upper manifesting as the red tongue, yellow and greasy tongue coating, rapid and slippery pulse. The ascending liver yang drives the qi and blood upward obstructing the orifices and channels manifesting as hemiplegia, deviation of the mouth and eye and aphasia. The disease is affecting the brain and is associated with the liver and kidney yin deficiency demonstrating a deficiency in the root and excess in the branch.

Diagnosis

TCM Diagnosis: Wind-strike due to hyperactivity of liver yang and obstruction in the collaterals

Western Medicine Diagnosis: Left-sided hemiplegia

Treatment

The pathomechanism of this case is mainly in ascendant hyperactivity of liver yang causing the qi and blood to flow upward and obstruct the channels and collaterals causing paralysis and weakness of the tendons and muscles leading to hemiplegia and speech disorder.

Principles:

- Subdue liver yang and extinguish internal wind
- Unblock channels and open orifices

Formula: Modified *Tiān Má Gōu Téng Tāng* (Gastrodia and Uncaria Decoction)

Ingredients:

天麻	*tiān má*	10 g	Rhizoma Gastrodiae
钩藤	*gōu téng*	15 g	Ramulus Uncariae Cum Uncis (decoct later)
石决明	*shí jué míng*	30 g	Concha Haliotidis (raw and decoct first)
夏枯草	*xià kū cǎo*	30 g	Spica Prunellae
黄芩	*huáng qín*	10 g	Radix Scutellariae
牛膝	*niú xī*	15 g	Radix Achyranthis Bidentatae
杜仲	*dù zhòng*	15 g	Cortex Eucommiae
桑寄生	*sāng jì shēng*	15 g	Herba Taxilli
山栀	*shān zhī*	10 g	Fructus Gardeniae
菊花	*jú huā*	10 g	Flos Chrysanthemi

Formula Analysis

In this formula, *tiān má, gōu téng* and *shí jué míng* are the chief medicinals and combined to calm the liver and extinguish wind. *Xià kū cǎo, shān zhī* and *huáng qín* are deputy medicinals, which can clear heat, purge fire and subdue liver hyperactivity. *Niú xī* leads blood downwards and combined with *dù zhòng* and *sāng jì shēng*, it can boost the liver and kidney. *Jú huā* serves to clear heat and calm the liver. These medicinals combined can achieve a heat clearing, liver calming and wind extinguishing effect.

Chinese Patent Medicine: The patent medicine of *Dà Huó Luò Dān* (Major Channel-Activating Elixir) was also prescribed with the formula taken warm, 1 pill 2 times a day. The patient was instructed to avoid raw, cold and greasy food.

Follow-up Consultations

On the 2nd consultation, after taking 15 packages of the decoction and patent medicine, the symptoms relieved slightly. The muscle strength of the right limbs reached the 3rd degree and he was able to walk by holding the walls. Based on the previous formula, *shēn jīn cǎo* (Herba Lycopodii) and Sichuan *mù guā* (Fructus Chaenomelis) were added.

On the 3rd consultation, after another 15 doses, the patient regained a 5th degree of muscle strength and his speech was fluent. The patient was released from the hospital and received physiotherapy care and took the patent formula of Major Channel-Activating Elixir. Three months later, the patient was able to look after his daily activities.

CASE STUDY 2: Right-sided Hemiplegia
By Dr. Shi Xue-min

Ms. Wu, 45 years old. 1st consultation: June 14th, 2006.

Main Complaint: Right-sided sensory disturbance of the body, inhibited movements of the limbs and poor balance for 3 years.

Medical History: Three years prior to consultation, the blood pressure of the patient rose to 180/120 mmHg due to stress at work which caused a cerebral hemorrhage with coma. An MRI scan of the brain showed a 10 ml bleeding in the left pons Varolii. The patient first received emergency care in a local hospital to lower intracranial pressure and lower the blood pressure. Afterwards, the patient regained consciousness but was suffering from right sided sensory disturbance, lack of flexibility of the limbs, a staggering gait, inability to perform fine motor movement with the fingers, diplopia, nystagmus, urine incontinence and irritability. The patient had received physiotherapy during the last three years which maintained a normal muscle tone of her limbs.

Presenting Symptoms: Numbness of the right limbs, vertigo, difficult gait, right side lower muscle strength, a dark red tongue with a scanty tongue coating, wiry and thin pulse.

Physical Examination: Right finger-nose test (+), right heel-knee-tibia test (+), Hoffmann sign (–), Babinski sign (+), muscle strength of the left extremities 5 degree, muscle strength of the right upper limbs 3 degree, muscle strength of the right lower limbs 4 degree.

Diagnosis

TCM Diagnosis: Post stroke sequelae due to qi and yin deficiency of the liver and kidney and essence deficiency not nourishing the brain

Western Medicine Diagnosis: Numbness of the right side of the body

Treatment

Principles:

- Open orifices and dredge the channels and collaterals
- Nourish liver yin and kidney essence
- Nourish the brain

Acupuncture Point Combination:

- PC 6 (*nèi guān*) (both sides), needled with the combine methods of twirling, lifting and thrusting for drainage.
- SP 6 (*sān yīn jiāo*), needled with the lifting and thrusting methods for supplementation.
- HT 1 (*jí quán*), LU 5 (*chǐ zé*) and BL 40 (*wěi zhōng*), needled with the lifting and thrusting methods for drainage.
- GB 20 (*fēng chí*), GB 12 (*wán gǔ*) and BL 10 (*tiān zhù*), needled with a small range and high frequency of twirling method for supplementation.
- The needle retention lasted over 20 mins per treatment, 2 times a day. Ten days defined 1 treatment course. 3 to 5 treatment courses are usually given for cases such as these.

In addition, applying the plum-blossom needling, cupping technique, *tui na* massage, and medicinal wash was applied as part of the physiotherapy techniques.

Chinese Patent Medicines: Patents were also prescribed, such as *Dān Qí Piān Tān Jiāo Náng* (Salvia-Astragalus Paralysis Capsules), and *Yì Shèn Yǎng Gān Hé Jì* (Kidney-Liver Nourishing Mixture) to supplement the acupuncture treatments.

Follow-up Consultations

30 days after the treatment, her muscle strength of the right extremities increased. Physical examination showed muscle strength of the left extremities 5 degree, muscle strength of the right upper limbs 4 degree, muscle strength of the right lower limbs 4 degree. Deep and superficial sensations had been partly resumed. The patient was asked to continue exercises for strengthening limbs and try to avoid contracting a cold and have light diet. Blood pressure should be monitored.

Clinical Analysis

The pathomechanism of post-stroke sequela is usually of complex nature with a combination of both severe deficiency and excess. Commonly, the excessive pathogenic factors of fire, phlegm, dampness, or blood stasis obstruct the collaterals causing the inhibited flow of qi and blood causing symptoms such as paralysis and weakness of limbs and face. The root patterns associated with wind-strike are deficiency of the liver blood and yin, kidney essence and spleen qi causing a severe malnourishment of the tendons and vessels. Therefore, when treating these complex patterns we must simultaneously strengthen the deficient qi and nourish essence and blood while moving the blood, soothing the liver and extinguishing wind, unblocking the channels and opening the orifices. While treating with acupuncture treatment, mainly choosing points on the *yangming* and *shaoyang* channels and the *Du* channel is more efficient. Specific acupuncture points are listed according to the pattern differentiation section. However, in case of coma PC 6 (*nèi guān*) and DU 26 (*shuǐ gōu*) are often used to treat the branch and open orifices, restore consciousness and regulate spirit. SP 6 (*sān yīn jiāo*) is targeted to treat the root by nourishing the liver and kidney, cultivating yin and subduing yang.

KEY CLINICAL POINTS

Generally, when a patient has a sudden attack of stroke, they first receive emergency care with western medicine to stabilize their blood pressure and prevent death. Afterwards, during the stage of recovery, acupuncture and Chinese medicine are combined to treat the sequelae which include a wide range of symptoms mainly due to obstruction of the channels and collaterals by phlegm, dampness, cold, blood stagnation. During this stage, it is primordial for the patient to perform physical exercise preferably within 4 hours after the acupuncture treatment for better results. In addition, the following points need to be considered:

1. Combination of Disease Differentiation for Prognosis

At the acute stage of cerebral hemorrhage, it is mostly manifested as wind striking the viscera with the block pattern of wind yang and phlegm-fire or wind striking the bowels with the pattern of bowel excess and static heat, though in some cases, there can be manifestations of desertion. For serious cases of wind striking the channels and collaterals, they are usually seen as cerebral infarction and cerebrovascular spasm. If the pattern of wind yang and phlegm fire occurs, though the patient is conscious, the doctor should observe carefully and prevent it from worsening.

2. Application of Unblocking the Bowels

The wind striking the bowels is due to internal obstruction of static heat, blocked bowel qi, upward disturbance of pathogenic heat and confused spirit, so the method of unblocking the bowels and discharging heat should be applied in time to help eliminate the pathogens downwards. As sometimes due to binding of pathogenic heat, the yang block pattern of wind striking the viscera with exuberant wind yang and phlegm fire that internally blocks the mind can also present symptoms of abdominal fullness, constipation, inhibited urination, yellow and greasy tongue coating, wiry and excess and forceful pulse. In such cases, the method of unblocking the bowels should also be combined to relax bowels and discharge phlegm heat, thus restoring consciousness and rescuing from critical conditions. However, it should not be applied to patients with obvious deficient healthy qi and desertion of original qi.

3. Combination of Cooling Blood and Dissolving Stasis for Wind-strike due to Hemorrhage

Cerebral hemorrhage and subarachnoid hemorrhage are referred to the blood syndromes. The mechanism of this kind of hemorrhage can often be binding of static heat and bleeding due to collateral impairment. Clinically, the manifestations will be cyanotic complexion and lips as well as dark purplish tongue veins. In such cases, the methods of cooling blood, dissolving stasis and arresting bleeding can be combined, prescribing *Xī Jiăo Dì Huáng Tāng* (Rhinoceros Horn and Rehmannia Decoction) as a basic formula to remove static heat and arrest bleeding.

4. The Treatment Method for Facial Palsy due to Wind-strike Sequela

Facial palsy due to wind-stroke sequela is often caused by wind-phlegm obstruction in the collaterals, which should be treated by dispelling wind, eliminating phlegm and unblocking collaterals. The recommended formula is *Qiān Zhèng Săn* (Symmetry-Correcting Powder).

BRIEF SUMMARY

The pathomechanism of wind-strike is complex and usually involves both deficiency and excess patterns. After the sudden attack has passed it is important to treat both the manifesting symptoms of paralysis and numbness of the limbs and facial muscles by opening the channels and removing the pathogenic factors of blood stasis, phlegm, fire or cold. We must also open the mind and remove obstruction in the mind and heart to uplift the spirit and remove confusion so that the patient may be able to return to their daily activities and become independent again. It is also important to strictly monitor the blood pressure to prevent a second episode of wind-strike as they are usually more severe with more complications.

COMPREHENSION QUESTIONS

1. What is the pathomechanism of wind-strike?
2. What are the channel and organ pattern differentiation and recommended formulas for wind-strike?
3. What are the differences between wind-strike, muscle atrophy syndrome (*wěi* 痿) and epilepsy?

4. Multiple choice questions:

1) Ms. Wang, 50 years old. The patient suffered from left-sided hemiplegia, weakness of the limbs, sallow complexion, occasional numbness of the body and limbs, a pale purple tongue with a thin whitish tongue coating and a thin, choppy and weak pulse. The recommended formula is:

A. *Sān Bì Tāng* (Three Impediments Decoction)
B. *Huáng Qí Guì Zhī Wǔ Wù Tāng* (Astragalus and Cinnamon Twig Five Substances Decoction)
C. *Táo Huā Tāng* (Peach Blossom Decoction)
D. *Bǔ Yáng Huán Wǔ Tāng* (Yang-Supplementing and Five-Returning Decoction)
E. *Dāng Guī Sì Nì Tāng* (Chinese Angelica Frigid Extremities Decoction)

2) Mr. Li, 56 years old. The patient suddenly suffered from coma, locked jaw, tight fists, constipation and urine retention, convulsions of the body and limbs, no vexation, cold limbs, excessive drooling, a white and greasy tongue coating with a deep, slippery and moderate pulse. The diagnosis is:

A. Wind-strike of yang pattern
B. Wind-strike of yin pattern
C. Wind-strike of depletion pattern
D. Wind-strike affecting the channels and collaterals
E. Sequela of wind-strike

Answers

1. The main cause of wind-strike is the uprising of pathogenic yang blocking the upper area of the body which can be triggered by various causes such as emotional excess, prolonged illness, phlegm blocking the collaterals and irregular diet. This counter flow of yang qi causes upsurging of qi and blood to the brain and a stagnation of qi and blood as well as pathogenic phlegm in the channels and collaterals causing symptoms of paralysis, aphasia, vertigo, fatigue, irritability, and so on. Usually, wind-strike affecting the channels and collaterals are mild; while wind-strikes affecting the viscera and bowels are more severe.

2. To make a concrete pattern differentiation of the disease of wind-strike we need to first identify the patterns affecting the channels and those affecting the organs. The patterns of wind strike affecting the channels will be relatively less severe in terms of sequelae with symptoms of hemiplegia, facial palsy, speech disorder and consciousness and will have a better prognosis. The patterns of wind-strike affecting the organs might have symptoms of unconsciousness or coma accompanied by paralysis of the limbs. Then, we need to identify if the symptoms present a deficiency or excess pattern. If the manifestations are unconsciousness, lockjaw, tight fists, convulsions of the body and limbs, we can classify it as an excessive pattern. If the symptoms present with unconsciousness, closed eyes and open mouth, loose and

cold limbs, paralysis, profuse cold sweating, fecal and urine incontinence, and low nasal breath, we can classify it under the deficiency pattern. The third aspect of the 8 guiding principles to identify the full complexity of the pattern is to identify the yin or yang features of the pattern. The yang patterns are due to phlegm fire, liver yang rising, and static heat that manifest as fever, redness of the face, heavy breathing, snoring, phlegm rattling sounds, constipation, yellow urine, yellow and greasy tongue coating, dry and crimson tongue, or curled tongue with a wiry, slippery and rapid pulse. The yin patterns are mainly due to obstruction of turbid phlegm manifesting as pale complexion, purple lips, exuberant phlegm and drool, cold limbs, white and greasy tongue coating, deep and slippery pulse. Here are a list of the patterns and their recommended formulas.

A. Patterns of wind-strike affecting the channels are:

- Sudden hyperactivity of liver yang: the recommended formula is *Tiān Má Gōu Téng Tāng* (Gastrodia and Uncaria Decoction) or *Líng Jiǎo Gōu Téng Tāng* (Antelope Horn and Uncaria Decoction)
- Wind-phlegm affecting the channels: the recommended formula is *Zhēn Fāng Bái Wán Zǐ* (Effective White Pill) or the combination of *Bàn Xià Bái Zhú Tiān Má Tāng* (Pinellia, Atractylodes Macrocephala and Gastrodia Decoction) and *Qiān Zhèng Sǎn* (Symmetry-Correcting Powder)
- Phlegm heat in the *fu* organs: the recommended formula is the combination of *Táo Hé Chéng Qì Tāng* (Peach Kernel Qi-Guiding Decoction) and *Dí Tán Tāng* (Phlegm-Flushing Decoction)
- Qi deficiency and blood stasis: the recommended formula is *Bǔ Yáng Huán Wǔ Tāng* (Yang-Supplementing and Five-Returning Decoction) or *Táo Hóng Sì Wù Tāng* (Peach Kernel and Carthamus Four Substances Decoction)
- Wind-strike due to yin deficiency: the recommended formula is *Zhèn Gān Xī Fēng Tāng* (Liver-Sedating and Wind-Extinguishing Decoction) or the combination of *Sì Wù Tāng* (Four Substances Decoction) and *Dà Dìng Fēng Zhū* (Major Wind-Stabilizing Pill)

B. Patterns of wind-strike affecting the organs are:

- Wind fire obstructing the heart: the recommended formula is the combination of *Tiān Má Gōu Téng Tāng* (Gastrodia and Uncaria Decoction) and *Zǐ Xuě Dān* (Purple Snow Elixir)
- Phlegm fire affecting the heart: the recommended formula is *Líng Yáng Jiǎo Tāng* (Antelope Horn Decoction) or *Qīng Qì Huà Tán Wán* (Qi-Clearing and Phlegm-Transforming Pill)
- Phlegm dampness obstructing the heart: the recommended formula is *Dí Tán Tāng* (Phlegm-Flushing Decoction) or *Sū Hé Xiāng Wán* (Storax Pill)
- Depletion of the original qi: the recommended formula is *Shēn Fù Tāng* (Ginseng and Aconite Decoction) or *Huí Yáng Jiù Jí Tāng* (Yang-Returning Emergency Decoction)

3. Wind-strike is a disease chiefly characterized as sudden coma, unconsciousness, with sequelae of hemiplegia, facial palsy and aphasia which can last from 3 months to a life time. Epilepsy is mainly characterized by the convulsion of the body and limbs, spasm of the nape and back followed by incontinence of urine and stool which have sequelae of memory loss and fatigue which last a few hours. *Wěi* syndrome manifests as a slow progression of weakness and paralysis of the limbs and is usually a chronic syndrome or twitching and muscular atrophy.

4. 1) D, 2) B.

3.3 Trembling Syndrome

The symptom of trembling is mainly characterized by involuntary shaking of the head or limbs. In mild cases, it manifests as slight shaking that can only sometimes be perceived by others. While in severe cases, there is constant involuntary and visible shaking of the head and limbs, with some sporadic spasms of the limbs which inhibit the patient to care for their daily activities. In western medicine, the symptom of trembling can be due to a metabolic pathology such as Parkinson's disease, liver degeneration, hyperthyroidism, neurological disorders such as multiple sclerosis or trauma to the brain.

In Chinese medicine, trembling appears when there is stirring up of the liver wind due to either a deficient or excessive pattern. The natural or excessive decline of the spleen and stomach qi fails to create the blood necessary to nourish the body. Deficiency of kidney essence and liver blood create a lack of nourishment to the sinews and tendons causing this internal wind manifesting as uncontrolled movement of the limbs and head. This deficiency can be done by the natural decline of the spleen and stomach qi, a prolonged illness, a severe loss of blood, surgery, overstrain and over stimulation of the senses. The severe damage of the spleen and stomach qi also causes a lack of transformation of the fluid causing an accumulation of dampness and phlegm which blocks the channels and also stirs up the internal wind. This blockage also inhibits the blood and qi to nourish the areas appropriately creating a malnourishment of the sinews and tendons. The main pathomechanism of the trembling syndrome is based in the liver, kidney and spleen with a deficient root and an apparent excess.

Clinically, the common patterns are internal stirring of wind, phlegm-heat retention and heat stagnation, phlegm retention, blood stagnation, qi and blood deficiency, deficiency of the marrow, and deficiency of yang qi.

CLINICAL PATTERNS DIFFERENTIATION AND TREATMENTS

1. Liver Wind Stirring Internally

Symptoms: Trembling of the head and limbs, vertigo with head distention, impatience and irritability, red complexion, dry mouth and tongue, tinnitus, a red tongue with a thin and yellow coating and a wiry, tight and rapid pulse.

Treatment Principle:

- Nourish blood and tonify qi

- Subdue liver yang and pacify liver wind

Main Acupuncture Points:

- EX-HN 1 (*sì shén cōng*): To open the orifices and awaken the mind
- SP 6 (*sān yīn jiāo*): To tonify liver and kidney, nourish yin and resolve painful muscular contractions
- GB 20 (*fēng chí*): To expel wind and clear heat, treat headaches and resolve hearing and vertigo
- SJ 5 (*wài guán*): *Luo* point of the *san jiao* to clear heat and benefit the head
- GB 34 (*yáng líng quán*): To relax sinews, benefit joints and treat lower limb weakness and pain
- LV 3 (*tài chōng*): *Yuan* point of the liver to clear heat, move qi, subdue yang and pacify wind, nourish blood and yin

Supporting Points: EX-HN 24 (*ān mián*): To calm the spirit, pacify the liver, treat insomnia

Recommended Formula: *Zī Shēng Qīng Yáng Tāng* (滋生青阳汤, Life-Cultivating and Yang-Subduing Decoction) from *The Refined in Medicine Remembered* (*Yī Chún Shèng Yì*, 医醇賸义)

Substitute Formulas:

- Combination of *Tiān Má Gōu Téng Tāng* (天麻钩藤汤, Gastrodia and Uncaria Decoction) and *Liù Wèi Dì Huáng Wán* (六味地黄丸, Six Ingredients Rehmannia Pill)
- *Zhèn Gān Xī Fēng Tāng* (镇肝熄风汤, Liver-Setting Wind-Extinguishing Decoction)

Patent Formula: *Qī Yè Shén Ān Piàn* (七叶神安片, Mind-Tranquilizing Tablet)

2. Liver and Kidney Yin Deficiency

Symptoms: Stiffness of the body, tremors and contraction of the limbs, stiff and uncoordinated movements, emaciation, vertigo, tinnitus, insomnia, dizziness, dreamful sleep, lower back and knee pain, night sweating, vexing heat in the five centers, dry mouth and tongue, constipation, a red tongue with scanty coating and a wiry, fine and rapid pulse.

Treatment Principle:

- Tonify liver yin and kidney essence
- Subdue internal wind and stop tremors

Main Acupuncture Points:

- KI 3 (*tài xī*): *Yuan* point of the kidney to nourish kidney yin, strengthen the lumbus and knees
- SP 6 (*sān yīn jiāo*): To tonify liver and kidney yin and resolve muscular contractions
- BL 23 (*shèn shù*): Back-*shu* point of the kidney to benefit the original qi and kidney yin
- GB 20 (*fēng chí*): To expel wind, clear heat, treat headaches and resolve tinnitus

and vertigo

- LV 3 (*tài chōng*): *Yuan* point of the liver to clear heat, pacify wind, nourish blood and yin
- BL 18 (*gān shù*): Back-*shu* point of the liver to spread liver qi, nourish blood, pacify wind and calm the spirit

Supporting Points:

- ST 4 (*dì cāng*): To expel wind and resolve facial paralysis
- EX-HN 3 (*yìn táng*): To calm the mind and improve sleep

Recommended Formula: *Dà Dìng Fēng Zhū* (大定风珠, Major Wind-Stabilizing Pill) from the *Systematic Differentiation of Warm Diseases* (*Wēn Bìng Tiáo Biàn*, 温病条辨)

Substitute Formula:

- *Zuǒ Guī Wán* (左归丸, Left-Restoring Pill)
- *Guī Lù Èr Xiān Gāo* (龟鹿二仙膏, Immortal Tortoise Shell and Deerhorn Glue Paste)

Patent Formula: *Liù Wèi Dì Huáng Wán* (六味地黄丸, Six Ingredients Rehmannia Pill)

3. Qi and Blood Deficiency

Symptoms: Chronic limb tremors, weak and tensed muscles, tendon spasms, pale complexion, fatigue, palpitations, shortness of breath, disinclination to speak, spontaneous sweating, vertigo, dizziness, poor appetite, loose stools, excessive salivation, a pale and enlarged tongue with a white tongue coating and a thready and weak pulse.

Treatment Principle:

- Tonify qi and nourish blood
- Expel wind and unblock collaterals

Main Acupuncture Points:

- ST 36 (*zú sān lǐ*): To tonify qi and invigorate blood, treat stroke and lower limb paralysis
- GB 20 (*fēng chí*): To expel wind, treat headaches and resolve balancing disorders
- BL 17 (*gé shù*): Influential point of the blood to activate and nourish blood, improve circulation and dispel stasis
- GB 34 (*yáng líng quán*): To relax sinews, benefit joints and treat lower limb weakness and pain
- LV 3 (*tài chōng*): *Yuan* point of the liver to pacify wind, nourish blood and spread liver qi, treat lower limb weakness
- RN 6 (*qì hǎi*): To tonify original qi and essence and resolve muscular weakness

Supporting Points:

- ST 4 (*dì cāng*): To expel wind and treat excessive salivation
- EX-HN 24 (*ān mián*): To calm the spirit, pacify the liver, resolve headaches and treat vertigo

Recommended Formulas: Combination of *Bā Zhēn Tāng* (八珍汤, Eight Gem Decoction) from the *Categorized Synopsis of the Whole* (*Zhèng Tǐ Lèi Yào*, 正体类要) and *Tiān Má Gōu Téng Tāng* (天麻钩藤汤, Gastrodia and Uncaria Decoction) from the *New Discussion on the Patterns and Treatment of Miscellaneous Disease* (*Zá Bìng Zhèng Zhì Xīn Yì*, 杂病证治新义)

Substitute Formulas:

- *Guī Pí Tāng* (归脾汤, Spleen-Restoring Decoction)
- *Rén Shēn Yǎng Róng Tāng* (人参养荣汤, Ginseng Supporting and Nourishing Decoction)

Patent Formula: *Bǔ Zhōng Yì Qì Wán* (补中益气丸, Center-Supplementing and Qi-Boosting Pill)

4. Phlegm Heat Retention Generating Wind

Symptoms: Tremors of the head or limbs, forward inclination of the head and thorax, yellow phlegm, excessive salivation, chest and epigastric stuffiness, abdominal fullness, poor appetite, slow movement, lethargy, obesity, dizziness, vertigo, heavy sensation of the head, irregular foul smelly stools, scanty and dark urine, a red or crimson tongue with yellow or greasy coating and a wiry and slippery or wiry and rapid pulse.

Treatment Principle:

- Clear heat and resolve wind
- Expel phlegm and dry dampness
- Strengthen spleen qi and soothe liver qi

Main Acupuncture Points:

- LI 11 (*qū chí*): To expel wind, resolve phlegm, clear heat and benefit upper limbs
- SP 3 (*tài bái*): *Yuan* point of the spleen to invigorate spleen, expel dampness, clear heat and promote digestion
- SJ 5 (*wài guán*): *Luo* point of the *san jiao* to clear wind and heat, benefit the upper limbs
- LV 3 (*tài chōng*): *Yuan* point of the liver to pacify wind, spread liver qi and treat lower limb weakness
- ST 40 (*fēng lóng*): Main point to transform phlegm and dampness
- BL 20 (*pí shù*): Back-*shu* point of the spleen to invigorate the spleen and resolve dampness

Supporting Points:

- BL 32 (*cì liáo*): To clear heat and resolve dampness, benefit the lumbus and lower limbs
- GB 34 (*yáng líng quán*): To relax sinews, benefit joints and treat lower limb numbness and pain

Recommended Formula: Combination of *Dǎo Tán Tāng* (导痰汤, Phlegm-Expelling Decoction) from the *Revised Yan's Prescriptions for Rescuing Lives* (*Chóng Dìng Yán Shì Jì*

Shēng Fāng, 重订严氏济生方) and *Líng Jiǎo Gōu Téng Tāng* (羚角钩藤汤, Antelope Horn and Uncaria Decoction) from the *Revised Popular Guide to Treatise on Cold Damage* (*Chóng Dìng Tōng Sú Shāng Hán Lùn*, 重订通俗伤寒论)

Substitute Formula:

- *Dí Tán Tāng* (涤痰汤,Phlegm-Flushing Decoction)
- Combination of *Huáng Lián Wēn Dǎn Tāng* (黄连温胆汤, Coptis Gallbladder-Warming Decoction) and *Tiān Má Gōu Téng Tāng* (天麻钩藤汤, Gastrodia and Uncaria Decoction)

5. Spleen and Kidney Yang Deficiency

Symptoms: Tremors of the head and limbs, spasms, aversion to cold, cold limbs, stiff expression, pale complexion, limb flaccidity, poor appetite, salivating, listlessness, shortness of breath, disinclination to speak, spontaneous sweating, profuse clear urination, impotence, spermatorrhea, a pale and big tongue with teeth marks with a thin white coating and a deep and thin pulse.

Treatment Principle:

- Warm and tonify spleen and kidney yang
- Move qi and dredge collaterals

Main Acupuncture Points:

- ST 36 (*zú sān lǐ*): To regulate qi, resolve phlegm and treat lower limb paralysis
- SP 6 (*sān yīn jiāo*): To tonify spleen and kidney, regulate urination, treat spermatorrhea and impotence, resolve painful muscular contractions
- RN 5 (*shí mén*): Front-*mu* point of the *san jiao* to invigorate spleen and kidney, regulate water passages and dredge collaterals
- BL 20 (*pí shù*): Back-*shu* point of the spleen to invigorate spleen, tonify qi and regulate the middle *jiao*
- BL 23 (*shèn shù*): Back-*shu* point of the kidney to tonify kidney and fortify yang, benefit urination and treat spermatorrhea and impotence
- RN 12 (*zhōng wǎn*): Front-*mu* point of the stomach to regulate spleen and stomach, harmonize the middle *jiao*

Supporting Points:

- BL 30 (*bái huán shù*): To warm the uterus, treat sexual dysfunction, resolve lumbar and lower limb pain
- ST 4 (*dì cāng*): To treat excessive salivation and facial paralysis

Recommended Formula: *Dì Huáng Yǐn Zǐ* (地黄饮子, Rehmannia Drink) from *An Elucidation of Formulas* (*Xuān Míng Lùn Fāng*, 宣明论方)

Substitute Formula: *Jīn Guì Shèn Qì Wán* (金匮肾气丸, Golden Cabinet's Kidney Qi Pill)

Patent Formula: *Jīn Guì Shèn Qì Wán* (金匮肾气丸, Golden Cabinet's Kidney Qi Pill)

Summary Chart for Trembling Syndrome

Patterns	Main Points	Supporting Points	Formulae
Liver Wind Stirring Internally	EX-HN 1, SP 6, GB 20, SJ 5, GB 34, LV 3	EX-HN 24 for irritability with headaches and vertigo	*Zī Shēng Qīng Yáng Tāng, Tiān Má Gōu Téng Tāng* plus *Liù Wèi Dì Huáng Wán* or *Zhèn Gān Xī Fēng Tāng*
Liver and Kidney Yin Deficiency	KI 3, SP 6, BL 23, GB 20, LV 3, BL 18	ST 4 for facial paralysis EX-HN 3 for insomnia	*Dà Dìng Fēng Zhū, Zuǒ Guī Wán* or *Guī Lù Èr Xiān Gāo*
Qi and Blood Deficiency	ST 36, GB 20, BL 17, GB 34, LV 3, RN 6	ST 4 for salivation EX-HN 24 for irritability with headaches and vertigo	*Bā Zhēn Tāng* and *Tiān Má Gōu Téng Tāng, Guī Pí Tāng* or *Rén Shēn Yǎng Róng Tāng*
Phlegm Heat Retention Generating Wind	LI 11, SP 3, SJ 5, LV 3, ST 40, BL 20	BL 32 for lumbago due to dampness GB 34 for tendon and joint stiffness	*Dǎo Tán Tāng* plus *Líng Jiǎo Gōu Téng Tāng, Dí Tán Tāng* or *Huáng Lián Wēn Dǎn Tāng* plus *Tiān Má Gōu Téng Tāng*
Spleen and Kidney Yang Deficiency	ST 36, SP 6, RN 5, BL 20, BL 23, RN 12	BL 30 for uterine cold and sexual dysfunction ST 4 for salivation	*Dì Huáng Yǐn Zǐ* or *Jīn Guì Shèn Qì Wán*

CASE STUDY 1: Parkinson's Disease

Mr. Song, 76 years old, retired.

Main Complaint: Involuntary trembling of the right hand and lower mandible for three years with aggravation for a year.

Medical History: The patient gradually suffered from involuntary shaking of the right hand and lower mandible for three years with unknown cause of onset. His trembling symptoms aggravated when he was still or felt excited and alleviated when the patient was moving. There were no paralysis of the limb, speech disorder, spontaneous salivation, unconsciousness, cough, nausea or vomiting. The symptoms slightly alleviated when taking *Liù Wèi Dì Huáng Wán* (Six-Ingredient Rehmannia Pill). The above symptoms gradually aggravated in the last year which made it impossible to hold objects in his right hand. Since the onset of the disease, there were also symptoms of dizziness, memory loss and general fatigue which were not alleviated by rest. His sleep was slightly poor, while his appetite, stool and urine were normal. The patient had no history of hypertension, hyperlipidemia, diabetes or coronary heart disease.

Presenting Symptoms: Involuntary shaking of the right hand and lower mandible causing the inability of holding objects in the right hand, poor spirit, lethargy, a thin red tongue with scanty coating and a thready and rapid pulse.

Physical Examination: The strength of the grip was normal on both hands with normal muscle strength of both the upper and lower limbs with normal tendon reflex. There were no abnormal findings in the CT scan of the brain.

Pattern Differentiation

The thin red tongue with a scanty coating as well as the thready pulse demonstrate a depletion of yin and blood. The deficient blood is unable to nourish the tendons and muscles causing tremors. The gradual progression of the syndrome also demonstrates a natural depletion of the kidney essence which can not nourish the tendons. This severe depletion of liver yin and kidney essence is causing internal wind to stir upward and cause the trembling of the right hand and lower jaw. The treatment approach for this pattern is to subdue internal wind as well as nourish liver yin and blood and kidney essence.

Diagnosis

TCM Diagnosis: Trembling syndrome due to liver and kidney deficiency stirring up internal wind

Western Medicine Diagnosis: Parkinson's disease

Treatment

Principles:

- Nourish liver blood and yin and subdue internal wind
- Strengthen kidney essence and unblock collaterals

Formula: Modified *Liù Wèi Dì Huáng Wán* (Six-Ingredient Rehmannia Pill)

Ingredients:

熟地黄	*shú dì huáng*	10 g	Radix Rehmanniae Praeparata
山茱萸	*shān zhū yú*	10 g	Fructus Corni
山药	*shān yào*	10 g	Rhizoma Dioscoreae
茯苓	*fú líng*	10 g	Poria
当归	*dāng guī*	10 g	Radix Angelicae Sinensis
白芍	*bái sháo*	10 g	Radix Paeoniae Alba
远志	*yuǎn zhì*	9 g	Radix Polygalae
阿胶	*ē jiāo*	10 g	Colla Corii Asini
鸡血藤	*jī xuè téng*	10 g	Caulis Spatholobi
枸杞子	*gǒu qǐ zǐ*	10 g	Fructus Lycii
地龙	*dì lóng*	10 g	Pheretima
炙甘草	*zhì gān cǎo*	6 g	Radix et Rhizoma Glycyrrhizae Praeparata cum Melle

Formula Analysis

The formula used is a modified *Liù Wèi Dì Huáng Wán* (Six-Ingredient Rehmannia Pill) used to nourish yin and supplement the kidney. The original formula is composed of 6 medicinals, in which *shú dì huáng* enriches the kidney yin and essence, *shān zhū yú* nourishes the liver and restrains the leakage of essence, while *shān yào* and *fú líng* are used to nourish qi and drain dampness to calm the mind. *Mǔ dān pí* and *zé xiè* are removed from the original formula since they are too cold in temperature for this case. *Bái sháo* is added to soften the liver to relax the sinews and muscles and treat muscle cramps causing pain. *Ē jiāo, dāng guī* and *jī xuè téng* nourish the blood and relax the sinews. *Dì lóng* invigorates blood and unblocks collaterals. *Gǒu qǐ zǐ* enriches and supplements the liver and kidney. All these medicinals are combined to supplement and boost the liver and kidney, extinguish wind and unblock the collaterals to treat tremors.

Follow-up Consultations

After 15 doses of the formula, the involuntary trembling of the right hand and lower mandible alleviated. Another 20 doses were given to consolidate the treatment and prevent a relapse. Afterwards the patient was asked to continue taking *Liù Wèi Dì Huáng Wán* (Six-Ingredient Rehmannia Pill) in pill form.

CASE STUDY 2: Involuntary Trembling

Mr. Jing Tian-jiu, 82 years old. 1st consultation on February. 13th, 2013.

Main Complaint: Involuntary trembling of the head and right hand for 2 years with aggravation for a day.

Medical History: The patient started suffering from involuntary trembling of the head and right hand 2 years ago with unknown cause of onset. The trembling was more obvious when he was still. At the time, he did not seek medical attention or treatment. Prior to these symptoms, the patient was diagnosed with diabetes mellitus twenty years ago and was presently treated with insulin injection before breakfast and dinner. He was also diagnosed with hypertension and hyper cholesterol ten years ago but did not take any medication to control it. The patient suffered from a stroke 3 years ago and had sequela of hemiplegia of the left limbs.

Presenting Symptoms: The day before the consultation, the trembling symptoms suddenly aggravated and the patient also suffered from abdominal distention and pain, nausea with the desire to vomit, dry mouth and soreness of the body. These symptoms did not reduce after rest. The patient was lethargic with slightly dry stools two to three times a day.

Physical Examination: Involuntary trembling of the head and the right hand. Deviated tongue to the left. The muscle strength of the left arm was grade 0, the left leg grade 3, and the right extremities grade 4. The Babinski sign was positive.

Diagnosis

TCM Diagnosis: Trembling syndrome due to phlegm-heat stirring internal wind
Western Medicine Diagnosis: Involuntary trembling

Treatment

Principles:

- Tonify qi and nourish blood
- Dissolve phlegm and unblock collaterals
- Extinguish wind and stop convulsion

Acupuncture Point Combination: DU 20 (*bǎi huì*), EX-HN 1 (*sì shén cōng*), GB 20 (*fēng chí*), LI 4 (*hé gǔ*), SJ 5 (*wài guān*), LV 3 (*tài chōng*), GB 34 (*yáng líng quán*).

Manipulations: Apply the tonifying method to DU 20 and *sì shén cōng* by twirling the needle with small range and high frequency. Apply the depleting method to LI 4, SJ 5 and LV 3 by lifting, thrusting and twirling the needle. Apply even method to GB 34 to nourish the gallbladder and subdue wind. Provide 1 acupuncture treatment a day and retain the needles for 30 minutes. Ten days make one treatment course and 1 to 3 courses are usually given for best results.

In addition, the Chinese medicinal formulas are added according to the affected pattern.

Point Analysis

In this case, the disease is located in the brain and the pathological organ is the liver. The points DU 20, *sì shén cōng* and GB 20 are chosen to raise the clear yang to the head, awaken the brain and calm the mind. LI 4 belongs to the *yangming* meridian and can unblock channels and collaterals and move blood. LV 3 and LI 4 needled together are the four gates which can move qi and blood, and harmonize yin and yang. GB 34 is the confluence of sinews and it can nourish blood, soften the sinews and unblock collaterals.

KEY CLINICAL POINTS

1. The location of the pathogens of the trembling syndrome is the sinews and it is closely related to the liver, spleen and kidney. Its main pathomechanism is the stirring upward of internal wind due to the lack of nourishment to the sinews by the blood and essence depletion. The liver stores the blood and governs the sinews, the spleen is the source of qi and blood production and governs the muscles and the kidney stores the essence and generates marrow. Deficiency of the liver, spleen and kidney leads to yin and essence insufficiency which fails to nourish the sinews causing the trembling of the limbs and body. Supplementing the liver and kidney treats the root of the syndrome while removing obstruction of the channels due to phlegm and blood stasis and subduing the internal wind treats the branch of the syndrome.

2. Since the trembling syndrome is a disease due to stirring up of internal wind, we can consider adding the following medicinals to subdue internal wind and unblock the channels: *gōu téng, bái jí lí, tiān má, zhēn zhū mǔ, shēng lóng gǔ, shēng mǔ lì, quán xiē, wú gōng* and *bái jiāng cán*. Among these medicinals, we have listed a few insect medicinals which are known to have effective results in extinguishing internal wind, treating tremor and unblocking collaterals. The famous doctor Ye Tian-shi from the Qing Dynasty said: "When treating prolonged illnesses, the pathogenic qi and healthy qi are mixed together and herbal products are not strong enough to separate them, so we need to use insect medicinals to unblock channels and dispel pathogens". The beneficial effects of these insects are also more effective taken fried in comparison to the boiled decoction.

BRIEF SUMMARY

The trembling syndrome is located in the sinews and the main pathomechanism is liver wind stirring up internally affecting the sinews causing involuntary tremors. The pattern usually has an underlining depletion of liver blood and yin as well as kidney yin and essence which fail to nourish the sinews and muscles. This blood and essence depletion also fails to nourish the sinews increasing the symptoms of tremors. The other pathological syndrome includes blood stasis and phlegm retention causing an obstruction of the channels and collaterals inhibiting the areas from being nourished by the qi and blood. The main treatment principles for tremors are to subdue internal wind, move and nourish blood, dissolve phlegm, unblock channels, clear heat, and stop tremors. Acupuncture and Chinese medicinals can be combined for better results in the course of treatment.

COMPREHENSION QUESTIONS

1. What is the main pathomecanism and treatment principles and reasoning of the trembling syndrome?

2. Name the common pattern differentiations of the trembling syndrome and their recommended formula patterns.

3. Multiple choice questions:

1) The patient has suffered from the trembling syndrome for many years with the accompanied symptoms of vertigo, dizziness, tinnitus, insomnia, profuse dreaming, weakness and numbness of the lumbar and legs, dementia, forgetfulness, slow reaction, a thin and dark red tongue with a scanty coating and a thready and wiry or deep and thin pulse. This trembling syndrome is due to:

A. Liver and kidney deficiency

B. Qi and blood deficiency

C. Phlegm heat retention with stirring wind

D. Qi stagnation and blood stasis
E. Ascendant hyperactivity of liver yang

2) The location of the trembling syndrome lies in:
A. The sinews
B. The lung
C. The liver
D. the heart
E. The large intestine

3) The patient suffers from trembling that is sometimes severe and sometimes mild, which he can sometimes control it. His accompanied symptoms include chest and epigastric oppression and stuffiness, dry mouth, vertigo, bitter taste in the mouth, yellow sputum, dry stool, dark yellow urine, a red tongue with yellow and greasy coating and a wiry and rapid pulse. This trembling syndrome is due to:
A. Hyperactivity of liver yang
B. Qi stagnation and blood stasis
C. Phlegm heat and wind stirring
D. Liver and kidney deficiency
E. Qi and blood deficiency

Answers

1. The location of the pathogens in the trembling syndrome is the sinews and it is closely related to the liver, spleen and kidney. Its main pathomechanism is the stirring of internal wind due to the lack of nourishment to the sinews by the blood and essence depletion. The liver stores the blood and governs the sinews, the spleen is the source of qi and blood production and governs the muscles and the kidney stores the essence and generates marrow. Deficiency of the liver, spleen and kidney leads to yin and essence insufficiency which fails to nourish the sinews causing the trembling of the limbs and body. Supplementing the liver and kidney treats the root of the syndrome while removing obstruction of the channels due to phlegm and blood stasis and subduing the internal wind treat the branch of the syndrome.

2. The treatment approaches for the commonly seen patterns of tremors are:

• Liver wind stirring internally pattern: recommended formula is *Zī Shēng Qīng Yáng Tāng* (Life-Cultivating and Yang-Subduing Decoction), or the combination of *Tiān Má Gōu Téng Tāng* (Gastrodia and Uncaria Decoction) and *Liù Wèi Dì Huáng Wán* (Six Ingredients Rehmannia Pill); or *Zhèn Gān Xī Fēng Tāng* (Liver-Setting Wind-Extinguishing Decoction).

• Liver and kidney yin deficiency pattern: recommended formula is *Dà Dìng Fēng Zhū* (Major Wind-Stabilizing Pill), *Zuǒ Guī Wán* (Left-Restoring Pill) or *Guī Lù Èr Xiān Gāo* (Immortal Tortoise Shell and Deerhorn Glue Paste).

• Qi and blood deficiency pattern: recommended formula is the combination of *Bā Zhēn Tāng* (Eight Gem Decoction) and *Tiān Má Gōu Téng Tāng* (Gastrodia and Uncaria Decoction); *Guī Pí Tāng* (Spleen-Restoring Decoction), or *Rén Shēn Yǎng Róng Tāng* (Ginseng Supporting and Nourishing Decoction).

• Phlegm heat retention generating wind pattern: recommended formula is the combination of *Dǎo Tán Tāng* (Phlegm-Expelling Decoction) and *Líng Jiǎo Gōu Téng Tāng* (Antelope Horn and Uncaria Decoction), *Dí Tán Tāng* (Phlegm-Flushing Decoction) or the combination of *Huáng Lián Wēn Dǎn Tāng* (Coptis Gallbladder-Warming Decoction) and *Tiān Má Gōu Téng Tāng* (Gastrodia and Uncaria Decoction).

• Spleen and kidney yang deficiency pattern: recommended formula is *Dì Huáng Yǐn Zǐ* (Rehmannia Drink) or *Jīn Guì Shèn Qì Wán* (Golden Cabinet's Kidney Qi Pill).

3. 1) A, 2) A, 3) C.

3.4 Epilepsy

Epilepsy is a disorder characterized by massive synchronous discharges in the brain neurones with symptoms of sudden loss of consciousness, seizures, upward staring of the eyes, foaming at the mouth, convulsions or screaming, hallucinations followed by incontinences of feces and urine, and severe fatigue. This disorder affects over 2% of the population.

The severity of epileptic seizures varies greatly. A mild case manifests as "petit mal" which is brief lapse of awareness or sudden unresponsiveness lasting only a few seconds but sometimes happening many times a day and night. A more severe case of epilepsy manifests as frequent, violent and debilitating attacks. A genetic link is the cause in over 40% of the epileptic patients. Other causes are trauma to the brain, brain tumour, aneurysms, infarction and side effect of some medication just to name a few.

In Chinese medicine, the main pathological factor of epilepsy is the retention of turbid phlegm. There is a common saying in Chinese medicine which states: "no phlegm, no epilepsy". Furthermore, epilepsy is classified in a yin seizure or a yang seizure. The classification is made according to the frequency, severity and duration of the seizures as well as the accompanied symptoms. If the seizures are mild with little or no convulsions, and no muscle contractions, the syndrome is a yin pattern. If the seizures are very violent and strong with excessive muscle contraction and screaming, the syndrome is a yang pattern. The cause of these seizures usually presents due to a combination of excess and deficiency pattern. There is usually a strong deficiency of the righteous qi with a pathogenic factor of phlegm retention, internal wind, blood stasis, or heat stagnation.

Here is a short summary of the commonly seen patterns with their treatment principles, recommended formulas and point prescriptions.

CLINICAL PATTERNS DIFFERENTIATION AND TREATMENTS

1. Wind Phlegm Obstructing the Mind

Symptoms: Vertigo, chest stuffiness and fatigue before seizures, sudden loss of consciousness after seizures, headaches with an aura, convulsing extremities, locked jaw, fixed upward gaze, drooling, screaming, urinary and fecal incontinence, temporary mental unclarity or trance-like states (milder cases), a white and greasy tongue coating and a wiry and slippery pulse.

Treatment Principle:

- Resolve phlegm and extinguish wind
- Open the mind and unblock orifices

Main Acupuncture Points:

- BL 18 (*gān shù*): Back-*shu* point of the liver to expel liver wind, regulate and smoothen the qi flow and resolve depression
- BL 15 (*xīn shù*): Back-*shu* point of the heart to treat heart pain and unbind the chest
- DU 20 (*bǎi huì*): To supplement and raise the qi, regulate liver yang, benefit the heart and calm the spirit
- RN 15 (*jiū wěi*): To treat epilepsy and manic psychosis
- ST 40 (*fēng lóng*): To expel phlegm and dampness
- DU 23 (*shàng xīng*): To clear the head and open the orifices

Supporting Points:

- PC 5 (*jiān shǐ*): To treat plum-stone qi sensation (globus hystericus)
- DU 26 (*shuǐ gōu*) and SI 3 (*hòu xī*): To resuscitate in case of loss of consciousness
- EX-HN 3 (*yìn táng*): To calm the mind and improve sleep

Recommended Formula: *Dìng Xián Wán* (定痫丸, Convulsion-Settling Pill) from the *Medical Revelations* (*Yī Xué Xīn Wù*, 医学心悟)

Substitute Formula: *Dǎo Tán Tāng* (导痰汤, Phlegm-Expelling Decoction)

Patent Formula: *Quán Tiān Má Jiāo Náng* (全天麻胶囊, Gastrodia Capsules)

2. Internal retention of Phlegm Fire

Symptoms: Sudden loss of consciousness, convulsing extremities, drooling, screaming, irritability, restlessness, insomnia, phlegm which is difficult to expectorate, dry mouth, halitosis, bitter taste in the mouth, constipation (remission stage), a red tongue with a yellow and greasy coating and a wiry, slippery, thready and rapid pulse.

Treatment Principle:

- Purge liver fire and resolve phlegm
- Unblock channels and open the orifices
- Clear pathogenic heat and calm the spirit

Main Acupuncture Points:

- GB 13 (*běn shén*): Main point for epilepsy and manic disorders
- BL 18 (*gān shù*): Back-*shu* point of the liver to clear liver and gall bladder fire, regulate and smoothen the qi flow and resolve depression
- ST 40 (*fēng lóng*): To expel phlegm and dampness, clear phlegm from the lung, heart and chest
- LV 2 (*xíng jiān*): To clear liver fire
- PC 6 (*nèi guān*): *Luo*-connecting point of the pericardium to regulate the heart and unbind the chest

Supporting Points:

- DU 26 (*shuǐ gōu*), KI 1 (*yǒng quán*) and EX-UE 11 (*shí xuān*): To treat acute stages
- LI 11(*qū chí*): To clear intestinal fire

Recommended Formula: *Huáng Lián Wēn Dǎn Tāng* (黄连温胆汤, Coptis Gallbladder-Warming decoction) from the *Important Formulas Worth a Thousand Gold Pieces for Emergency* (*Bèi Jí Qiān Jīn Yào Fāng*, 备急千金要方)

Substitute Formula:

- Combination of *Dí Tán Tāng* (涤痰汤, Phlegm-Flushing Decoction) and *Lóng Dǎn Xiè Gān Tāng* (龙胆泻肝汤, Gentian Liver-Draining Decoction)
- *Dāng Guī Lóng Huì Wán* (当归龙荟丸, Chinese Angelica, Gentian, and Aloe Pill)

Patent Formula:

- *Niú Huáng Qīng Xīn Wán* (牛黄清心丸, Bovine Bezoar Heart-Clearing Pill)
- *Méng Shí Gǔn Tán Wán* (礞石滚痰丸, Chlorite Phlegm-Removing Pill)

3. Heart and Kidney Deficiency

Symptoms: Sudden loss of consciousness or loss of awareness and dream-like state of consciousness, insomnia, phlegm which is difficult to expectorate, poor memory, palpitations, dizziness, blurry vision, lumbago, mental fatigue, a thin and greasy tongue coating and a thready and weak pulse.

Treatment Principle:

- Tonify the heart blood and kidney essence
- Strengthen the spleen and resolve phlegm

Main Acupuncture Points:

- BL 15 (*xīn shù*): Back-*shu* point of the heart to treat heart pain and unbind the chest
- BL 23 (*shèn shù*): Back-*shu* point of the kidney to benefit the original qi and kidney yin
- BL 20 (*pí shù*): Back-*shu* point of the spleen to invigorate the spleen and resolve dampness
- KI 3 (*tài xī*): *Yuan*-source point of the kidney to nourish kidney and strengthen the lumbus
- GB 20 (*fēng chí*): To treat epilepsy
- ST 40 (*fēng lóng*): To expel dampness and phlegm

Supporting Points:

- PC 4 (*xì mén*): *Xi*-cleft point of the pericardium to dispel stasis and cool blood
- SI 19 (*tīng gōng*) and SJ 3 (*zhōng zhǔ*): To treat dizziness
- HT 5 (*tōng lǐ*): To treat heart pain with arrhythmia

Recommended Formula: *Dà Bǔ Yuán Jiān* (大补元煎, Major Yuan-Supplementing Decoction) from *The Complete Works of [Zhang] Jing-yue* (*Jǐng Yuè Quán Shū*, 景岳全书)

Substitute Formula: *Zuǒ Guī Wán* (左归丸, Left-Restoring Pill)

Patent Formula:

- *Liù Wèi Dì Huáng Wán* (六味地黄丸, Six Ingredients Rehmannia Pill)
- *Dà Bŭ Yīn Wán* (大补阴丸, Major Yin-Supplementing Pill)

4. Blood Stasis Obstructing the Orifices

Symptoms: Sudden loss of consciousness, convulsing extremities, irritability, restlessness, insomnia, bleeding of the nose, dark spots on the face and body, easily bruised skin, dry mouth, constipation (remission stage), dark or purple tongue with a thin coating, wiry, slippery, thready and choppy pulse.

Treatment Principle:

- Move blood and remove stasis
- Unblock channels and open the orifices

Main Acupuncture Points:

- GB 13 (*běn shén*): Main point for epilepsy and manic disorders
- DU 20 (*băi huì*): To supplement and raise the qi, regulate liver yang, move qi and blood in the local area
- BL 18 (*gān shù*): Back-*shu* point of the liver to regulate and smoothen the qi flow
- BL 15 (*xīn shù*): Back-*shu* point of the heart to nourish and move heart blood
- BL 20 (*pí shù*): Back-*shu* point of the spleen to invigorate the spleen qi and resolve dampness
- PC 6 (*nèi guān*): *Luo*-connecting point of the pericardium regulates the heart to unbind the chest and treat heart pain

Supporting points:

- DU 26 (*shuĭ gōu*), KI 1 (*yŏng quán*) and EX-UE 11 (*shí xuān*): To treat during acute stages
- EX-HN 1 (*sì shén cōng*): To improve poor memory, resolve insomnia and awaken the mind

Recommended formula: *Tōng Qiào Huó Xuè Tāng* (通窍活血汤, Orifice-Soothing Blood-Activating Decoction) from the *Correction of Errors in Medical Works* (*Yī Lín Găi Cuò*, 医林改错)

Substitute Formula:

- *Diān Kuáng Mèng Xĭng Tāng* (癫狂梦醒汤, Mind-Clearing Decoction)
- *Xuè Fŭ Zhú Yū Tāng* (血府逐瘀汤, Blood Stasis Expelling Decoction)

Patent Formula: *Xuè Fŭ Zhú Yū Jiāo Náng* (血府逐瘀胶囊, Blood Stasis Expelling Capsules)

Summary Chart for Epilepsy

Patterns	Main Points	Supporting Points	Formulae
Wind Phlegm Obstructing the Mind	BL 18, BL 15, DU 20, RN 15, ST 40, DU 23	PC 5 for plum-stone qi DU 26 and SI 3 for loss of consciousness EX-HN 3 for poor sleep	*Dìng Xián Wán* or *Dăo Tán Tāng*

Continued

Patterns	Main Points	Supporting Points	Formulae
Internal Retention of Phlegm Fire	GB 13, BL 18, ST 40, LV 2, PC 6	DU 26, KI 1 and EX-UE 11 for acute stages LI 11 for intestinal fire	*Huáng Lián Wēn Dǎn Tāng*, the combination of *Dí Tán Tāng* and *Lóng Dǎn Xiè Gān Tāng* or *Dāng Guī Lóng Huì Wán*
Heart and Kidney Deficiency	BL 15, BL 23, BL 20, KI 3, GB 20, ST 40	PC 4 for heart blood stasis due to heat SI 19 and SJ 3 for dizziness HT 5 for heart pain with arrhythmia	*Dà Bǔ Yuán Jiān* or *Zuǒ Guī Wán*
Blood Stasis Obstructing the Orifices	GB 13, DU 20, BL 18, BL 15, BL 20, PC 6	DU 26, KI 1 and EX-UE 11 for acute stages EX-HN 1: for poor memory, insomnia	*Tōng Qiào Huó Xuè Tāng*, *Diān Kuáng Mèng Xǐng Tāng* or *Xuè Fǔ Zhú Yū Tāng*

CASE STUDY 1: Chronic Epilepsy

Mrs. Zhao, 22 years old. Teacher.

Main Complaint: Recurrent epilepsy for 18 years.

Medical History: At 4 years old, the patient had a grand map seizure and suddenly fell to the ground in convulsion with foaming at the mouth without known cause. The medical EEG was abnormal and the patient was diagnosed with epilepsy and received regular western medicine treatment which did not fully control the symptoms and the patient continued having seizures. During every seizure, there was foaming at the mouth, clenched jaws, convulsions of the body and limbs and urinary incontinence. The seizures came about two or three times a year and lasted for two or three minutes. Other than the seizures, the patient was slightly obese, had a good appetite, normal sleep, dry stool and normal urination.

Presenting Symptoms: Occasional epileptic seizures for 18 years with loss of consciousness lasting a few seconds to one minute, weakness and somnolence after the seizures with lethargic mental state, a light red tongue with thin coating and a wiry pulse.

Physical Examination: Temperature: 36.1 ℃, pulse: 73 bpm, respiration: 20 bpm, and blood pressure: 120/75 mmHg. The patient was conscious with a poor spirit. She spoke clearly with pertinent answers. Her reaction was slightly slow. Nervous system examination showed cranial nerves (–), normal muscular tension and strength and the tendon reflex was symmetrical. The EEG was moderately abnormal and the cerebral CT showed no obvious abnormalities.

Pattern Differentiation

The patient had very deep fear during her childhood which caused the qi to sink leading to the abnormal flow of qi and impairing the spleen and stomach. This deficiency of the spleen and stomach inhibited the natural function of transformation and caused the formation and accumulation of phlegm and dampness in the body clouding the mind and obstructing the orifices causing the epileptic seizures. This pattern is due to obstruction of the orifice and mind by phlegm and qi stagnation with depletion of the spleen and stomach. The location of the disease is in the brain, and the spleen, stomach and liver are involved in the root.

Diagnosis

TCM Diagnosis: Epilepsy due to binding of wind phlegm and qi
Western Medicine Diagnosis: Epilepsy

Treatment

In this case, the pathomechanism is mainly the phlegm obstructing the orifices and causing the seizures while the spleen fails to transport the fluids causing the accumulation of dampness and phlegm in the body. The retention of phlegm is then affected by emotional stimuli which affects the upper and clouds the mind.

Principles:

- Dissolve phlegm and open orifices
- Resolve internal wind and stop seizures
- Strengthen the spleen qi and soothe the flow of qi

Formula: Modified *Tiān Má Gōu Téng Yǐn* (Gastrodia and Uncaria Beverage) combined with *Wēn Dǎn Tāng* (Gallbladder-Warming Decoction)

Ingredients:

天麻	*tiān má*	12 g	Rhizoma Gastrodiae
钩藤	*gōu téng*	10 g	Ramulus Uncariae Cum Uncis
胆南星	*dǎn nán xīng*	10 g	Arisaema cum Bile
茯苓	*fú líng*	10 g	Poria
僵蚕	*jiāng cán*	8 g	Bombyx Batryticatus
天竹黄	*tiān zhú huáng*	10 g	Concretio Silicea Bambusae
丹参	*dān shēn*	15 g	Radix et Rhizoma Salviae Miltiorrhizae
枳实	*zhǐ shí*	10 g	Fructus Aurantii Immaturus
竹茹	*zhú rú*	10 g	Caulis Bambusae in Taenia
远志	*yuǎn zhì*	8 g	Radix Polygalae
浙贝母	*zhè bèi mǔ*	10 g	Bulbus Fritillariae Thunbergii
白芍	*bái sháo*	12 g	Radix Paeoniae Alba
炙甘草	*zhì gān cǎo*	10 g	Radix et Rhizoma Glycyrrhizae Praeparata cum Melle

20 doses were given. The decoction was taken once in the morning and once in the evening respectively.

Formula Analysis

This is a case of epilepsy due to the binding of phlegm and qi which have been intertwining for many years causing severe stagnation and obstruction of the channels. To treat such a chronic and severe case of seizures, we need to promote the circulation of qi flow, unblock the channels and resolve the phlegm. The formula used is a combination of *Tiān Má Gōu Téng Yǐn* and *Wēn Dǎn Tāng*. *Tiān Má Gōu Téng Yǐn* is used to calm the liver, extinguish wind, and promote the circulation of qi. It is often used when the internal wind affects the upper areas of the body. *Wēn Dǎn Tāng* serves to tonify qi and resolve phlegm, open the orifices and awaken the spirit. *Jiāng cán* is added to unblock collaterals and expel wind more thoroughly. *Tiān zhú huáng* and *dǎn nán xīng* are used to strengthen the effect of resolving the phlegm. The combination of these medicinals promotes the free flow of qi, resolves phlegm, extinguishes wind and treats convulsion.

Follow-up Consultations

After 20 doses of the formula, the frequency of the onset of epilepsy reduced from once every two to three days to once every one to two months. The patient continued to take the formula for two months. A follow-up visit three months later showed that the patient only had one epileptic seizure in the last three months.

CASE STUDY 2: Acute Convulsion

Ms. Deng Xia-wei, 25 years old. 1st consultation on December. 18th, 2008.

Main Complaint: Fever with loss of consciousness and convulsions for 2 days.

Medical History: Five days ago, the patient caught a cold, and then had stuffy and runny nose, dry, sore and itchy throat but did not seek medical attention. Two days ago, the condition of the patient aggravated because of exhaustion and she developed a fever of 39.2 ℃. The patient was given intravenous drip infusion at a local of "Andrographolide" and "Ceftriaxone Sodium", but the symptoms did not resolve and the patient fainted twice with violent convulsion, opisthotonos, clenched jaws, wheezing with phlegm in larynx, no urinary or fecal incontinence, foaming at the mouth and hemiplegia. The presenting symptoms above lasted for three minutes and then the patient woke up with a dull expression, slow movements and could not remember the event. The patient felt sleepy, weak, giddy and mentally unclear.

Physical Examination: Temperature: 39.2 ℃, pulse: 108 bpm, respiration: 20 bpm, blood pressure: 110/70 mmHg. Nervous system examination showed normal muscle strength and tension with symmetrical tendon reflex, a light red tongue with white coating, wiry and slippery pulse.

Pattern Differentiation

The patient had a weak constitution and was susceptible to catch cold. In this time, the patient contracted wind-cold pathogen externally, which entered the interior to transform heat. Meanwhile, weak spleen and stomach produced phlegm-turbidity that bound with the heat, obstructing the brain orifice and depriving its spirit manifesting as epilepsy.

The root of this case is impairment of the head spirit and its branch lies in *zang-fu* dysfunction. The key of pathomechanism is spiritual involvement and disorder. The disease location is in the brain and the disease nature is root deficiency with a branch excess.

Diagnosis

TCM Diagnosis: Epilepsy due to spleen and lung depletion with turbid phlegm obstructing the brain

Western Medicine Diagnosis: Acute epilepsy

Treatment

Principles:

- Dissolve phlegm and remove turbidity
- Unblock the collaterals to relieve epilepsy

Acupuncture Point Combination: PC 6 (*nèi guān*), DU 26 (*shuǐ gōu*), DU 1 (*cháng qiáng*), DU 8 (*jīn suō*), RN 15 (*jiū wěi*), GB 34 (*yáng líng quán*), ST 40 (*fēng lóng*), SP 6 (*sān yīn jiāo*), LI 4 (*hé gǔ*) and LU 7 (*liè quē*).

Manipulations: Needle DU 26 (*shuǐ gōu*) towards the nasal septum deeply and strongly. Do not retain the needle in DU 1 (*cháng qiáng*). Perform bloodletting on RN 15 (*jiū wěi*). Apply routine needling methods for the other points while retaining the needles for 30 minutes per treatment. Provide an acupuncture treatment once a day, 10 days make one course of treatment, perform three to five courses of treatment consecutively. Inform the patient to avoid overly stimulating situation, excessive stressful situation and over exhaustion.

Notes

Epilepsy is mostly due to innate pathogenic injury due to excessive emotions, especially excessive fright, external injury due to skull injuries and improper diet. Other causes are sometimes seen when a pregnant woman suffers a sudden or excessive fright, high fever, improper medication, and emotional excess and overstrain. These pathological conditions cause the constriction of the liver qi and deplete the spleen and kidney qi and essence causing the sudden uprising of liver yang mixed with the internal pathological phlegm seen as the epileptic seizures.

The therapeutic principles are to reinforce the healthy qi by strengthening the spleen and kidney, dispel pathogenic phlegm and wind. We need to treat the root and branch simultaneously, while eliminating phlegm to open the orifices, extinguishing wind to stop seizure, strengthening liver, spleen and kidney, and tonifying qi and nourishing the blood. Therefore, using acupuncture points on yin channels and *du mai* is appropriate. The points PC 6 (*nèi guān*), DU 26 (*shuǐ gōu*), DU 1 (*cháng qiáng*), DU 8 (*jīn suō*), and ST 40 (*fēng lóng*) are applied to awaken spirit and open the orifices, dissolve phlegm and extinguish wind to treat the branch, and SP 6 (*sān yīn jiāo*) is used to enrich and nourish the liver and kidney yin and subdue yang to treat the root.

KEY CLINICAL POINTS

1. Identifying the symptoms of Epilepsy

The symptoms of epilepsy are complex and diverse. Getting familiar with the variety of symptoms is important to the pattern differentiation. Epilepsy often has the following symptoms: ① typical absence of seizure with aura, suddenly falling down, unconsciousness, upward staring of the eyes, screaming with squeeking sounds, convulsions, apnea, pallid or purple complexion, foaming at the mouth, incontinence of urine, coming back to consciousness by themselves with no recollection of the event; ② paroxysmal mild seizure without falling down but stopping activities suddenly, upward staring of the eyes, unresponsive, holding things down; ③ local twitching of the mouth, eyelids or fingers and toes, or transient aphasia, or the sense of paroxysmal numbness and electrical shock in the mouth, tongue and fingers and toes, visual hallucinations, or the sense of regarding old things as new; ④ performing unconscious and repetitious actions, such as sucking, chewing, licking lips, shaking hands and caressing face, unbuttoning, stripping, wandering, aimless walking with no memory of the event.

2. Distinguish the severity of the condition

It is clinically very significant to identify the severity of the case while providing treatment to a patient with epilepsy. Generally, the duration of the attacks and the length of time between the attacks are significant to monitor the prognosis and efficacy of the treatment. Longer duration of attacks with shorter intervals is regarded as increasing in severity, whereas shorter duration with longer intervals between the attacks indicates the symptoms are improving. By observing the level of severity of the clinical manifestations, we can directly relate it to the depth and severity of the internal pathological turbid phlegm and condition of healthy qi.

3. Treatment approach of epilepsy

Since epilepsy is a paroxysmal transient disease, we are mostly able to treat it after the onset and between the attacks. The aim of the treatment is to stop the reoccurrence of the attacks. However, if you are faced with an epileptic attack you will need to tend to the symptoms and treat the branch. Usually we are treating between the attacks by eliminating phlegm to unblock the channels with acrid-warm medicinals, clearing and dissolving phlegm-heat, and eliminating internal wind. Treatments usually last a relatively long time to be able to remove the root of the disease. Monitoring the length of the attacks and the lapse of time between them will monitor your results.

BRIEF SUMMARY

The basic pathogenesis of epilepsy is phlegm, fire, blood stasis and innate cause leading to disorder of qi and blood and clouding the brain. The therapeutic principles are to eliminate phlegm and open the orifices, unblock channels and collaterals, and enrich and nourish liver, spleen and kidney. PC 6 (*nèi guān*), DU 26 (*shuǐ gōu*), DU 1 (*cháng qiáng*), DU 8 (*jīn suō*), and ST 40 (*fēng lóng*) are applied to dissolve phlegm and extinguish wind, and awaken spirit and open the orifices to treat the branch, and SP 6 (*sān yīn jiāo*) is used to enrich and nourish the liver and kidney, and subdue yang to treat the root.

COMPREHENSION QUESTIONS

1. What is the pathomechanism of epilepsy?
2. What are the common pattern differentiation and their recommended formulas?
3. Multiple choice questions:

1) Which is the most important pathogenic factor in epilepsy?
A. Fire
B. Qi
C. Wind
D. Phlegm
E. Stasis

2) Which is not a clinical feature of epilepsy?
A. Sudden attack
B. Unconsciousness
C. Foaming at the mouth
D. Upward staring of the eyes
E. Spasms and rigidity of limbs

3) The representative formula of epilepsy "deficiency of both the heart and spleen" is:
A. *Dìng Xián Wán* (Convulsion-Settling Pill)
B. *Lóng Dǎn Xiè Gān Tāng* (Gentian Liver-Draining Decoction) and *Dí Tán Tāng*

(Phlegm-Flushing Decoction)

C. *Tōng Qiào Huó Xuè Tāng* (Orifices-Unblocking and Blood-Moving Decoction)

D. *Liù Jūn Zǐ Tāng* (Six Gentlemen Decoction) and *Guī Pí Tāng* (Spleen-Restoring Decoction)

E. *Zuǒ Guī Wán* (Left-Restoring Pill) and *Tiān Wáng Bǔ Xīn Dān* (Celestial Emperor Heart-Supplementing Elixir)

Answers

1. The pathomechanism of epilepsy is mostly attributed to externally-contracted six pathogenic factors, internal damage caused by emotions, congenital insufficiency, improper diet, overwork, or fright causing pathogenic turbid phlegm to cloud the brain and obstruct the channels and collaterals.

2. The patterns for epilepsy and their recommended formulas are:

- For wind phlegm obstructing the mind, the recommended formula is *Dìng Xián Wán* (Convulsion-Settling Pill) or *Dǎo Tán Tāng* (Phlegm-Expelling Decoction);
- For internal retention of phlegm fire, the recommended formula is *Huáng Lián Wēn Dǎn Tāng* (Coptis Gallbladder-Warming Decoction), the combination of *Dí Tán Tāng* (Phlegm-Flushing Decoction) and *Lóng Dǎn Xiè Gān Tāng* (Gentian Liver-Draining Decoction), or *Dāng Guī Lóng Huì Wán* (Chinese Angelica, Gentian, and Aloe Pill);
- For heart and kidney deficiency, the recommended formula is *Dà Bǔ Yuán Jiān* (Major Yuan-Supplementing Decoction) or *Zuǒ Guī Wán* (Left-Restoring Pill);
- For blood stasis obstructing the orifices, the recommended formula is *Tōng Qiào Huó Xuè Tāng* (Orifice-Soothing Blood-Activating Decoction), *Diān Kuáng Mèng Xǐng Tāng* (Mind-Clearing Decoction) or *Xuè Fǔ Zhú Yū Tāng* (Blood Stasis Expelling Decoction).

3. 1) D, 2) E, 3) D.

3.5 Bipolar Disorder (*Diān Kuáng*)

Diān kuáng is a common mental disorder resembling what is known as bipolar disorder or manic depression. The term "*diān*" is characterized by mental and emotional depression, indifference to life, quiet behaviour, incoherent speech, and disconnectedness from reality. The term "*kuáng*" is characterized by being overly excited or stimulated, restlessness, noisy behaviour, unreasonably irritable, yelling and cursing without reason, acting out of control and breaking things. Bipolar patients demonstrate these two behaviours alternatively changing from one to the other in a regular basis in cycles of hours, days, weeks or months. This condition is most commonly seen in mainly young and middle-aged adults and usually the disease presents itself in people with a genetic trace and is found to be triggered by food allergies, emotional stress or a strong mental or emotional shock.

In Chinese medicine, this emotional imbalance and extremes changes are associated with a combination of excessive and deficiency patterns. Pathogenic phlegm, heat, blood and qi stagnation cloud the mind and disrupt the healthy flow of qi and blood affecting the depleted organs of the heart, spleen, liver, gallbladder and kidney causing this combination of emotional excesses and physical exhaustion.

Here is a detailed list of the pattern differentiation and related treatment principles and methods.

CLINICAL PATTERNS DIFFERENTIATION AND TREATMENTS

1. Phlegm Qi Stagnation

Symptoms: Depression, lethargy, heaviness of the body, lack of vitality, incoherent or erratic speech, excessive mood swings, irrational behaviour, white foam at the mouth especially when screaming, poor appetite, greasy tongue coating, wiry and slippery pulse.

Treatment Principle:

- Regulate qi and resolve stagnation
- Expel phlegm and open the orifices

Main Acupuncture Points:

- BL 18 (*gān shù*): Back-*shu* point of the liver to regulate and smoothen the qi flow and harmonize the liver
- BL 20 (*pí shù*): Back-*shu* point of the spleen to control the blood

- ST 40 (*fēng lóng*): To expel phlegm and dampness from the lung, heart and chest
- LV 3 (*tài chōng*): *Yuan*-source point of the liver to relieve chest congestion and irritability
- DU 24 (*shén tíng*): To clear the head and open the orifices
- RN 12 (*zhōng wǎn*): To regulate qi and invigorate spleen

Supporting Points:

- LI 14 (*bì nào*): To treat excessive phlegm-heat accumulation
- LV 14 (*qī mén*): Front-*mu* point of the spleen to spread liver and regulate qi, harmonize liver and spleen

Recommended Formula: *Shùn Qì Dǎo Tán Tāng* (顺气导痰汤, Qi-Regulating and Phlegm-Expelling Decoction) from *the Mirror for Medicine by Li* (*Lǐ Shì Yī Jiàn*, 李氏医鉴)

Substitute Formula: *Xiāo Yáo Sǎn* (逍遥散, Free Wanderer Powder) plus *Èr Chén Tāng* (二陈汤, Two Matured Substances Decoction)

Patent Formula: *Xiāo Yáo Wán* (逍遥丸, Free Wanderer Pill)

2. Deficiency of Heart and Spleen

Symptoms: Palpitations, susceptibility to fright, crying for no reason, fatigue, poor appetite, a pale tongue and a thready and weak pulse.

Treatment Principle:

- Tonify the spleen qi and nourish the heart blood
- Soothe the qi and move the blood
- Open the orifice and calm the mind

Main Acupuncture Points:

- HT 6 (*yīn xì*): *Xi*-cleft point of the heart to benefit the heart and calm the spirit
- PC 6 (*nèi guān*): *Luo*-connecting point of the pericardium to regulate qi and unbind the chest
- BL 15 (*xīn shù*): Back-*shu* point of the heart to nourish the heart and calm the spirit
- BL 18 (*gān shù*): Back-*shu* point of the liver to regulate and smooth the qi flow and harmonize the liver
- BL 20 (*pí shù*): Back-*shu* point of the spleen to nourish the spleen and benefit the qi
- SP 9 (*yīn líng quán*): To regulate the spleen and eliminate dampness

Supporting Points:

- ST 36 (*zú sān lǐ*): To invigorate the spleen, tonify qi and invigorate blood
- EX-CA 5 (*wèi shàng*): To tonify and raise the middle qi

Recommended Formula: *Guī Pí Tāng* (归脾汤, Spleen-Restoring Decoction) from the *Formulas to Aid the Living* (*Jì Shēng Fāng*, 济生方)

Substitute Formula:

- *Rén Shēn Yǎng Róng Tāng* (人参养荣汤, Ginseng Supporting and Nourishing Decoction)

• Combination of *Yǎng Xīn Tāng* (养心汤, Heart-Tonifying Decoction) and *Yuè Jú Wán* (越鞠丸, Constraint-Resolving Pill)

Patent Formula: *Guī Pí Wán* (归脾丸, Spleen-Restoring Pill)

3. Phlegm Fire Disturbing the mind

Symptoms: Sudden irritability and mood swings, headache, insomnia, flushed face, red eyes, aggression, poor appetite, poor sleep, a dark red tongue with a yellow, greasy coating, and a big, wiry, slippery and rapid pulse.

Treatment Principle:

- Calm the mind and open orifice
- Clear liver fire and smooth the flow of qi
- Support the spleen and expel phlegm

Main Acupuncture Points:

- DU 16 (*fēng fǔ*): To nourish the sea of marrow and calm the mind
- LV 2 (*xíng jiān*): To clear liver fire and treat irritability
- PC 6 (*nèi guān*): *Luo*-connecting point of the pericardium to clear fire and calm the spirit
- ST 40 (*fēng lóng*): To expel phlegm and dampness
- DU 14 (*dà zhuī*): To clear heat, activate the yang to regulate qi and calm the spirit
- 12 *jing*-well points: To clear fire and open the orifice (in sudden acute attacks)

Supporting Points:

- EX-HN 1 (*sì shén cōng*): To calm the spirit and clear the head
- EX-HN 24 (*ān mián*): To calm the spirit, treat insomnia, vertigo and mental disorders

Recommended Formula: *Shēng Tiě Luò Yǐn* (生铁落饮, Iron Flakes Beverage) from the *Medical Revelations* (*Yī Xué Xīn Wù*, 医学心悟)

Substitute Formula:

- *Méng Shí Gǔn Tán Wán* (礞石滚痰丸, Chlorite Phlegm-Removing Pill)
- *Ān Gōng Niú Huáng Wán* (安宫牛黄丸, Peaceful Palace Bovine Bezoar Pill)

Patent Formula:

- *Qīng Xīn Gǔn Tán Wán* (清心滚痰丸, Heart-Clearing and Phlegm-Transforming Pill)
- *Ān Nǎo Wán* (安脑丸, Brain Tranquilizing Pill)

4. Excessive Fire Damaging Yin

Symptoms: Excessive talking, anxious, susceptibility to fright, restlessness, rapid weight loss, red cheeks, tongue ulcers, insomnia, night sweat, a red tongue with scanty coating and a thready and rapid pulse.

Treatment Principle:

- Nourish yin and clear fire
- Calm the mind and soothe qi

Main Acupuncture Points:

- DU 16 (*fēng fǔ*): To clear heat, nourish the marrow and calm the spirit
- DU 24 (*shén tíng*): To clear heat, calm the spirit and benefit the heart
- HT 7 (*shén mén*): *Yuan*-source point of the heart to regulate and tonify the original qi of the heart, calm the spirit and treat tongue ulcers
- SP 6 (*sān yīn jiāo*): To nourish yin and invigorate blood
- KI 2 (*rán gǔ*): To clear deficient fire
- HT 6 (*yīn xì*): *Xi*-cleft point of the heart to alleviate night sweats, clear heart fire and calm the spirit

Supporting Points:

- EX-HN 24 (*ān mián*): To calm the spirit, treat insomnia, vertigo and mental disorders
- LV 2 (*xíng jiān*): To clear liver fire

Recommended Formula: *Èr Yīn Jiān* (二阴煎, Two Yin Brew) from *The Complete Works of [Zhang] Jing-yue* (*Jǐng Yuè Quán Shū*, 景岳全书)

Substitute Formula:

- *Ān Shén Bǔ Xīn Wán* (安神补心丸, Mind-Tranquilizing and Heart-Tonifying Pill)
- *Hǔ Pò Yǎng Xīn Dān* (琥珀养心丹, Amber Nourishing the Heart Elixir)

Summary Chart of Bipolar Disorder

External Patterns	Main Points	Supporting Points	Formulae
Phlegm Qi Stagnation	BL 18, BL 20, ST 40, LV 3, DU 24, RN 12	LI 14 for excessive phlegm-heat accumulation LV 14 for spleen and liver disharmony	*Shùn Qì Dǎo Tán Tāng* or *Xiāo Yáo Sǎn*
Deficiency of both the heart and spleen	HT 6, PC 6, BL 15, BL 18, BL 20, SP 9	ST 36 for qi and blood insufficiency EX-CA 5 for middle qi sinking	*Guī Pí Tāng*, *Rén Shēn Yǎng Róng Tāng* or combination of *Yǎng Xīn Tāng* and *Yuè Jú Wán*
Phlegm-fire disturbing the mind	DU 16, LV 2, PC 6, ST 40, DU 14, 12 *jing*-well points	EX-HN 1 for mental unclarity and irritability EX-HN 24 for insomnia and mental disorders	*Shēng Tiě Luò Yǐn*, *Méng Shí Gǔn Tán Wán* or *Ān Gōng Niú Huáng Wán*
Exuberant fire damaging yin	DU 16, DU 24, HT 7, SP 6, KI 2, HT 6	EX-HN 24 for insomnia LV 2 for liver fire	*Èr Yīn Jiān*, *Ān Shén Bǔ Xīn Wán* or *Hǔ Pò Yǎng Xīn Dān*

CASE STUDY 1: Schizophrenia

Mr. Zhao, 59 years old, farmer.

Main Complaint: Sudden incoherent speech and mental confusion for 3 days with aggravation for a day.

Medical History: The patient quarrelled with a fellow villager 3 days prior and afterwards he suffered from disordered speech, mental disorder, murmuring to himself, paranoia, anxiety, nervous, and fear of staying at home alone. He was brought to a local health center and was given an intravenous drip of the formula *Dān Shēn Zhù Shè Yè* (Salvia Solution) and oral intake of Estazolam in pill form which relieved his symptoms temporarily. The day before the consultation, the patient started to get very irritable and restless while yelling loudly. The patient had a history of hypertension for over 12 years reaching up to 150/90 mmHg which was under control with a daily dose of Indapamide.

Presenting Symptoms: Dysphoria, nervousness, irrational yelling, paranoia, fatigue, lack of strength, slow reaction, poor spirit, obesity, low appetite, insomnia, dry stool, normal urination, a red tongue with yellow greasy coating and a slippery, thin and weak pulse.

Physical Examination: Temperature: 36.5 ℃, pulse: 89 bpm, respiration: 21 bpm, blood pressure: 130/85 mmHg. The patient demonstrated an extremely poor spirit and was non-cooperative even if he had a clear speech and responded well to the medical intake. The test of the nervous system showed normal muscle tone and strength, symmetrical tendon reflex with normal deep and superficial sensations.

Pattern Differentiation

After the quarrel, the patient felt extremely angry and depressed which affected the liver and caused a severe liver qi constraint as well as liver fire rising upward affecting the mind. When the liver fails to control the healthy circulation of qi, it affects the mind directly and causes emotional imbalance. The anger induces fire of the liver and gallbladder which rises upward affecting the heart and brain causing confusion and irrational behaviour. The sudden episode of anger affected the mind and body of the patient and caused temporary mental unclarity and imbalance. While the disease location is in the brain and mind, it also involves the depletion of the kidney yin and essence which was unable to control the uprising of liver fire, as well as the depletion of the spleen and stomach qi which was unable to stabilize the pathogenic fire and maintain a healthy balance. The nature of disease pattern in this case is a deficiency in the root with an excess in the branch.

Diagnosis

TCM Diagnosis: *Kuáng* syndrome due to liver qi constraint and phlegm-fire harassing the mind

Western Medicine Diagnosis: Schizophrenia

Treatment

The pathomechanism of this syndrome is the sudden and excessive anger harming the flow of liver qi and causing liver phlegm and fire to rise and harass the mind causing irrational behaviour and emotions. This case also demonstrates a depletion in the liver and kidney yin unable to restrain the uprising of liver fire and long standing spleen qi depletion causing an internal retention of dampness and phlegm.

Principles:

- Soothe the liver and rectify qi
- Strengthen the spleen and expel dampness
- Clear heat and dissolve phlegm

Formula: A modification of *Chái Hú Shū Gān Săn* (Bupleurum Liver-Soothing Powder) combined with *Huáng Lián Wēn Dăn Tāng* (Coptis Gallbladder-Warming Decoction)

Ingredients:

柴胡	*chái hú*	10 g	Radix Bupleuri
川芎	*chuān xiōng*	10 g	Rhizoma Chuanxiong
香附	*xiāng fù*	10 g	Rhizoma Cyperi
茯苓	*fú líng*	10 g	Poria
枳实	*zhĭ shí*	8 g	Fructus Aurantii Immaturus
黄连	*huáng lián*	10 g	Rhizoma Coptidis
竹茹	*zhú rú*	10 g	Caulis Bambusae in Taenia
陈皮	*chén pí*	10 g	Pericarpium Citri Reticulatae
瓜蒌	*guā lóu*	10 g	Fructus Trichosanthis
石菖蒲	*shí chāng pú*	10 g	Rhizoma Acori Tatarinowii
远志	*yuăn zhì*	8 g	Radix Polygalae
龙骨	*lóng gŭ*	15 g	Fossilia Ossis Mastodi (raw)
牡蛎	*mŭ lì*	15 g	Concha Ostreae
磁石	*cí shí*	15 g	Magnetitum (raw)
炙甘草	*zhì gān căo*	10 g	Radix et Rhizoma Glycyrrhizae Praeparata cum Melle

Formula Analysis

The original formula of *Chái Hú Shū Gān Săn* (Bupleurum Liver-Soothing Powder) is to soothe the liver qi and clear the liver fire rising and affecting the emotional state of the patient with anxiety and irritability. It is combined with the formula *Huáng Lián Wēn Dăn Tāng* (Coptis Gallbladder-Warming Decoction) to further clear the liver fire and drain the phlegm while clearing the mind. The combination of these two formulas targets the liver phlegm fire rising upward harassing the mind causing irrational emotions.

The patient was asked to avoid stimulating food, such as seafood, mutton, spicy and oily foods as well as alcohol. He was also advised to avoid over exhaustion and emotional and mental stress.

Follow-up Consultations

After 15 doses, the patient was less agitated and did not scream anymore. He felt less anxious and nervous. The patient continued the same formula for another 15 doses and his mood came back to normal. A follow-up consultation 3 months afterwards confirmed there was no relapse of the condition.

CASE STUDY 2: Chronic Schizophrenia

Ms. Chen, 34 years old. 1st consultation on March 13th, 2010.

Main Complaint: Irregular and unstable mental and emotional state for a year with increasing imbalance for 3 days.

Medical History: The family members said the temper of the patient changed drastically about 1 year ago without known cause. The patient often instigated quarrels with others for no reasons while screaming angrily. She often murmured to herself and her sleep was poor. She was diagnosed with schizophrenia and got better after taking Chlorpromazine. Three days ago, the patient experienced a severe relapse with no known trigger.

Presenting Symptoms: Irritability, paranoia, dry mouth, normal appetite, insomnia, normal urination and stool. Physical examination showed normal reflex in the four limbs, a red tongue body and a rapid and wiry pulse.

Diganosis

TCM Diagnosis: "*Diān*" due to yin deficiency and exuberant fire

Western Medicine Diagnosis: Schizophrenia

Principles:

- Nourish yin and subdue empty fire
- Open orifices and calm the mind

Acupuncture Point Combination: DU 20 (*bǎi huì*), DU 24 (*shén tíng*), *yìn táng* (EX-HN 3), HT 7 (*shén mén*), BL 15 (*xīn shù*), LV 3 (*tài chōng*), PC 6 (*nèi guān*), KI 3 (*tài xī*), SP 6 (*sān yīn jiāo*).

Manipulations: Insert the needles subcutaneously backwards for DU 20 and DU 24 and sedate. Insert the needle obliquely towards the spine for BL 15 and sedate. Use the depletion method for LV 3 and supplementing method for KI 3 and SP 6. Use the balancing methods for the other points. The acupuncture treatment was provided 6 times a week with a needle retention of 30 minutes during each treatment.

Notes

This disease is often caused by excessive emotional frustration which interrupts the free flow of liver qi causing a severe stagnation. In time, this stagnation turns into retention of pathogenic fire which congeals the body fluids creating phlegm stagnation. The internal pathogenic fire raises this pathogenic phlegm and heat upward which obstructs and clouds the mind causing uncontrollable behaviour and emotional outbursts. Therefore, to treat this condition we need to simultaneously subdue the liver fire while draining the turbid phlegm, activate the qi and blood circulation while removing stasis, opening the orifices and calming the mind. Acupuncture points on the pericardium and liver channels and the *du mai* are appropriate. DU 20 and DU 24 are combined to raise the clear yang to the head, open orifices and awaken the mind. DU 26 and *yìn táng* are combined to calm and awaken the mind. LV 3 and LI 4 are combined to move qi, activate blood and remove stasis. HT 7 and PC 6 are used to open the chest, clear heat and calm the mind.

KEY CLINICAL POINTS

1. Precursory Symptoms

Before the onset of severe psychosis or bipolar disorder, there are often some noticeable abnormal changes of the spirit. The Spiritual Pivot (*Líng Shū*, 灵枢) states: "At the beginning of *diān kuáng*, the patient is depressed." In the beginning of the syndrome, the patient experiences an introverted personality with some level of depression. When the patient demonstrates a state of severe indifference, silence, irritability, moodiness, restlessness, insomnia or dreamful sleep, appetite changes or lack of appetite, the patient should be taken to a neurological hospital for early diagnosis and treatment. If appropriate treatment is given at the initial stage, prognosis is positive and often prevents a severe relapse of the condition.

2. Application of Expelling Phlegm Medicinals by Inducing Vomiting and Defecation

The primordial pathological factor of *diān kuáng* is phlegm, or phlegm accumulation and qi stagnation, or phlegm accumulation transforming fire. Therefore, when treating a psychosic patient with a strong constitution and a good appetite in the initial stage of the disease, vomiting and defecation are induced to eliminate the turbid phlegm and fire stagnation with medicinals such as *dà huáng* (Radix et Rhizoma Rhei), *méng shí* (Chlorite-schist), *máng xiāo* (Natrii Sulfas), and *yuán huā* (Flos Genkwa). If the turbid phlegm is prominent with excessive production of drool, chest oppression and a slippery, large and forceful pulse, using *Sān Shèng Săn* (Three Sages Powder) to induce vomiting and eliminate the phlegm can be considered. If the patient appears weak after inducing vomiting the practitioner needs to modify the treatment approach to appropriately nourish the spleen qi. Another formula to expel excessive turbid phlegm with salivation by promoting vomiting and defecation is *Lóng Hŭ Wán* (Dragon-Tiger Pill). It is an empirical formula consisting of *niú huáng* (Calculus Bovis), *bā dòu shuāng* (Semen Crotonis Pulveratum), *zhū shā* (Cinnabaris), *bái fán* (Alumen) and rice powder. Though this formula is seldom used, we should know it and use it when the presenting case needs it in clinic.

3. Application of Blood Activating and Stasis Removing Formula

During the Qing Dynasty, the famous doctor Wang Qing-ren wrote in the *Correction of Errors in Medical Works* (*Yī Lín Găi Cuò*, 医林改错) that: "Patients with moodiness, screaming and singing to strangers are afflicted by qi and blood stagnation in the brain with the brain qi failing to interact with the qi of *zang-fu* organs; they are living as if in a dream." This condition of psychosis is due to qi and blood stasis in the brain. Applying the formula *Diān Kuáng Mèng Xĭng Tāng* (Psychosis Awakening Decoction) is suitable to treat this syndrome. In modern times, both the retention of turbid phlegm intertwined with pathologic fire and blood stasis in the brain are regarded as the main pathogenesis of *diān kuáng*. Phlegm and blood have the same root in the body fluids and can influence each other very closely. Phlegm retention will cause static blood and vice versa. The retention of turbid phlegm and blood stasis can affect both the organs and the channels to become a lingering severe disease. They are often triggered by emotional stress and manifest as mental disorders. The common treatment approach to treat these conditions is to activate blood and resolve stasis, strengthen the spleen qi and resolve phlegm with the recommended formulas listed in the summary above.

4. Application of Opening Orifices

In addition to the previously mentioned pathogenesis, we must consider that the stagnated blood and phlegm is obstructing the mind and clouding the spirit. In this case, adding medicinals to open the orifices and clear the mind is important such as formulas like *Sū Hé Xiāng Wán* (Storax Pill) to warmly open the orifices or *Ān Gōng Niú Huáng Wán* (Peaceful Palace Bovine Bezoar Pill) and *Zhì Băo Dān* (Supreme Jewel Elixir) to cool and open the orifices.

BRIEF SUMMARY

Diān kuáng mainly occurs due to internal damage caused by the seven emotions with the retention of phlegm disturbing the mind and stagnation of qi and blood as the pathomechanism. Its location involves the brain and the organs involved are the liver, gallbladder, heart and spleen. The treatment principles for this disease are to move qi and activate blood, dissolve phlegm and subdue fire, open orifices and calm the mind. Acupuncture and Chinese medicinal formulas are combined to bring more effective results.

COMPREHENSION QUESTIONS

1. What is the main pathomechanism of *diān kuáng*?
2. What are the differences between *diān* and *kuáng*?
3. What are the main differentiation patterns and corresponding treatment approaches of *diān kuáng*?
4. Multiple choice questions:

1) The patient presents with symptoms of absent-minded, palpitations, easily frightened, susceptible to sadness, weakness, poor appetite and digestion, a pale red tongue with a thin and white coating and a deep, thin and feeble pulse. Select the recommended formula:

A. Combination of *Xiāo Yáo Sǎn* (Free Wanderer Powder) and *Dǎo Tán Tāng* (Phlegm-Expelling Decoction)
B. Combination of *Yǎng Xīn Tāng* (Heart Nourishing Decoction) and *Yuè Jú Wán* (Constraint-Resolving Pill)
C. Combination of *Wēn Dǎn Tāng* (Gallbladder-Warming Decoction) and *Bái Jīn Wán* (White Metal Pill)
D. Combination of *Diān Kuáng Mèng Xǐng Tāng* (Diān Kuáng Awakening Decoction) and *Zhū Shā Ān Shén Wán* (Cinnabar Spirit-Calming Pill)
E. Combination of *Èr Yīn Jiān* (Bi-Yin Decoction) and *Hǔ Pò Yǎng Xīn Dān* (Amber Heart Nourishing Elixir)

2) A male patient yells and breaks things in a fury anger. He presents with a flushed face, red eyes, no appetite, insomnia, phlegm rales in the throat, no stool for a week, a deep red tongue with a yellow greasy coating and a wiry, slippery and rapid pulse. All the following formulas can be applied EXCEPT:

A. *Shēng Tiě Luò Yǐn* (Iron Flakes Beverage)
B. *Méng Shí Gǔn Tán Wán* (Chlorite Phlegm-Removing Pill)
C. *Xiǎo Chéng Qì Tāng* (Minor Purgative Decoction)
D. *Ān Gōng Niú Huáng Wán* (Peaceful Palace Bovine Bezoar Pill)
E. *Hǔ Pò Yǎng Xīn Dān* (Amber Heart Nourishing Decoction)

3) *Diān Kuáng Mèng Xǐng Tāng* (Diān Kuáng Awakening Decoction) is often applied to treat *kuáng* with:

A. Phlegm retention and qi constraint
B. Phlegm fire disturbing the spirit
C. Stagnation of phlegm and heat
D. Deficiency of both spleen and heart
E. Exuberant fire impairing yin

Answers

1. The primordial pathological factor of *diān kuáng* is phlegm, or phlegm accumulation and qi stagnation, or phlegm accumulation transforming into fire. Therefore, when treating a patient with a strong constitution and a good appetite in the initial stage of the disease, vomiting and defecation can be induced to eliminate the turbid phlegm. The second important pathological factor is qi and blood stasis in the brain. Phlegm and blood have the same root in the body fluids and can influence each other very closely in the body. Phlegm retention will cause static blood and vice versa. The retention of turbid phlegm and blood stasis can affect both the organs and the channels to become a lingering severe disease. They are often triggered by emotional stress and manifest as mental disorders. The common treatment approach to treat these conditions is to activate blood and resolve stasis, strengthen the spleen qi and resolve phlegm. The last important factor is to consider the obstruction of the mind disturbing the spirit.

2. *Diān* and *kuáng* are two aspects of emotional and mental disorders. The *diān* aspect of the disorder pertains to the yin aspect of the mental instability and is mainly characterized by depression, paranoia, abnormally tranquil, excluding themselves from a group or from society, incoherent speech, phobia of meeting people, irregular crying or laughing, and low voice. The *kuáng* aspect pertains to the yang aspect and is mainly characterized by acting and speaking overly loud and excessively emotional with irregular mental reasoning including excessive anger, screaming with a high pitched voice, running taking off clothing and so on.

3. The commonly seen patterns and treatment formulas of bipolar disorders are:

- For phlegm qi stagnation, the recommended formula is: *Shùn Qì Dǎo Tán Tāng* (Qi-Regulating and Phlegm-Expelling Decoction) or *Xiāo Yáo Sǎn* (Free Wanderer Powder) plus *Èr Chén Tāng* (Two Matured Substances Decoction)
- For heart and spleen deficiency, the recommended formula is: *Guī Pí Tāng* (Spleen-Restoring Decoction), *Rén Shēn Yǎng Róng Tāng* (Ginseng Supporting and Nourishing Decoction) or the combination of *Yǎng Xīn Tāng* (Heart Tonifying Decoction) and *Yuè Jú Wán* (Constraint-Resolving Pill)
- For phlegm fire disturbing the mind, the recommended formula is: *Shēng Tiě Luò Yǐn* (Iron Flakes Beverage), *Méng Shí Gǔn Tán Wán* (Chlorite Phlegm-Removing Pill), or *Ān Gōng Niú Huáng Wán* (Peaceful Palace Bovine Bezoar Pill)
- For excessive fire damaging the yin, the recommended formula is: *Èr Yīn Jiān* (Two Yin Brew), *Ān Shén Bǔ Xīn Wán* (Mind-Tranquilizing and Heart-Tonifying Pill) or *Hǔ Pò Yǎng Xīn Dān* (Amber Nourishing the Heart Elixir)

4. 1) B, 2) E, 3) C.

3.6 Depression

Depression is a global disease that has been plaguing humans since the beginning of time with an increasing rate affecting twice the amount of women than men. Statistics also confirm that depression is affecting the developed countries more severely than the developing countries. There are over 8 different types of depression in western medicine characterized with their types of symptoms, length of disease and various intensity and severity. Depression usually appears with symptoms of an oppressed emotional state, unstable emotions, irritability, low spirit, chest oppression or stiffness, distention in the rib-side, susceptible to sadness and crying, plum qi stagnation sensation in the throat, dislike to speak and might be inclined to harm themselves.

In Chinese medicine, this disease mainly results from internal impairment of the healthy flow of qi due to an excess of the seven emotions or due to a depletion of the qi causing the liver qi to stagnate. Long standing qi constraint can transform to pathological fire which also stagnates and harms the body fluids causing phlegm heat stagnation and blood stasis. Excessive grief and anxiety can impair the lung and spleen qi, leading the spleen to fail in its main function of transporting and transforming the nutrients, thus creating poor digestion, as well as food, dampness and phlegm retention. These pathological factors will also cause internal heat stagnation affecting the emotions and causing depression. Emotional disorders are often linked to digestive disorders.

The location of disease is in the heart, spleen, liver, and kidney. In the early stage, this disease is mainly characterized by qi stagnation and pertains to an excessive syndrome. However, in time, chronic depression will affect the qi, blood, body fluids and become a deficiency or a complex deficiency and excess syndrome.

There are six commonly seen patterns of depression in Chinese medicine. Here is a list of their presenting symptoms with their recommended acupuncture and Chinese medicinal treatment approaches.

CLINICAL PATTERNS DIFFERENTIATION AND TREATMENTS

1. Liver Depression and Qi Stagnation

Symptoms: Mental depression, restlessness, anxiety, fidgeting, frequent sighing, chest stuffiness and fullness, glomus sensation under the heart, belching, abdominal distension, poor appetite, vomiting, irregular defecation, irregular menstruation, dark tongue body with thin and greasy coating and a wiry pulse.

Treatment Principle:

- Soothe liver and resolve depression
- Regulate qi to move stagnation

Main Acupuncture Points:

- BL 18 (*gān shù*): Back-*shu* point of the liver to regulate qi flow and resolve depression
- BL 15 (*xīn shù*): Back-*shu* point of the heart to calm the spirit, regulate emotions and unbind the chest
- LV 14 (*qī mén*): Front-*mu* point of the liver to spread liver and regulate qi, harmonize liver and stomach
- LV 3 (*tài chōng*) and LI 4 (*hé gŭ*): To promote qi and blood circulation, regulate emotions and stop pain
- RN 17 (*dàn zhōng*): Front-*mu* point of the pericardium and influential point of qi, to unbind the chest and invigorate qi

Supporting Points:

- SP 4 (*gōng sūn*): To regulate the middle *jiao* qi
- SP 6 (*sān yīn jiāo*): To regulate liver and spleen, invigorate blood and harmonize menstruation

Recommended Formula: *Chái Hú Shū Gān Săn* (柴胡疏肝散, Bupleurum Liver-Soothing Powder) from *The Complete Works of [Zhang] Jing-yue* (*Jĭng Yuè Quán Shū*, 景岳全书)

Substitute Formula:

- *Yuè Jú Wán* (越鞠丸, Constraint-Resolving Pill)
- *Xiāo Yáo Săn* (逍遥散, Free Wanderer Powder)

Patent Formula: *Xiāo Yáo Wán* (逍遥丸, Free Wanderer Pill)

2. Liver Depression and Spleen Deficiency

Symptoms: Low spirits, grief, compulsive thinking, pessimism, frequent sighing, chest and rib-side distention and fullness, glomus sensation under the heart, poor appetite, abdominal distension, belching, emaciation, fatigue, sloppy or dry stools, pale red tongue body with thin white coating and a wiry and thin pulse.

Treatment Principle:

- Soothe liver and resolve depression
- Tonify spleen and rectify qi

Main Acupuncture Points:

- BL 18 (*gān shù*): Back-*shu* point of the liver to regulate qi flow and resolve depression
- BL 20 (*pí shù*): Back-*shu* point of the spleen to invigorate spleen and qi, control blood, harmonize middle *jiao* and resolve abdominal distention

- LV 3 (*tài chōng*): *Yuan*-source point of the liver to spread liver qi, regulate menstruation and relieve depression
- LV 14 (*qī mén*): Front-*mu* point of the liver to spread liver and regulate qi, harmonize liver and stomach
- ST 36 (*zú sān lǐ*): To harmonize spleen and stomach, tonify correct qi and invigorate blood
- SP 6 (*sān yīn jiāo*): To regulate liver and spleen, invigorate blood and harmonize menstruation

Supporting Points:

- EX-HN 3 (*yìn táng*): To calm the mind and treat insomnia
- DU 20 (*bǎi huì*): To raise clear liver yang, calm the spirit and nourish the sea of marrow

Recommended Formula: *Xiāo Yáo Sǎn* (逍遥散, Free Wanderer Powder) from the *Beneficial Formulas from the Taiping Imperial Pharmacy* (*Tài Píng Huì Mín Hé Jì Jú Fāng*, 太平惠民和剂局方)

Substitute Formula:

- *Chái Hú Shū Gān Sǎn* (柴胡疏肝散, Bupleurum Liver-Soothing Powder) plus *Bàn Xià Hòu Pò Tāng* (半夏厚朴汤, Pinellia and Officinal Magnolia Bark Decoction)
- *Dān Zhī Xiāo Yáo Sǎn* (丹栀逍遥散, Cortex Moutan and Gardenia Free Wanderer Powder)

Patent Formula: *Xiāo Yáo Wán* (逍遥丸, Free Wanderer Pill)

3. Heart and Spleen Deficiency

Symptoms: Palpitations, timidity, excessive thinking, insomnia, forgetfulness, lusterless complexion, dizziness, fatigue, vertigo, loose stools, poor appetite, fatigue, abdominal distension, pale tongue and a thready and weak pulse.

Treatment Principle:

- Invigorate spleen and tonify qi
- Nourish heart and calm the mind

Main Acupuncture Points:

- BL 15 (*xīn shù*): Back-*shu* point of the heart to calm the spirit, clear fire and unbind the chest
- BL 20 (*pí shù*): Back-*shu* point of the spleen to invigorate spleen and qi, control blood, harmonize middle *jiao* and resolve abdominal distension
- SP 6 (*sān yīn jiāo*): To regulate liver and spleen, invigorate blood and harmonize menstruation
- ST 36 (*zú sān lǐ*): To harmonize spleen and stomach, tonify correct qi and invigorate blood
- HT 7 (*shén mén*): *Yuan*-source point of the heart to tonify the original qi of the heart, treat insomnia and calm the spirit
- PC 6 (*nèi guān*): *Luo*-connecting point of the pericardium to unbind the chest and

calm the spirit

Supporting Points:

- EX-HN 24 (*ān mián*): To calm the spirit, pacify the liver and resolve insomnia
- EX-HN 1 (*sì shén cōng*): To calm the spirit, improve sleep and resolve vertigo

Recommended Formula: *Guī Pí Tāng* (归脾汤, Spleen-Restoring Decoction) from the *Formulas to Aid the Living* (*Jì Shēng Fāng*, 济生方)

Substitute Formula: *Rén Shēn Yǎng Róng Tāng* (人参养荣汤, Ginseng Supporting and Nourishing Decoction)

Patent Formula: *Guī Pí Wán* (归脾丸, Spleen-Restoring Pill)

4. Liver Depression and Phlegm Obstruction

Symptoms: Low spirits, plum-pit syndrome, chest fullness and distension, vertigo, fatigue, poor appetite, frequent sighing, nausea, vomiting of phlegm and stomach fluids, hypochondriac pain, white and greasy tongue coating and a wiry and slippery pulse.

Treatment Principle:

- Soothe liver and resolve depression
- Dissolve phlegm and soften hardness

Main Acupuncture Points:

- BL 18 (*gān shù*): Back-*shu* point of the liver to regulate qi flow and resolve depression
- BL 20 (*pí shù*): Back-*shu* point of the spleen to invigorate spleen and qi, control blood, harmonize middle *jiao* and resolve abdominal distension
- LV 3 (*tài chōng*): *Yuan*-source point of the liver to spread liver qi, regulate menstruation and relieve depression
- SP 6 (*sān yīn jiāo*): To regulate liver and spleen, invigorate blood and harmonize menstruation
- ST 40 (*fēng lóng*): To transform phlegm and dampness
- RN 17 (*dàn zhōng*): Front-*mu* point of the pericardium and influential point of qi to unbind the chest and invigorate qi

Supporting Points:

- RN 22 (*tiān tū*): To transform phlegm, resolve plum-pit syndrome and throat disorders
- PC 6 (*nèi guān*): *Luo*-connecting point of the pericardium to unbind the chest and calm the spirit

Recommended Formula: *Bàn Xià Hòu Pò Tāng* (半夏厚朴汤, Pinellia and Officinal Magnolia Bark Decoction) from the *Essentials from the Golden Cabinet* (*Jīn Guì Yào Lüè*, 金匮要略)

Substitute Formula: *Èr Chén Tāng* (二陈汤, Two Matured Substances Decoction) plus *Chái Hú Shū Gān Sǎn* (柴胡疏肝散, Bupleurum Liver-Soothing Powder)

5. Disharmony between Heart and Kidney

Symptoms: Low spirits, palpitations, restlessness, forgetfulness, profuse dreaming, vertigo, tinnitus, emaciation, painful lower back and knees, hot palms and soles, dry mouth, night sweating, spermatorrhea, a red or dark red tongue with thin coating and a thin and rapid pulse.

Treatment Principle:

- Tonify kidney and nourish yin
- Nourish heart and calm the mind

Main Acupuncture Points:

- BL 15 (*xīn shù*): Back-*shu* point of the heart to calm the spirit, clear heat and unbind the chest
- BL 23 (*shèn shù*): Back-*shu* point of the kidney to tonify kidney, regulate water passages and treat spermatorrhea
- KI 3 (*tài xī*): *Yuan*-source point of the kidney to nourish kidney yin, strengthen the lumbus and knees
- SP 6 (*sān yīn jiāo*): To regulate the kidney, invigorate blood and harmonize liver
- ST 36 (*zú sān lǐ*): To harmonize spleen and stomach, tonify correct qi and invigorate blood
- HT 7 (*shén mén*): *Yuan*-source point of the heart to tonify the original qi of the heart, stop palpitations and calm the spirit

Supporting Points:

- BL 40 (*wěi zhōng*): To benefit the lumbar region and knees
- DU 20 (*bǎi huì*): To raise clear liver yang, calm the spirit and nourish the sea of marrow

Recommended Formula: *Tiān Wáng Bǔ Xīn Dān* (天王补心丹, Celestial Emperor Heart-Supplementing Elixir) from the *Corrections and Annotations to Fine Formulas for Women* (*Jiào Zhù Fù Rén Liáng Fāng*, 校注妇人良方)

Substitute Formula:

- *Huáng Lián Ē Jiāo Tāng* (黄连阿胶汤, Coptis and Donkey-Hide Gelatin Decotion) plus *Jiāo Tài Wán* (交泰丸, Peaceful Interaction Pill)
- *Bǎi Zǐ Yǎng Xīn Wán* (柏子养心丸, Arborvitae Seed Heart-Nourishing Pill)

Patent Formula: *Tiān Wáng Bǔ Xīn Dān* (天王补心丹, Celestial Emperor Heart-Supplementing Elixir)

6. Heart and Gallbladder Qi Deficiency

Symptoms: Low spirits, palpitations, timidity, low self-esteem, despair, restlessness, insomnia with profuse dreaming, shortness of breath, fatigue, a pale tongue with a thin white coating and a deep and thin or weak pulse.

Treatment Principle:

- Tonify qi and nourish yin
- Nourish the heart qi and warm the gallbladder
- Calm the mind and open orifices

Main Acupuncture Points:

- HT 7 (*shén mén*): *Yuan*-source point of the heart to tonify the original qi of the heart, stop palpitations and calm the spirit
- SP 6 (*sān yīn jiāo*): To regulate liver and spleen, invigorate blood and harmonize liver
- ST 36 (*zú sān lǐ*): To tonify correct qi, stop palpitations and treat insomnia
- BL 15 (*xīn shù*): Back-*shu* point of the heart to regulate the heart, calm the spirit, clear heat and unbind the chest
- BL 19 (*dǎn shù*): Back-*shu* point of the gallbladder to clear gallbladder heat, tonify yin and clear the liver

Supporting Points:

- BL 43 (*gāo huāng*): To tonify all the *zang*-organs, nourish yin and clear heat
- EX-HN 3 (*yìn táng*): To calm the mind and treat insomnia

Recommended Formula: *Ān Shén Dìng Zhì Wán* (安神定志丸, Mind-Tranquilizing Pill) from the *Medical Revelations* (*Yī Xué Xīn Wù*, 医学心悟)

Substitute Formula:

- *Gān Mài Dà Zǎo Tāng* (甘麦大枣汤, Licorice, Wheat and Jujube Decoction)
- *Hǔ Pò Yǎng Xīn Dān* (琥珀养心丹, Amber Nourishing the Heart Elixir)

Patent Formula: *Hǔ Pò Ān Shén Wán* (琥珀安神丸, Chrysophoron Spirit-Calming Pill)

Summary Chart for Depression

Patterns	Main Points	Supporting Points	Formulae
Liver Depression and Qi Stagnation	BL 18, BL 15, LV 14, LV 3, LI 4, RN 17	SP 4 for middle *jiao* qi disorders SP 6 for liver and spleen disharmony	*Chái Hú Shū Gān Sǎn* or *Yuè Jú Wán* or *Xiāo Yáo Sǎn*
Liver Depression and Spleen Deficiency	BL 18, BL 20, LV 3, LV 14, ST 36, SP 6	EX-HN 3 for insomnia DU 20 for yang collapse	*Xiāo Yáo Sǎn* or *Chái Hú Shū Gān Sǎn* plus *Bàn Xià Hòu Pò Tāng* or *Dān Zhī Xiāo Yáo Sǎn*
Heart and Spleen Deficiency	BL 15, BL 20, SP 6, ST 36, HT 7, PC 6	EX-HN 24 for insomnia EX-HN 1 for insomnia with vertigo	*Guī Pí Tāng* or *Rén Shēn Yǎng Róng Tāng*
Liver Depression and Phlegm Obstruction	BL 18, BL 20, LV 3, SP 6, ST 40, RN 17	RN 22 for throat obstruction or qi stagnation sensation PC 6 for chest oppression	*Bàn Xià Hòu Pò Tāng* or *Èr Chén Tāng* plus *Chái Hú Shū Gān Sǎn*

Continued

Patterns	Main Points	Supporting Points	Formulae
Disharmony between Heart and Kidney	BL 15, BL 23, KI 3, SP 6, ST 36, HT 7	BL 40 for lumbus and knee pain DU 20 for yang collapse	*Tiān Wáng Bǔ Xīn Dān* or *Huáng Lián Ē Jiāo Tāng* plus *Jiāo Tài Wán* or *Bǎi Zǐ Yǎng Xīn Wán*
Heart and Gallbladder Qi Deficiency	HT 7, SP 6, ST 36, BL 15, BL 19	BL 43 for heat due to yin deficiency EX-HN 3 for insomnia	*Ān Shén Dìng Zhì Wán* or *Gān Mài Dà Zǎo Tāng* or *Hǔ Pò Yǎng Xīn Dān*

CASE STUDY 1: Depression

Ms. Liang, 34 years old, civil servant.

Main Complaint: Low spirits and insomnia for 7 years with aggravation for a month.

Medical History: Seven years ago, the patient suffered from low spirits, deep sadness, anxiety, susceptible to cry, and insomnia. She started taking lorazepam intermittently and her symptoms varied from mild to severe without known cause. These symptoms aggravated about a month ago without known triggers. In the past week, the patient could hardly fall asleep and was extremely restless with low spirits while taking Lorazepam. She did not suffer from hypertension, diabetes mellitus or coronary disease.

Presenting Symptoms: Depression, sadness, irritability, unwillingness to speak, conscious but in poor spirit, flustered complexion, poor appetite, insomnia, dry stool, normal urination, a light red tongue with white coating and a slippery, thready, and rapid pulse.

Physical Examination: Temperature: 36.2 ℃, pulse: 75 bpm, respiration: 20 bpm, blood pressure: 125/70 mmHg. The patient spoke clearly and responded well. Her breath was steady and she was cooperative with the physical examination. The neurological examination showed cranial nerves (–), normal strength and muscles tone of hand grip and extremities and symmetrical tendon reflex. The patient took the Hamilton Depression Scale (21 items) and scored 25 indicating a mild depression.

Pattern Differentiation

The main complaint of the patient is low spirits and insomnia for 7 years with aggravation for a month diagnosed as depression. The binding constraint of liver qi, and the liver failing to govern the smooth circulation of qi caused the symptom of low spirit. Meanwhile, the heart qi and blood deficiency and the kidney yin depletion resulted in the lack of nourishments causing the symptoms of flusteredness, light red tongue, white coating, and slippery, thready, and rapid pulse. In conclusion, the pathomechanism is the binding constraint of liver qi, with heart qi and blood depletion. The disease location is in the brain and the affected organs in this case are the liver, heart, and kidney. The nature of disease is a complex syndrome of depletion in the root with an excess in the branch.

Diagnosis

TCM Diagnosis: Constraint syndrome due to the stagnation liver qi with heart qi and blood and kidney yin depletion

Western Medicine Diagnosis: Chronic depression

Treatment

The patient suffered from depression, uneasiness, chest fullness and oppression, migratory rib-side distending pain, oppression in the stomach cavity, belching, and no desire to eat. The diagnosis is constraint syndrome due to liver qi stagnation affecting the function of the spleen and stomach. This syndrome has been affecting the patient for many years resulting in a depletion in the heart qi and blood.

Principles:

- Soothe liver qi and resolve constraint
- Strengthen the spleen and stomach qi
- Rectify qi to loosen the middle *jiao*

Formula: Modified *Chái Hú Shū Gān Săn* (Bupleurum Liver-Soothing Powder)

Ingredients:

柴胡	*chái hú*	10 g	Radix Bupleuri
川芎	*chuān xiōng*	10 g	Rhizoma Chuanxiong
香附	*xiāng fù*	10 g	Rhizoma Cyperi
白芍	*bái sháo*	10 g	Radix Paeoniae Alba
陈皮	*chén pí*	10 g	Pericarpium Citri Reticulatae
郁金	*yù jīn*	15 g	Radix Curcumae
菖蒲	*chāng pú*	10 g	Rhizoma Acori
龙骨	*lóng gŭ*	30 g	(decocted first) Os Draconis
牡蛎	*mŭ lì*	30 g	(decocted first) Concha Ostreae
远志	*yuăn zhì*	10 g	Radix Polygalae
葛根	*gé gēn*	12 g	Radix Puerariae Lobatae
丹参	*dān shēn*	15 g	Radix et Rhizoma Salviae Miltiorrhizae
合欢皮	*hé huān pí*	15 g	Cortex Albiziae
炙甘草	*zhì gān căo*	6 g	Radix et Rhizoma Glycyrrhizae Praeparata cum Melle

Formula Analysis

In this case the modified formula of *Chái Hú Shū Gān Săn* is used to move liver qi and remove constrain, strengthen spleen and stomach qi. In the formula, *chái hú*, *xiāng fù*, and *chén pí* are combined to soothe the liver and resolve constraint, and rectify qi to loosen the middle *jiao*. *Yù jīn* and *hé huān pí* serve to regulate qi and resolve constraint. *Chuān xiōng* and *dān shēn* can rectify qi and invigorate blood. *Bái sháo* and *gān cǎo* cool and nourish the blood and soften the liver and remove tension. *Chāng pú* and *yuǎn zhì* can dissolve phlegm to open the orifices. In addition, the patient was asked to avoid spicy, oily food, sea food and mutton. She was also asked to avoid over exhaustion as well as emotional and mental stress.

Follow-up Consultations

After taking 15 doses of the decoction, the patient experienced a more relaxed and smoother mood. She also openly communicated with others happily. She was asked to take another 15 doses of the listed formula which was later replaced by *Xiāo Yáo Wán* (Free Wanderer) since her symptoms had completely resolved. The follow-up visit 3 months later confirmed that the symptoms of depression were completely resolved.

CASE STUDY 2: Chronic Depression

Mr. Li, 38 years old. 1st consultation on January 14th, 2010.

Main Complaint: Depression and dysphoria accompanied by insomnia for 5 years with aggravation for 3 months.

Medical History: The patient suffered from unexplained agitation and depression accompanied by insomnia which began 5 years ago. In severe conditions, he remained awake all night and felt dizzy, flustered, vexed, and unable to concentrate. He was diagnosed with depression from Xi'an Jiao Tong University Hospital. However, the medication did not bring any significant improvement of the above symptoms and his memory sharply decreased. His symptoms aggravated three months ago and all kinds of treatments were unsuccessful. He was hospitalized again for 28 days where he was administered Seroxat, Doxepin, Mirtazapine, Clonazepam and some Chinese patent medicines which alleviated his symptoms. He denied any disturbance of consciousness, headache, visual distortion, nausea, vomiting, numbness, paralysis, obvious chest tightness, and shortness of breath. After being released from the hospital, the patient wanted to continue to take medication to prevent a relapse of his symptoms.

Presenting Symptoms: Poor spirit, difficulty in falling asleep, dreamful sleep with poor quality, alternating normal to low appetite, normal stool and urination, a dark tongue with yellow coating and a slippery, thin and weak pulse.

Physical Examination: Cranial nerves (–), normal strength and muscle tone of the hands and extremities and symmetrical tendinous reflex with normal superficial and deep sensations. No pathologic reflex was induced.

Diagnosis

TCM Diagnosis: Constraint syndrome due to phlegm-heat obstructing the orifices
Western Medicine Diagnosis: Depression

Treatment

Principles:

- Soothe the liver and resolve constraint
- Clear heat and dissolve phlegm
- Calm the heart and open orifices

Acupuncture Point Combination: DU 20 (*bǎi huì*), HT 7 (*shén mén*), PC 7 (*dà líng*), PC 6 (*nèi guān*), LV 14 (*qī mén*), BL 15 (*xīn shù*), LI 4 (*hé gǔ*), LV 3 (*tài chōng*), ST 40 (*fēng lóng*), and SP 6 (*sān yīn jiāo*).

Manipulations: Insert the needle transversely backwards for DU 20 and twirl the needle rapidly at about 200 times per minute. Apply the depleting technique to ST 40, LV 3 and LI 4. Apply the even method to all the other points. Retain the needles for 30 minutes, and treat every day, 6 times per week during 6 weeks.

Combine by taking *Xǐng Nǎo Jiě Yù Jiāo Náng* (Brain Awakening and Depression Resolving Capsule) Chinese medicinal patent orally.

Clinical Analysis

In a broad sense, the constraint syndrome includes the constraint caused by both external pathogens and internal factors which correspond mostly to emotional factors. Externally, emotional shock or mental stress can cause our liver qi to stagnate and cause the constraint syndrome. Internally, qi stagnation can also be due to a physical trauma where the stagnation of blood influences the circulation of qi and might cause the constraint syndrome such as in post stroke, dementia, paralysis patients. In a narrow sense, it refers to the stagnation caused only by keeping emotions blocked inside or by overly indulging in the emotional body without expressing it outwards. Simply put, anger damages the liver which fails to govern the free flow of qi causing liver qi constraint. This liver qi stagnation oppresses the spleen which can not complete its function of transporting nutrients and transforming dampness. The stagnation of dampness creates internal retention of rheum and phlegm which then transforms into heat moving upwards harassing the mind.

We need to take all of these different aspects into consideration during our treatment approach by soothing the liver and resolving constraint, fortifying the spleen and benefiting the stomach, clearing heat and dissolving phlegm, and calming the heart and opening orifices. The points are mainly selected from the heart, spleen, stomach, pericardium, and liver channels. LV 3 (*tài chōng*) and LI 4 (*hé gǔ*) are applied to soothe the liver and resolve constraint. SP 6 (*sān yīn jiāo*) is the intersecting point of the spleen, liver and kidney channels, so it can fortify spleen, supplement liver, nourish kidney, and regulate and rectify qi and blood. HT 7 (*shén mén*) is the *yuan*-source point of the heart channel to calm the heart, PC 7 (*dà líng*) is the *yuan*-source point of the pericardium channel to clear the upper heat, and their combination can regulate and rectify the heart. PC 6 (*nèi guān*), the *luo*-connecting point of the pericardium channel, can open the chest and resolve constraint.

KEY CLINICAL POINTS

1. When treating a liver constraint syndrome, we must first differentiate if the case belongs to a deficiency or an excess pattern. Generally speaking, the constraint syndrome mainly involves the liver and heart, but might also involve the spleen and kidney, qi and blood, internal rheum and phlegm. Its excess pattern is characterized by an acute onset, depression, distending pain in the chest and rib-side, blockage sensation in the pharynx and frequent sighing. While its deficiency pattern features as long course of disease, lethargy, indifference towards life, restlessness of the heart spirit and thin or thin and rapid pulse.

2. The main aspect of the treatment should be focused on soothing the liver and clearing liver heat while other treatment principles might be focused on moving blood, strengthening the spleen and nourishing the heart blood and kidney essence. Chinese medicinal herbs can be combined with acupuncture treatments according to the diagnosis for best results.

3. Depression is a severe widespread condition that greatly affects the emotions and the perception of life. Combining the treatment with some psychological support is recommended in severe cases or in life threatening cases.

BRIEF SUMMARY

The main pathomechanism of constraint syndrome is the liver failing to govern the free flow of qi, the spleen failing to transport nutrients, and the heart lack of nourishment, and disharmony of yin-yang and qi and blood in *zang-fu* organs. The location of disease is mainly in the liver. However, the heart and the spleen can be involved. In the early stage, it mainly presents as an excess syndrome with six kinds of constraints, qi constraint as the leading one. If it lasts over a long period of time, the excess syndrome will change into a deficient one, rendering deficiency of qi, blood, yin, and essence of the heart, spleen, liver, and kidney. Clinically, deficiency-excess complex of it is also common. So the treatment principles are to soothe the liver and resolve constraint, clear heat and dissolve phlegm, calm the heart and spirit, and fortify the spleen and boost the stomach. LV 3 (*tài chōng*) and LI 4 (*hé gǔ*) are selected to soothe the liver and resolve constraint. SP 6 (*sān yīn jiāo*) can fortify the spleen, supplement liver, nourish the kidney, and rectify qi and blood. HT 7 (*shén mén*), PC 7 (*dà líng*), and PC 6 (*nèi guān*) serve to calm the heart and spirit, loosen the chest and resolve constraint.

COMPREHENSION QUESTIONS

1. Why is it important to rectify the flow of liver qi in the constraint syndrome?
2. Illustrate the key diagnostic points of the constraint syndrome.
3. Multiple choice questions:

1) Depression is primarily due to which pathological factor:

A. Blood constraint
B. Fire constraint
C. Phlegm constraint
D. Food constraint
E. Qi constraint

2) Although depression is related to all five *zang*-organs, which main organs does it involve:

A. The heart, liver, and kidney
B. The liver, heart, and spleen
C. The lung, heart, and liver
D. The lung, spleen, and kidney
E. The heart, lung, and kidney

3) The optimum formula for the constraint syndrome due to qi stagnation transforming into fire pattern is:

A. *Zhī Bǎi Dì Huáng Wán* (Anemarrhena, Phellodendron and Rehmannia Pill)
B. *Qīng Jīn Huà Tán Wán* (Lung Clearing and Phlegm Resolving Decoction)
C. *Dān Zhī Xiāo Yáo Sǎn* (Moutan and Gardeniae Free Wanderer Powder)
D. *Xiè Xīn Tāng* (Heart-Draining Decoction)
E. *Lóng Dǎn Xiè Gān Tāng* (Gentian Liver-Draining Decoction)

Answers

1. The etiopathology of the constraint syndrome is an internal impairment caused by emotional disorders or external pathogens causing the stagnation of liver qi. This stagnation of liver qi oppresses the spleen and stomach not permitting them to perform their natural action of transforming and transporting food and fluid causing a retention of rheum and fluid and inhibiting the formation of blood causing a blood depletion not nourishing the heart. This qi stagnation and retention of dampness and phlegm often transform into fire surging upward blocking the orifices and misting the mind causing depression. The location of disease is the mind and the affected organs include the liver, spleen, heart and kidney. The pathological nature is usually an excess pattern at the early stage, and with time, it becomes a deficient or deficiency-

excess pattern in chronic cases.

2. The main clinical manifestations of the constraint syndrome are low mood, depression, emotional restlessness and distention, fullness and pain in the chest and rib-side, occasionally accompanied by irritability, easily angry and sad, blockage sensation in the throat that is unable to be swallowed or coughed up. Most patients also have a history of emotional instability or emotional excesses such as worry, anxiety, sadness, fear, and resentment. Once the constraint syndrome is corrected, close attention needs to be taken to avoid a relapse of the disease.

3. 1) E, 2) B, 3) C.

3.7 Hypochondriac Distention

Hypochondriac distention and pain is clinically marked by right rib-side distending and pain caused by qi constraint in the gallbladder or digestive problems. The symptoms can be due to an excessive pattern or a deficiency pattern. If the hypochondriac distention and pain is due to a disorder of the gallbladder, it often occurs from the age of 40 to 65 while it is more common in women than men especially when overweight. Hypochondriac distention is commonly seen in diseases such as chronic cholecystitis, chronic cholangitis, gastritis and gallstone.

In Chinese medicine, hypochondriac pain is caused by either an excess, deficiency or a combination of excess and deficiency pattern. Internal damage due to emotions can also cause the symptoms of hypochondriac distension and pain especially when there is extreme grief, anxiety, anger and violent rage. Externally contracted pathogens such as damp-heat or damp cold can also invade the body causing stagnation of qi and blood in the area. Deficiency patterns are sometimes due to the weakness, overstrain, and exhaustion of the spleen and stomach as well as the liver and gallbladder. These pathogenic factors, whether they are internal or external, deficiency or excess, will lead to qi stagnation of the gallbladder which sometimes transforms into fire causing pain and distension of the rib side area. The related organs for this disease are the gallbladder, liver and stomach. In chronic cases, the pathogenic qi will damage the healthy qi and the lingering phlegm-turbidity and damp-heat might damage the spleen and stomach. Insufficiency of qi and blood produced by the spleen and stomach further weakens the healthy qi, which leads to liver and kidney yin deficiency or spleen and kidney yang deficiency, being ultimately a pattern of healthy qi deficiency with pathogenic excess.

There are four common patterns: qi stagnation of the liver and gallbladder, damp heat stagnation in the liver and gallbladder, blood stasis in the meridians and malnutrition of the liver meridian.

CLINICAL PATTERNS DIFFERENTIATION AND TREATMENTS

1. Qi Stagnation of the Liver and Gallbladder

Symptoms: distending or wandering hypochondriac pain which is often triggered by emotional outbursts, chest stuffiness, shortness of breath, poor appetite, frequent belching, a thin tongue coating and a wiry pulse.

Treatment Principle:

- Soothe the liver and regulate qi
- Strengthen spleen and harmonize stomach

Main Acupuncture Points:

- BL 18 (*gān shù*): Back-*shu* point of the liver to spread liver qi, regulate emotions and stop pain
- LV 14 (*qī mén*): Front-*mu* point of the liver to spread liver and regulate qi, harmonize liver and stomach
- GB 43 (*xiá xī*): To stop hypochondriac pain, clear heat and calm the spirit
- PC 6 (*nèi guān*): To regulate liver and spleen, invigorate blood and harmonize menstruation
- SJ 6 (*zhī gōu*): To stop chest and hypochondriac pain and regulate qi by unblocking the stools

Supporting Points:

- GB 40 (*qiū xū*): To treat jaundice due to damp-heat accumulation
- LV 2 (*xíng jiān*): To treat qi stagnation transforming to fire

Recommended Formula: *Chái Hú Shū Gān Săn* (柴胡疏肝散, Bupleurum Liver-Soothing Powder) from *The Complete Works of [Zhang] Jing-yue* (*Jĭng Yuè Quán Shū*, 景岳全书)

Substitute Formula: *Xiāo Yáo Săn* (逍遥散, Free Wanderer Powder)

Patent Formula: *Chái Hú Shū Gān Wán* (柴胡舒肝丸, Bupleurum Liver-Soothing Pill)

2. Damp-Heat Retention in the Liver and Gallbladder

Symptoms: Hypochondriac pain, bitter taste, chest stuffiness, poor appetite, nausea, vomiting, red or yellow eyes, icteric skin, dark urine, a yellow and greasy tongue coating and a wiry, slippery and rapid pulse.

Treatment Principle:

- Clear heat and drain dampness
- Soothe the liver and nourish the gallbladder
- Move qi and blood and stop pain

Main Acupuncture Points:

- LV 14 (*qī mén*): Front-*mu* point of the liver to spread liver and regulate qi, harmonize liver and stomach
- LV 3 (*tài chōng*): *Yuan*-source point of the liver to clear liver heat and gallbladder damp heat, stop pain and clear the eyes
- SJ 6 (*zhī gōu*): To stop chest and hypochondriac pain and regulate qi
- GB 34 (*yáng líng quán*): To clear liver and gallbladder damp-heat, spread qi and stop hypochondriac pain
- GB 24 (*rì yuè*): Front-*mu* point of the gallbladder to resolve hypochondriac pain, expel damp-heat and benefit the gallbladder

- ST 36 (*zú sān lǐ*): To resolve dampness, stop pain and regulate qi

Supporting Points:

- SJ 5 (*wài guān*) and GB 39 (*xuán zhōng*): To treat alternating fever and chills
- DU 9 (*zhì yáng*): To treat jaundice

Recommended Formula: *Lóng Dǎn Xiè Gān Tāng* (龙胆泻肝汤, Gentian Liver-Draining Decoction) from the *Secrets from the Orchid Chamber* (*Lán Shì Mì Cáng*, 兰室秘藏)

Substitute Formula: *Yīn Chén Wǔ Líng Sǎn* (茵陈五苓散, Five Substances Powder with Poria and Virgate Wormwood)

Patent Formula:

- *Lóng Dǎn Xiè Gān Wán* (龙胆泻肝丸, Gentian Liver-Draining Pill)
- *Lì Dǎn Pái Shí Piàn* (利胆排石片, Gallbladder-Disinhibiting Stone-Expelling Tablet)

3. Qi and Blood Stasis Obstructing the Meridians

Symptoms: Stabbing and fixed pain which aggravates at night, dark purple spider veins over the ribs, low-grade night fever, palpable masses under rib-sides, dry mouth and throat with no desire to drink, dry skin, dark circles under eyes, purple lips, a dark-purple tongue and a deep and choppy pulse.

Treatment Principle:

- Invigorate blood and eliminate stagnation
- Regulate qi and stop pain

Main Acupuncture Points:

- LV 14 (*qī mén*): Front-*mu* point of the liver to spread liver and regulate qi, harmonize liver and stomach
- LV 13 (*zhāng mén*): Front-*mu* point of the spleen to spread liver qi, invigorate spleen and stop pain
- BL 17 (*gé shù*): Influential point of the blood to promote blood circulation and unbind the chest
- SP 10 (*xuè hǎi*): To promote blood flow and dispel blood stasis
- GB 34 (*yáng líng quán*): To clear liver and gallbladder damp-heat, spread qi and stop hypochondriac pain
- GB 24 (*rì yuè*): Front-*mu* point of the gallbladder to resolve hypochondriac pain, expel damp-heat and benefit the gallbladder

Supporting Points:

- SP 21 (*dà bāo*): To unbind the chest, stop coastal pain and treat asthma
- LV 2 (*xíng jiān*): To treat blood stasis transforming to fire

Recommended Formula: *Xuè Fǔ Zhú Yū Tāng* (血府逐瘀汤, Blood Stasis Expelling Decoction) from the *Correction of Errors in Medical Works* (*Yī Lín Gǎi Cuò*, 医林改错)

Substitute Formula: *Táo Hóng Sì Wù Tāng* (桃红四物汤, Peach Kernel and Carthamus Four Substances Decoction)

Patent Formula: *Xuè Fǔ Zhú Yū Jiāo Náng* (血府逐瘀胶囊, House of Blood Stasis

Expelling Capsule)

4. Malnutrition of the Liver Meridian

Symptoms: Dull and lingering hypochondriac pain which aggravates with fatigue, dry mouth and throat, heat sensation in the chest, dizziness, blurry vision, lower back and knees pain and soreness, a red tongue with scanty coating and a thready, wiry and rapid pulse.

Treatment Principle:

- Nourish liver yin and heart blood
- Soothe liver qi and move blood

Main Acupuncture Points:

- LV 14 (*qī mén*): Front-*mu* point of the liver to spread liver and regulate qi, harmonize liver and stomach
- LV 8 (*qū quán*): To spread liver qi and invigorate blood
- LV 3 (*tài chōng*): *Yuan*-source point of the liver to spread liver qi, nourish liver blood and yin, clear eyes resolve chest congestion
- BL 18 (*gān shù*): Back-*shu* point of the liver to spread liver qi, regulate emotions and stop pain
- BL 23 (*shèn shù*): Back-*shu* point of the kidney to tonify liver and kidney yin, stop lumbus and knee pain, and benefit eyes
- SP 6 (*sān yīn jiāo*): To harmonize the liver and tonify the kidney

Supporting Points:

- KI 3 (*tài xī*): To treat liver and kidney yin deficiency, tinnitus and deafness
- DU 21 (*qián dǐng*): To clear head and eyes, treat dizziness and subdue liver yang

Recommended Formula: *Yī Guàn Jiān* (一贯煎, Effective Integration Decoction) from the *[Wei] Liu-zhou's Discourse on Medicine* (*Liǔ Zhōu Yī Huà*, 柳州医话)

Substitute Formula: *Liù Wèi Dì Huáng Tāng* (六味地黄汤, Six Ingredients Rehmannia Decoction)

Patent Formula: *Liù Wèi Dì Huáng Wán* (六味地黄丸, Six Ingredients Rehmannia Pill)

Summary Chart for Hypochondriac Distention

Patterns	Main Points	Supporting Points	Formulae
Liver-Qi Stagnation	BL 18, LV 14, GB 43, PC 6, SJ 6	GB 40 for jaundice LV 2 for stagnation transforming to fire	*Chái Hú Shū Gān Sǎn* or *Xiāo Yáo Sǎn*
Dampness-Heat in the Liver and Gallbladder	LV 14, LV 3, SJ 6, GB 34, GB 24, ST 36	SJ 5 and GB 39 for alternating fever and cold DU 9 for jaundice	*Lóng Dǎn Xiè Gān Tāng* or *Yīn Chén Wǔ Líng Sǎn*

Continued

Patterns	Main Points	Supporting Points	Formulae
Stagnant Blood Obstructing the Meridians	LV 14, LV 13, BL 17, SP 10, GB 34, GB 24	SP 21 for local coastal pain and asthma LV 2 for blood stasis transforming to fire	*Xuè Fŭ Zhú Yū Tāng* or *Táo Hóng Sì Wù Tāng*
Malnutrition of the Liver Meridian	LV 14, LV 8, LV 3, BL 18, BL 23, SP 6	KI 3 for tinnitus and deafness DU 21 for dizziness due to liver yang rising	*Yī Guàn Jiān* or *Liù Wèi Dì Huáng Tāng*

CASE STUDY 1: Bilateral Hypochondriac Pain

Ms. Ma, 39 years old.

Main Complaint: Icteric eyes and body skin, and bilateral rib-side pain for a week.

Medical History: A week ago, the patient suffered from bilateral hypochondriac pain that was more severe on the right side, accompanied by high fever, chest oppression, nausea, desire to vomit, and constipation. Two days later, her eyes and body became icteric so she went to a hospital for treatment. The patient was diagnosed with acute cholecystitis due to gallstone. After taking some Western medicine, the hypochondriac pain was slightly relieved. The following day she was released from the hospital and came for a Chinese medicine consultation.

Presenting Symptoms: Alternating chills and fever, bright jaundiced eyes and body, right sided hypochondriac pain radiating to the shoulder and back, nausea, bitter taste in the mouth, constipation, difficulty in defecation, scanty and dark yellow urine, a red tongue with a yellow coating and a wiry and rapid pulse.

Physical Examination: Temperature: 39.6 ℃, obvious pain with percussion over the hepatic region. The liver and the spleen were not enlarged. Murphy's sign was positive. An ultrasound confirmed the acute cholecystitis and gallstone. White blood cell is 12.3×10^9/L, neutrophil 85%. Liver functions were normal.

Pattern Differentiation

Alternating chills and fever is a consequence of pathogenic constraint in the *shao yang* layer that causes a struggle between the healthy qi and pathogenic qi. As gallstones obstruct the biliary tract, the gallbladder is blocked and the bile is extracted within the body and is shown in the icteric colouring of the skin and eyes as jaundice. The gallbladder is located under the right rib side and its channel runs along the shoulder and the back. If the vessel of the gallbladder is obstructed, qi stagnates and causes severe pain in the right rib side radiating to the shoulder and upper back. Gallbladder heat harassing the upper body and the disharmony of the stomach lead to bitter taste in the mouth, nausea and vomiting. Internal blazing of pathogenic heat, and inhibited movement of qi in the intestines cause constipation and difficulty in defecation. Heat harassing the urinary bladder leads to the disturbance of qi transformation seen in the scant and dark urine. The red tongue with yellow coating as well as the rapid pulse all indicates internal heat excess. The wiry quality of the pulse indicates there is stagnation or a liver and gallbladder disorder.

Diagnosis

TCM Diagnosis: Hypochondriac pain due to liver and gallbladder retention of damp-heat

Western Medicine Diagnosis: Jaundice due to cholecystitis and gallstone

Treatment

The pathogenesis in this case is liver and gallbladder retention of damp-heat causing a stagnation of qi and heat in the rib side area.

Principles:

- Soothe liver and promote gallbladder function
- Clear heat and remove dampness
- Strengthen the spleen and unblock the bowels

Formula: Modified *Dà Chái Hú Tāng* (Major Bupleurum Decoction).

Ingredients:

柴胡	*Chái Hú*	10 g	Radix Bupleuri
黄芩	*huáng qín*	10 g	Radix Scutellariae
茵陈	*yīn chén*	30 g	Herba Artemisiae Scopariae
黄连	*huáng lián*	3 g	Rhizoma Coptidis
金银花	*jīn yín huā*	15 g	Flos Lonicerae Japonicae
枳实	*zhǐ shí*	10 g	Fructus Aurantii Immaturus
郁金	*yù jīn*	9 g	Radix Curcumae
白芍	*bái sháo*	12 g	Radix Paeoniae Alba
金钱草	*jīn qián cǎo*	30 g	Herba Lysimachiae
川楝子	*chuān liàn zǐ*	9 g	Fructus Toosendan
延胡索	*yán hú suǒ*	9 g	Rhizoma Corydalis
山栀	*shān zhī*	9 g	Fructus Gardeniae
半夏	*bàn xià*	3 g	Rhizoma Pinelliae
甘草	*gān cǎo*	3 g	Radix et Rhizoma Glycyrrhizae
生大黄	*dà huáng*	9 g	Radix et Rhizoma Rhei (added later)

Formula Analysis

This modified version of *Dà Chái Hú Tāng* is given to strengthen the function of clearing heat binding. *Chái Hú* is the chief medicinal and when it is combined with *huáng qín,* it expels pathogenic heat in the *shao yang* layers by harmonizing.

Dà huáng and *zhǐ shí* serve to internally drain *yang ming* heat binding, move qi and disperse *pǐ. Huáng qín, dà huáng,* and *zhǐ shí* are assistant medicinals.

Bái sháo softens the liver, relaxes cramps, cools blood and relieves pain. When it is combined with *dà huáng,* it can relieve excessive pattern causing pain in the abdominal area. Combined with *zhǐ shí,* they can rectify qi and harmonize blood in order to eliminate pain and fullness below the heart. *Bàn xià* harmonizes the stomach and directs counterflow downward. Meanwhile, it is combined with medicinals which can soothe the liver, promote gallbladder qi, and move qi to relieve pain.

Chinese Patent Medicine: *Xiāo Yán Lì Dǎn Fēn Sàn Piàn* (Antiphlogistic Gallbladder-Benefiting tablet) was also given to the patient by taking orally 3 tablets, 3 times a day. The patient was also advised not to eat raw, cold, and greasy food.

Follow-up Consultations

After 7 doses of the formula, the hypochondriac pain significantly relieved, the jaundice gradually faded away, and the defecation became normal. The patient continued to take another 14 doses of the same formula and the hypochondriac pain resolved completely and the appetite, urination and defecation were normal. She took another 7 doses to recover completely.

CASE STUDY 2: Chronic Cholecystitis with Gallstones
By Dr. Li Shou-shan

Mr. Yang, 36 years old. 1st consultation on October 7th, 1976.

Main Complaint: Chronic cholecystitis with gallbladder stone for 3 years.

Medical History: The patient frequently suffered from distending pain in the right side of the abdomen, back and hypochondriac areas for 3 years. Recently, he consumed a lot of alcohol and greasy food which induced an acute severe pain in the upper right abdominal area radiating to the rib sides. His eyes and body were icteric. He had dark yellow urine and constipation. An ultrasound and CT confirmed the blockage of the bile duct by gallstones and cholecystitis. His body temperature was above average at 38.5 ℃. A course of antibiotics put the symptoms in remission and he was discharged from the hospital. Three day later, the patient experienced sudden and sharp pain in the hypochondriac and abdominal regions with a high fever.

Presenting Symptoms: Severe pain in the upper right abdominal, hypochondriac and back areas with a sudden onset, vomiting of sour and bitter liquid, constipation, scant and dark yellow urine resembling soy sauce, icteric eyes and body, skin itching, a wiry, slippery and rapid pulse and a red tongue with yellow, greasy and dry coating.

Physical Examination: Temperature: 38.5 ℃. There was a tenderness and rebound tenderness in the right upper abdomen and an ultrasound confirmed the chronic cholecystitis with gallstones in the bile duct area.

Diagnosis

TCM Diagnosis: Hypochondriac distention and pain due to damp heat retention in the gallbladder

Western Medicine Diagnosis: Cholecystitis with gallstones in the bile duct area

Treatment

This syndrome of dampness and heat retention in the liver and gallbladder areas was triggered by the consummation of alcohol and excessive intake of greasy food. The patient already had a preexisting retention of dampness and heat in the liver and gallbladder and in combination with poor life habits, it led to the sudden and severe pain in the hypochondriac and abdominal areas. When the pathogenic dampness and heat inhibited the function of the gallbladder, the bile spilled out of the gallbladder and caused icteric eyes and body. At this time the stomach also failed to harmonize and descend the food content manifested as vomiting. The inhibited flow of *gu* qi and the retention of dampness and heat also lead to constipation. In addition, the yellow tongue coating and rapid pulse confirm internal accumulation of dampness and heat as well.

Principles:

- Clear heat and drain dampness from the liver and gallbladder
- Purge the stools and relax bowels

Formula: Modified *Sì Nì Săn* (Frigid Extremities Powder) combined with *Dà Chéng Qì Tāng* (Major Purgative Decoction) and *Yīn Chén Hāo Tāng* (Virgate Wormwood Decoction)

Ingredients:

柴胡	*chái hú*	15 g	Radix Bupleuri
枳实	*zhĭ shí*	10 g	Fructus Aurantii Immaturus
赤芍	*chì sháo*	10 g	Radix Paeoniae Rubra
香附	*xiāng fù*	15 g	Rhizoma Cyperi
郁金	*yù jīn*	15 g	Radix Curcumae
茵陈	*yīn chén*	30 g	Herba Artemisiae Scopariae
大黄	*dà huáng*	15 g	Radix et Rhizoma Rhei (decoction in the end)
川朴	*chuān pò*	10 g	Cortex Magnoliae Officinalis
芒硝	*máng xiāo*	15 g	Natrii Sulfas (melted in decoction)
甘草	*gān căo*	10 g	Radix et Rhizoma Glycyrrhizae
金钱草	*jīn qián căo*	30 g	Herba Lysimachiae

Follow-up Consultations

Two weeks later, the patient returned for a second consultation and said that after taking the first dose of the formula, he defecated three times which slightly relieved the epigastric and hypochondriac pain. After another 2 doses, the pain was further relieved, vomiting disappeared and the fever also resolved. His body temperature was 36.9 ℃. It indicated the formula was right for his pattern. However, his tongue and pulse conditions and icteric skin remained the same. The previous formula was given again for 3 more days and his icteric skin slightly reduced and the epigastric and hypochondriac pain resolved. The tongue coating became normal while the pulse was wiry and thin. The changes of symptoms demonstrated that the damp heat retention in the gallbladder had been cleared. Therefore, *máng xiāo* was removed from the formula and the dosage of *dà huáng* and *yīn chén* were reduced, while *mù xiāng* and *gān jiāng* were added to resolve qi stagnation and dampness constraint by warming and unblocking. After taking this formula, the remaining icteric skin was completely alleviated and his appetite, urination and defecation were normal. This formula was modified again with the addition of *Xiāo Shí Să* (Stone Eliminating Powder) for 20 additional days and the gallstones were discharged. Afterwards, the patient stopped taking the decoction and corrected his diet and life habits. Two weeks afterwards, he went back to work and there was no relapse within the following 6 months.

Clinical Analysis

This is a case of hypochondriac distension due to dampness and heat retention in the liver and gallbladder with jaundice and constipation. The treatment principle was to purge heat and dampness through the bowels as well as soothe the liver and gallbladder. The formula *Sì Nì Săn* was used to soothe the liver and gallbladder qi, *Dà Chéng Qì Tāng* was used to purge the dampness and heat by the way of the bowels, and *Yīn Chén Hāo Tāng* was used to resolve jaundice by clearing damp-heat. *Xiāng fù, yù jīn* and *jīn qián căo* were combined with *Xiāo Shí Săn* to move qi, remove stasis and dissolve stone. This formula is often used to treat cholecystitis and gallstone in modern times.

CASE STUDY 3: Acute Pancreatitis with Gallstones
By Dr. Zhang Ren

Mr. Lin, 61 years old. 1st consultation on August 16th, 1984.

Main Complaint: Repeated episodes of acute hypochondriac pain for over 1 year.

Medical History: The patient suddenly experienced right sided hypochondriac and abdominal pain with vomiting and fever in the mid-April, 1983. He was sent to the emergency room of the Shanghai Hua Shan Hospital and was diagnosed with an acute onset of gallstone as well as an acute condition of pancreatitis. The symptoms were relieved after receiving western medical treatment. However, the patient had some reoccurring pain after overindulging in his diet and sought Chinese medicine for a cure.

Presenting Symptoms: Soreness and dull pain in the hypochondriac area, a light red tongue with a slightly yellow and greasy coating and wiry pulse. An ultrasound confirmed a rough gallbladder wall without obvious thickening, several strong echoes with sound shadow in the neck of gallbladder, peak diameter 6mm. There was no dilated common bile duct.

Diagnosis

TCM Diagnosis: Hypochondriac distension due to damp heat retention in the liver and gallbladder

Western Medicine Diagnosis: Reoccurring pangreatitis with gallstones

Treatment

Principles:

- Clear heat and drain dampness
- Sooth the liver and subdue the gallbladder
- Move qi and relieve pain.

Ear Acupuncture Points:

Shoulder (*jiān*)	Pancreas and Gallbladder (*yí dǎn*)	Duodenum (*shí èr zhǐ cháng*)
Root of Ear Vagus (*ěr mí gēn*)	Liver (*gān*)	

Body Acupuncture Points:

- GB 24 (*rì yuè*): The front-*mu* point of gallbladder to drain damp heat from the gallbladder
- GB 40 (*qiū xū*): The *yuan*-source point of gallbladder to tonify the gallbladder qi and dredge the meridian

Manipulations: Apply vaccaria seeds on each of the listed ear points and tape them to the chosen locations. Ask the patient to press each ear point for 5 min every 20 min four times a day, more specifically after having meals and before sleep. Needle one ear during the acupuncture treatment and maintain the other ear to place the vaccaria seeds. Two acupuncture treatments a week is required. Apply the draining method to GB 24 and GB 40 for 2 minutes without retaining the needles. For any additional body acupuncture points chosen, only points of the right side are necessary.

Notes

The patient suffered from repeated attacks of pancreatitis secondary to multiple gallstones. Since the biggest of the gallbladder stones has a diameter of 0.6cm, the doctor used ear acupressure as the main treatment approach. The treatment showed to be effective in releasing multiple small sized gallbladder stones.

In addition to the stones, the patients had the clinical manifestations of hypochondriac pain, dry and bitter taste in the mouth, incomplete defecation and greasy tongue coating demonstrating that the case is due to the retention of damp-heat obstructing the collaterals and leading to the qi stagnation of the liver and gallbladder. GB 24, the front-*mu* point of gallbladder, and GB 40, the *yuan*-source point of gallbladder, are needled to clear heat and drain dampness, soothe the liver and gallbladder, and strengthen the unblocking function of the ear point.

Gallbladder distension was initially described in the *Yellow Emperor's Inner Classic* (*Huáng Dì Nèi Jīng*, 黄帝内经). For example, *The Spiritual Pivot – Discussion on Distension* (*Líng Shū - Zhàng Lùn*, 灵枢·胀论) records that: "Patients with gallbladder distension have hypochondriac pain and distension, bitter taste in the mouth and frequent sighing", which accurately describes the symptoms presented in the listed patients.

KEY CLINICAL POINTS

Generally speaking, the treatment principles for gallbladder distension are soothing the liver and benefiting the gallbladder, purging dampness and heat retention and relaxing the bowels. The treatment should be modified in accordance with the presentation of the changing symptoms in both the deficiency and excess patterns. For an excess pattern, the treatment is to soothe the liver, benefit the gallbladder and relax bowels. For a deficiency pattern, we need to consider supplementing the middle and moving qi, assisted by warming the yang qi or nourishing yin, so as to effectively remove the pathogenic blockage and restore health.

1. Various Sorts of Hypochondriac Pain

One of the specific hypochondriac pain especially characterized by right rib-side pain due to qi constraint in the gallbladder, and gallbladder failing to release bile causes gallbladder distension. It is often accompanied with nausea, vomiting, bitter taste in the mouth, and belching due to the uprising of the gallbladder and stomach qi. It is often caused or triggered by taking too much alcohol or greasy food. However, general hypochondriac pain is mainly due to the disorders of the liver qi stagnation, causing heat or dampness and heat retention or local qi and blood stagnation.

2. Differentiation of Deficiency, Excess, Chronic and Acute

The excess pattern of hypochondriac distention and pain is characterized by an acute onset, a severe painful sensation and usually a short disease course. In some occasions, the acute onset stems from a long disease course, but is triggered and has a sudden response. The symptoms normally include constant distending pain which is aggravated by pressure with symptoms of bitter taste in the mouth, fever, thick tongue coating and excess pulse quality.

The deficiency pattern is characterized by a chronic onset with a long disease course. The symptoms include intermittent dull and mild rib-side distending pain, easily induced by fatigue, scanty coating and deficient pulse quality.

The acute condition is characterized by severe spastic hypochondriac pain, alternating chills and fever, frequent vomiting, a yellow tongue coating and a rapid pulse.

The chronic condition is characterized by mild pain, no fever, vomiting and jaundice.

3. Transmission from Excess to Deficiency and Formation of Deficiency-excess Complex

The excess pattern is usually due to qi stagnation at the initial stage which rapidly transforms into heat constraint or damp-heat retention causing local pain and affecting the spleen and stomach functions. In time, the lingering heat consumes the fluids which leads to liver and kidney yin deficiency. In addition, over indulgence of cold and greasy food and alcohol can overstrain the spleen and stomach which have already been impaired and further damage the yang qi causing a more severe deficiency accompanying the excess pattern. Delayed or mistreatment of such a case can be life threatening and will consume body fluids and yang qi resulting in syncope.

4. Prognosis

In acute cases, when the healthy qi is strong and the constitution of the patient is good, this disease has a good prognosis considering the patient will receive appropriate treatment in a timely manner. However, if the pathogenic factors linger within the body for a long time and the patient is administered the incorrect treatment, the prognosis is not favorable.

COMPREHENSION QUESTIONS

1. What are the etiopathology of the hypochondriac distension?
2. How can you differentiate the gallbladder distension from stomachache?
3. What are the treatment principles of hypochondriac distension?
4. Multiple choice questions:

1) Mr. Li, 45 years old. Presenting symptoms are right hypochondriac distension, fullness and pain radiating to the right shoulder which worsens when agitated, chest oppression, epigastric distension, frequent sighing and belching, acid reflux, a thin and greasy tongue coating, and a wiry and forceful pulse. Select the recommended formula:

A. *Shēng Mài Sǎn* (Pulse-Engendering Powder)
B. *Chái Hú Shū Gān Sǎn* (Bupleurum Liver-Soothing Powder)
C. *Yī Guàn Jiān* (Effective Integration Decoction)
D. *Qīng Dǎn Tāng* (Gallbladder-Clearing Decoction)

E. *Yīn Chén Hāo Tāng* (Virgate Wormwood Decoction)

2) Ms. Xu, 56 years old. Presenting symptoms are right hypochondriac burning distension, bitter taste in the mouth, dry throat, constipation, scanty and dark yellow urine, vexation, insomnia, irritability, a red tongue with a yellow, thick and dry coating and a wiry and rapid pulse. The disease pattern is:

A. Qi stagnation and blood stasis
B. Yin deficiency constraint
C. Liver and gallbladder damp-heat retention
D. Liver and gallbladder qi constraint
E. Constraint heat in the gallbladder

3) There are symptoms of distending pain in the hypochondriac area without any precise location while the sensation changes according to the emotion state, chest oppression, abdominal distension, frequent belching, poor appetite, bitter taste in the mouth, a thin and white coating and a wiry pulse. The pattern differentiation is:

A. Liver constraint and qi stagnation
B. Damp-heat retention in the liver and gallbladder
C. Static blood obstructing the network vessels
D. Lack of nourishment of the liver collaterals
E. Liver blood deficiency

4) Ms. Zhang, 45 years old. Presenting symptoms are distending and migratory pain in the hypochondriac area changing with the emotion state, chest oppression and abdominal distension, poor appetite, bitter taste in the mouth, a thin coating and a wiry pulse. What is the recommended formula?

A. *Chái Hú Shū Gān Săn* (Bupleurum Liver-Soothing Powder)
B. *Dān Zhī Xiāo Yáo Săn* (Peony Bark and Gardenia Free Wanderer Powder)
C. *Lóng Dăn Xiè Gān Tāng* (Gentian Liver-Draining Decoction)
D. *Yī Guàn Jiān* (Effective Integration Decoction)
E. *Huà Gān Jiān* (Liver-Soothing Decoction)

Answers

1. Hypochondriac distension is caused by the effect of indigenous pathogenic factors such as the excessive intake of greasy and fatty food and alcohol combined with excessive emotions such as anxiety or anger harming the internal function of the liver and gallbladder as well as the stomach and spleen. Some externally contracted pathogens such as dampness, heat, cold combined with overstrain, fatigue and stress can influence the stagnation of dampness and heat in the liver and gallbladder and cause hypochondriac pain and gallbladder stone.

2. Gallbladder distension is mainly characterized by hypochondriac distending

pain accompanying bitter taste in the mouth and belching. Stomachache is mainly characterized by pain in the epigastric area accompanied by nausea, vomiting and acid regurgitation and can occur at any age.

3. The treatment principles for the hypochondriac distension are soothing the liver and benefiting the gallbladder, harmonizing qi and benefitting the spleen and stomach qi, opening orifices and nourishing *fu*-organs. Clinically, the treatment should vary according to a specific case presenting with a deficiency, excess or a combination of deficiency and excess pattern. For an excess pattern, focus should be given to soothing the liver, benefiting the gallbladder, draining dampness and clearing heat from the bowels. In a deficiency pattern, the focus should be on supplementing the middle and unblocking organs, warming the yang and opening orifices.

4. 1) B, 2) E, 3) A, 4) A.

3.8 Liver Cancer

Liver cancer is a malignant disease characterized by painful and hard swelling in the right hypochondriac area, emaciation, poor appetite, lack of strength, or with jaundice, or coma. Its disease root is deficiency of qi, blood and *zang-fu* organs, while the branch is the binding constriction of qi, blood, dampness, heat and toxins in the liver, gradually leading to the stasis and accumulation of these pathogenic factors. The liver cancer is a malignant disease difficult to treat affecting 8 males to 1 female more commonly seen in the age between 31 and 50 in China. The specific types of liver cancer are listed as massive, tubercular, diffused and small cancerous cells. The massive type is more common than others.

According to Chinese medicine understanding, this disease mainly results from the binding constraint of qi, blood, dampness, heat and toxins creating a severe stasis combined with the severe deficiency of qi, blood and *zang-fu* organs. It is also often combined with the internal damage caused by excess of the seven emotions combined with depressed emotion, or dampness gatherings and phlegm-damp coagulation due to spleen deficiency. In the early stages, the nature of disease is mainly excess, such as qi stagnation, blood stasis, and damp-heat retention. As the disease progresses and in chronic conditions, the pathogenic factors are accompanied by deficiency of qi, blood, yin and yang, becoming a deficiency-excess complex with root deficiency and branch excess. The pathomechanism development of liver cancer is complex, while the disease location is the liver, the spleen and kidney are also involved and might transform into tympanites. If the pathogenic toxin becomes exuberant, the pericardium will also be clouded, resulting in coma.

CLINICAL PATTERNS DIFFERENTIATION AND TREATMENTS

1. Liver Depression and Spleen Deficiency

Symptoms: Right sided distending hypochondriac pain, chest stuffiness, depression, frequent sighing, epigastric distension and fullness, belching, emaciation, poor appetite, loose stools, pale enlarged tongue with white and greasy coating, thready or soggy pulse.

Treatment Principle:

- Soothe the liver and resolve depression
- Tonify spleen and invigorate qi

- Move blood and remove stasis

Main Acupuncture Points:

- RN 16 (*zhōng tíng*): To unbind the chest and regulate qi
- BL 18 (*gān shù*): Back-*shu* point of the liver to regulate and smoothen the qi flow and harmonize the liver
- LV 14 (*qī mén*): Front-*mu* point of the liver to spread liver qi and harmonize the middle
- GB 43 (*xiá xī*): To clear damp-heat from the gallbladder channel and reduce swelling
- BL 20 (*pí shù*): Back-*shu* point of the spleen to invigorate spleen, regulate and harmonize the middle *jiao*

Supporting Points:

- LV 3 (*tài chōng*) and LI 4 (*hé gǔ*): To regulate qi circulation, calm emotional outbursts and resolve depression
- DU 20 (*bǎi huì*): To supplement and raise the qi and calm the spirit

Recommended Formula: *Xiāo Yáo Sǎn* (逍遥散, Free Wanderer Powder) from the *Beneficial Formulas from the Taiping Imperial Pharmacy* (*Tài Píng Huì Mín Hé Jì Jú Fāng*, 太平惠民和剂局方)

Substitute Formula: *Chái Hú Shū Gān Sǎn* (柴胡疏肝散, Bupleurum Liver-Soothing Powder)

Patent Formula: *Gān Fù Lè Piàn* (肝复乐片, Liver-Restoring Tablet)

2. Qi Stagnation and Blood Stasis

Symptoms: Distension and fullness under the ribs, painful masses in the right hypochondriac area, fixed pain which dislikes pressure, abdominal distension and oppression, emaciation, fatigue, belching, acid reflux, irregular stools, a dark red tongue or tongue with petechiae, a thin white tongue coating and a thready and choppy pulse.

Treatment Principle:

- Soothe the liver and regulate qi
- Invigorate blood and resolve stasis

Main acupuncture points:

- LV 8 (*qū quán*): To spread liver qi, alleviate pain and invigorate blood
- SP 10 (*xuè hǎi*): To promote blood flow and dispel blood stasis
- SP 6 (*sān yīn jiāo*): To regulate spleen and resolve dampness, invigorate blood and improve digestion
- BL 17 (*gé shù*): Influential point of the blood to activate circulation of blood, unbind the chest, nourish and harmonize blood and descend rebellious qi
- SP 21 (*dà bāo*): *Luo*-connecting point of the spleen to regulate qi and blood, unbind the chest and invigorate spleen
- RN 6 (*qì hǎi*): To harmonize blood and regulate qi

Supporting Points:

• ST 20 (*chéng mǎn*): To descend rebellious qi, harmonize the middle *jiao* and alleviate pain

• RN 3 (*zhōng jí*): Front-*mu* point of the bladder to dispel stagnation and harmonize the lower *jiao*, benefit the uterus and regulate menstruation

Recommended Formula: *Chái Hú Shū Gān Sǎn* (柴胡疏肝散, Bupleurum Liver-Soothing Powder) from *The Complete Works of [Zhang] Jing-yue* (*Jǐng Yuè Quán Shū*, 景岳全书) combined with *Táo Hóng Sì Wù Tāng* (桃红四物汤, Peach Kernel and Carthamus Four Substances Decoction) from the *Golden Mirror of the Medical Tradition* (*Yī Zōng Jīn Jiàn*, 医宗金鉴)

Substitute Formula:

• *Xiāo Yáo Sǎn* (逍遥散, Free Wanderer Powder) combined with *Gé Xià Zhú Yū Tāng* (膈下逐瘀汤, Expelling Stasis Below the Diaphragm Decoction)

• *Xuè Fǔ Zhú Yū Tāng* (血府逐瘀汤, Blood Stasis Expelling Decoction) combined with *Biē Jiǎ Jiān Wán* (鳖甲煎丸, Turtle Shell Decocted Pill)

Patent Formula: *Xuè Fǔ Zhú Yū Jiāo Náng* (血府逐瘀胶囊, Blood Stasis Expelling Capsule) combined with *Biē Jiǎ Jiān Wán* (鳖甲煎丸,Turtle Shell Decocted Pill)

3. Damp-Heat Retention with Stagnant Toxins

Symptoms: Right-sided hard solid masses under the ribs or a drum-like tight and distended abdomen, icteric of the body and eye, dark complexion, scaly skin, high fever, vexation, thirst, bitter taste, dry throat, dark urine and stools, a dark red tongue with petechiae with a yellow greasy coating and a thready and rapid or choppy pulse.

Treatment Principle:

• Clear heat and expel dampness

• Move liver qi and activate blood

• Remove toxins and resolve stasis

Main Acupuncture Points:

• LV 14 (*qī mén*): Front-*mu* point of the liver to spread liver qi, alleviate abdominal distension, stop pain and harmonize the middle

• GB 24 (*rì yuè*): Front-*mu* point of the gallbladder to expel damp-heat, descend rebellious qi, alleviate chest distension and stop hypochondriac pain

• GB 34 (*yáng líng quán*): *He*-sea point of the gallbladder to clear liver and gallbladder damp- heat, regulate qi and stop pain

• LV 3 (*tài chōng*): *Yuan*-source point of the liver to benefit qi, clear liver and gallbladder damp heat, regulate menstruation and unbind the chest

• SJ 6 (*zhī gōu*): To clear heat, activate circulation and benefit the chest

• SP 9 (*yīn líng quán*): *He*-sea point of the spleen to expel damp-heat and resolve abdominal pain and distention

Supporting Points:

• SP 10 (*xuè hǎi*): To clear blood heat, expel dampness, promote circulation and dispel blood stasis

- SP 21 (*dà bāo*): To unbind the chest and stop coastal pain and body aches

Recommended Formula: *Yīn Chén Hāo Tāng* (茵陈蒿汤, Virgate Wormwood Decoction) from the *Treatise on Cold Damage* (*Shāng Hán Lùn*, 伤寒论) combined with *Gé Xià Zhú Yū Tāng* (膈下逐瘀汤, Expelling Stasis Below the Diaphragm Decoction) from the *Correction of Errors in Medical Works* (*Yī Lín Gǎi Cuò*, 医林改错)

Substitute Formula: *Lóng Dǎn Xiè Gān Tāng* (龙胆泻肝汤, Gentian Liver-Draining Decoction) combined with *Biē Jiǎ Jiān Wán* (鳖甲煎丸, Turtle Shell Decocted Pill)

Patent Formula:

- *Fù Fāng Bān Máo Jiāo Náng* (复方斑蝥胶囊, Compound Cantharis Capsule)
- *Fù Fāng Chán Chú Wán* (复方蟾蜍丸, Compound Toad Pill)

4. Liver and Kidney Yin Deficiency

Symptoms: Enlarged and distended abdomen, dull hypochondriac pain, dizziness, tinnitus, low grade fever, night sweating, vexing heat in the five centers, emaciation, fatigue, limp pain in the lumbus and knees, scanty urine, dry stools, red tongue with scanty coating, thready and rapid pulse.

Treatment Principle:

- Nourish the liver and kidney yin
- Warm yang to produce body fluids
- Cool blood and expel toxins

Main Acupuncture Points:

- HT 6 (*yīn xì*): *Xi*-cleft point of the heart to clear deficient heat, alleviate night sweats, and calm the spirit
- BL 18 (*gān shù*): Back-*shu* point of the liver to clear liver heat, nourish liver blood and spread the qi
- SP 10 (*xuè hǎi*): To cool blood heat, promote circulation and dispel blood stasis
- SP 6 (*sān yīn jiāo*): To tonify liver and kidney, invigorate blood
- BL 20 (*pí shù*): Back-*shu* point of the spleen to invigorate spleen and harmonize the middle *jiao*
- BL 23 (*shèn shù*): Back-*shu* point of the kidney to tonify liver and kidney yin, stop lumbus and knee pain, regulate lower *jiao* and water passage

Supporting Points:

- ST 25 (*tiān shū*): To treat abdominal distension, pain, dizziness and lumbago
- KI 7 (*fù liū*): To tonify kidney, arrest night sweating, benefit lumbus and regulate water passage

Recommended Formula: *Qǐ Jú Dì Huáng Wán* (杞菊地黄丸, Lycium Berry, Chrysanthemum and Rehmannia Pill) from the *Precious Mirror for the Advancement of Medicine* (*Yī Jí Bǎo Jiàn*, 医级宝鉴)

Substitute Formula:

- *Yī Guàn Jiān* (一贯煎, Effective Integration Decoction)

- *Zī Shuǐ Qīng Gān Yǐn* (滋水清肝饮, Water-Enriching Liver-Clearing Beverage)

Patent Formula: *Biē Jiǎ Jiān Wán* (鳖甲煎丸,Turtle Shell Decocted Pill)

Summary Chart for Liver Cancer

Patterns	Main Points	Supporting Points	Formulae
Liver Depression and Spleen Deficiency	RN 16, BL 18, LV 14, GB 43, BL 20	LV 3 and LI 4 for depression DU 20 for qi collapse	*Xiāo Yáo Sǎn* or *Chái Hú Shū Gān Sǎn*
Qi Stagnation and Blood Stasis	LV 8, SP 10, SP 6 BL 17, SP 21, RN 6	ST 20 for rebellious qi RN 3 for irregular menstruation	*Chái Hú Shū Gān Sǎn* plus *Táo Hóng Sì Wù Tāng* or *Xiāo Yáo Sǎn* or *Xuè Fǔ Zhú Yū Tāng* plus *Biē Jiǎ Jiān Wán*
Damp-Heat and Stasis Toxin	LV 14, GB 24, GB 34, LV 3, SJ 6, SP 9	SP 10 for blood heat SP 21 for local coastal pain	*Yīn Chén Hāo Tāng* plus *Gé Xià Zhú Yū Tāng* or *Lóng Dǎn Xiè Gān Tāng* plus *Biē Jiǎ Jiān Wán*
Liver-Kidney Yin Deficiency	HT 6, BL 18, SP 10, SP 6, BL 20, BL 23	ST 25 for abdominal disorders KI 7 for night sweating	*Qǐ Jú Dì Huáng Wán* or *Yī Guàn Jiān* or *Zī Shuǐ Qīng Gān Yǐn*

CASE STUDY 1: Liver Cancer

Mr. Sun, 56 years old.

Main Complaint: Distending pain in the upper right abdominal area for over one year.

Medical History: The patient felt a sudden oppressive pain in the hypochondriac area on February 23th, 1974. He could not tolerate the severe pain and was sent to the hospital. The electrocardiogram showed anterior wall myocardial infarction. After being hospitalized the symptoms resolved. However, shortly afterwards he suffered from a distending mass in the upper abdomen, a fever of 38 ℃ and icteric sclera and skin with abnormal blood test results. The patient was treated with anti-inflammatory medication which had no effect on the syndrome and the mass in the liver area increased gradually. Further examinations showed lesion in the liver. An ultra-scan of the liver, chest X-ray and blood test results confirmed liver cancer. The patient then received the Western treatment for the liver cancer and showed symptoms of intermittent fever. He refused the chemotherapy treatments and turned to Chinese medicine for treatment.

Presenting Symptoms: Distending pain in the upper right abdominal area, fever, poor appetite, a wiry pulse, a dull-red tongue with a mirror coating.

Physical Examination: Temperature: 38.3 ℃, pulse: 88 bpm, respiration: 20 bpm, blood pressure: 125/80 mmHg. The patient demonstrated a poor mental state with icteric sclera and skin. The liver could be felt below the rib cage of a 2-finger width and the mass was below the xiphoid process of a 5-finger width. The AFP test was positive and the GGT was 390 units.

Pattern Differentiation

This case is due to blood stasis in the liver and spleen, binding constraint of damp-heat, liver and spleen disharmony, qi stagnation, and static blood retention below the rib-side, becoming gradually enlarged mass below the rib-side. Internal damp-heat accumulation leads to bile failing to run the normal duct and overflowing to the skin, so there are icteric skin and eyes. Internal damp-heat exuberance causes fever.

Diagnosis

TCM Diagnosis: Hypochondriac pain due to toxic heat retention in the liver binding into masses

Western Medicine Diagnosis: Liver cancer

Treatment

The pathomechanism of this case is mainly blood, dampness, heat and toxin stasis in the liver and liver and spleen disharmony. Therefore, the treatment is to invigorate blood, dissolve stasis, clear heat, and resolve toxins.

Principles:

- Invigorate blood and dissolve stasis
- Clear heat and dredge dampness
- Resolve toxins and dispel mass
- Smooth liver qi and harmonize the spleen

Ingredients:

丹参	*dān shēn*	60 g	Radix et Rhizoma Salviae
赤芍	*chì sháo*	10 g	Radix Paeoniae Rubra
郁金	*yù jīn*	10 g	Radix Curcumae
川楝子	*chuān liàn zǐ*	10 g	Fructus Toosendan
草河车	*cǎo hé chē*	15 g	Rhizoma Paridis; Rhizoma Bistortae
山豆根	*shān dòu gēn*	15 g	Radix et Rhizoma Sophorae
白花蛇舌草	*bái huā shé shé cǎo*	30 g	Herba Hedyotis Diffusae
蒲公英	*pú gōng yīng*	30 g	Herba Taraxaci
茵陈	*yīn chén*	30 g	Herba Artemisiae Scopariae
犀黄丸	*xī huáng wán*	6 g	Rhinoceros Bezoar Pill

Formula Analysis

In the formula, *dān shēn* and *chì sháo* are added to invigorate blood and dissolve stasis. *Yù jīn* and *chuān liàn zǐ* serve to soothe the liver, rectify qi, and resolve constraint promoting qi flow to move the blood. *Bái huā shé shé cǎo, cǎo hé chē, shān dòu gēn, yīn chén,* and *xī huáng wán* are included to clear heat, resolve toxins and remove dampness.

Follow-up Consultations

After 7 doses of this formula, the fever remitted. After another 18 doses, all symptoms resolved. After taking this formula for 2 months, the jaundice resolved, his appetite improved and body weight increased by 1.5 kg. The liver gradually softened and decreased to a 3-finger width below the xiphoid process. At this time, the patient felt numbness in the lumbus and legs, so *nǚ zhēn zǐ* and *niú xī* were added to the previous formula. He took the formula for 2 more months and all the symptoms resolved. The edge of the liver was two centimeters under the xiphoid process. His condition was stable and the reexamination showed that the AFP was negative. The isotope liver scan reported that the pathological changes of right lobe were obviously relieved. The left lobe was slightly larger and tests showed alkaline phosphatase 5 units, rocket electrophoresis 20 μg/L, GGT 76 units, and ALT 255 units. At this time the patient stopped taking the formula and started taking patent medicine of Polygonati Pill (*huáng jīng wán),* Rehmannia Pill (*dì huáng wán),* Liver Soothing and Pain Relieving Pill (*shū gān zhǐ tòng wán*), compound phospholipase, and vitamin C. The next reexamination in January 1975 showed negative AFP, rocket electrophoresis 20 μg/L, GGT 111 units, normal ALT, negative flocculation test, musk turbidity 4 units, and there were no subjective symptoms. The patient could return to work while he continued to have regular check-ups every three to six months without relapse.

CASE STUDY 2: Liver Cancer
By Dr. Gao Hui-yuan

Mr. Li, 44 years old. 1st consultation on August 10th, 1986.

Main Complaint: Distending pain in the liver area for over half a year.

Medical History: The patient began to feel generalized weakness and soreness at the beginning of 1986 which inhibited him from going back to work. He had an aversion to greasy food and was fond of cold drinks and food. His daily food intake was about 250-300 g in average.

Presenting Symptoms: The patient suffered from occasional abdominal distension, dry mouth, poor sleep, distending pain in the liver area, and slightly dry stool. His tongue was red with thin and yellow coating and his pulse was thready and rapid.

Physical Examination: The patient experienced confusion, poor mental state, and had a tender mass in the right costal margin of the abdominal area. An ultrasound confirmed an enlarged liver with an abnormal external shape, a local protuberance in both the exterior and interior aspect of the left lobe and the right costal margin. The diagnosis of the ultrasound was hepatic multiple substantial occupying lesions. The

AFP was above 25.

Diagnosis

TCM Diagnosis: Liver mass due to qi and blood deficiency with blood and toxin stasis

Western Medicine Diagnosis: Liver cancer

Treatment

The pathomechanism of this case is mainly qi and blood deficiency, liver and spleen disharmony, and blood and toxins stasis.

Principles:

- Fortify the spleen and harmonize the stomach
- Move blood and dispel stasis
- Soften hardness and dissipate masses

Formula: Modified *Wŭ Wèi Yì Gōng Săn* (Five-Ingredient Special Achievement Powder)

Ingredients:

太子参	*tài zĭ shēn*	10 g	Radix Pseudostellariae
白术	*bái zhú*	10 g	Rhizoma Atractylodis Macrocephalae
茯苓	*fú líng*	10 g	Poria
陈皮	*chén pí*	8 g	Pericarpium Citri Reticulatae
炙甘草	*zhì gān căo*	5 g	Radix et Rhizoma Glycyrrhizae Praeparata cum Melle
赤芍	*chì sháo*	10 g	Radix Paeoniae Rubra
柴胡	*chái hú*	10 g	Radix Bupleuri
三棱	*sān léng*	10 g	Rhizoma Sparganii
白花蛇舌草	*bái huā shé shé căo*	15 g	Herba Hedyotis Diffusae
薏苡仁	*yì yĭ rén*	5 g	Semen Coicis
莪术	*é zhú*	10 g	Rhizoma Curcumae
土茯苓	*tŭ fú líng*	20 g	Rhizoma Smilacis Glabrae
肉苁蓉	*ròu cōng róng*	10 g	Herba Cistanches
黄芪	*huáng qí*	15 g	Radix Astragali
天冬	*tiān dōng*	10 g	Radix Asparagi

Follow-up Consultations

After taking 7 doses of the formula, the pain in the right abdomen and hypochondriac area slightly resolved. His appetite improved, stool became normal and his weight stopped decreasing. His tongue coating was thin and yellow, and the pulse was thready, rapid and wiry. The same formula was given for another week.

After one more week of the formula, the patient was less fatigued, but right sided back pain was occasionally felt, so *yán hú suǒ* 10 g was added to the previous formula.

After taking one more week of the formula, his appetite improved that he could eat about 500 g of food daily. The symptoms of general aching and fatigue resolved and the distending pain in the liver area was also milder. But the tongue and pulse conditions remained the same. The patient was then discharged from the hospital and continued to take the medicine at home.

The patient persisted on taking the formula which was sometimes slightly modified according to the changing symptoms until the end of 1988. At that time, the patient demonstrated a normal mental state and a good appetite. There was mild ascites and occasional distending pain in the liver area. He could work half days and care for himself.

CASE STUDY 3: Liver Cancer
By Dr. Zhu Ru-gong

Mrs. Yu, 38 years old. First consultation on June 16th, 1981.

Main Complaint: The presence of a mass in the right upper abdominal area for over a month.

Present Condition: The patient had no appetite and was fatigue since 1978. She originally considered it as the result of the daily stress and paid little attention to these symptoms. A general physical examination in 1979 showed normal liver function without any swelling. On April 22nd, 1981, she suddenly felt severe pain in the right upper abdomen which aggravated when walking or bending her knees sometimes causing sudden unconsciousness. She went to a local hospital for examination which showed AFP>1000 ng/ml and normal liver function. At the beginning of June, she was transferred to the Shanghai Tumor Hospital for treatment and was diagnosed with liver cancer. She had then took some Chinese medicine and was asked to go back to her hometown but she stayed at the hospital and sought acupuncture and moxibustion treatment.

Presenting Symptoms: General weakness, dry mouth, normal stools and urination, abdominal distension and dull pain in the liver region.

Physical Examination: The patient was obviously emaciated. She had experienced paroxysmal severe pain with unconsciousness three times since May that year which lasted one to two minutes each time. She had poor appetite, eating about 50 g to 100 g per meal. She had no history of hepatitis or bilharziasis, and no family history of tumors. The radiographic test showed enlargement of the frontal aspect of the liver of 6cm below the rib and 14cm below the xiphoid process of abnormal shape with uneven distribution.

Diagnosis

TCM Diagnosis: Abdominal mass due to stagnation of liver qi

Western Medicine Diagnosis: Liver cancer

Principles:

- Soothe the liver and resolve qi stagnation
- Move blood and resolve mass

Acupuncture Point Combination:

Points for acupuncture: bilateral LI 10 (*shǒu sān lǐ*), ST 36 (*zú sān lǐ*), PC 6 (*nèi guān*), LI 4 (*hé gǔ*), LV 3 (*tài chōng*), RN 6 (*qì hǎi*), LV 5 (*lí gōu*), and SP 9 (*yīn líng quán*). Apply even needling method and retain the needles for 30 minutes.

Points for indirect moxibustion:

- RN 10 (*xià wǎn*) and right LV 14 (*qī mén*)
- RN 13 (*shàng wǎn*) and right LV 14 (*qī mén*)
- RN 12 (*zhōng wǎn*) and right LV 14 (*qī mén*)
- RN 6 (*qì hǎi*) and right LV 14 (*qī mén*)

Manipulations: Above four groups of points are applied in turn, using one group of points at a time. For the moxibustion method, scatter some *dīng xiāng* and *ròu guì* on the point and then cover it with a dry slice of aconite. Apply indirect moxibustion using 3 moxa cones for each point.

Follow-up Consultations

On the second visit, on 18th of June, there was no change in the condition. The same points were needled and moxa was applied on RN 13 (*shàng wǎn*) and right LV 14 (*qī mén*). A Chinese patent medicine of *Shuāng Bàn Hé Jì* (Half-Half Mixture) was given to the patient.

On the third visit, on 20th June, the same points were needled and indirect moxibustion was given on RN 12 (*zhōng wǎn*) and right LV 14 (*qī mén*).

On the fourth visit, on 23rd of June, the patient felt more energized and her appetite improved. The same acupuncture points were used and indirect moxibustion was given on RN 6 (*qì hǎi*) and right LV 14 (*qī mén*).

On the fifth visit, on 2nd of July. The overall symptoms improved greatly and the same acupuncture points were used while indirect moxibustion was applied on RN 10 (*xià wǎn*) and the right LV 14(*qī mén*).

On the sixteenth visit, on 21st of July. The appetite of the patient improved greatly and she felt energized. The same acupuncture points were needled and indirect moxibustion was performed on RN 6 (*qì hǎi*) and right LV 14 (*qī mén*).

On the twentieth visit, on 30th of July. The patient had no residual symptoms and had a strong appetite, eating from 100 g to 150 g of food per meal. Her disease condition was stable.

Clinical Analysis

Liver cancer belongs to the "concretions and accumulations" in Chinese medicine. The concretions and accumulations of this case lie in the liver. Dr. Zhu emphasizes the acupuncture treatment to dredge the meridian and the location of the disease while paying attention to the cause of disease by soothing and resolving the stagnated qi. He usually selects the points of the liver, spleen, and the heart channels. According to the theories which state: "warming the qi to smooth the circulation of blood" and "treating congealed obstruction by warming qi", he treats the patient by warming-needle moxibustion or indirect moxibustion applied locally to warm the meridians and dissipate mass.

In this case, the mass and stagnation is located in the right lobe of the liver at the level of the *yangming* and *taiyin* channels. This explains the selected points being LI 4 (*hé gǔ*), LI 10 (*shǒu sān lǐ*), ST 36 (*zú sān lǐ*), and SP 9 (*yīn líng quán*), which are selected to unblock these channels. In addition, PC 6 (*nèi guān*), LV 5 (*lí gōu*) and LV 3 (*tài chōng*) are simultaneously treated to soothe liver and resolve the stagnation of qi of the heart and liver channels. Then moxibustion warming technique is applied on LV 14 (*qī mén*), RN 13 (*shàng wǎn*), RN 12 (*zhōng wǎn*) and RN 10 (*xià wǎn*) to treat the local area of the disease, invigorate blood and dissolve stasis. RN 6 (*qì hǎi*) is the sea of generating qi and applying moxibustion on RN 6 benefits the original qi and activates the blood circulation.

KEY CLINICAL POINTS

1. The important excess syndrome of qi stagnation, blood stasis, and damp-heat retention affects the free flow of qi and hinders the spleen function of transportation and transformation which causes a low appetite, enlargement of the liver and jaundice. In severe cases, it also can cause coma and tympanites.

2. The treatment should be determined according to the disease differentiation and the general condition of the patient to strengthen the healthy qi and remove the pathogenic factors, by purging and supplementing appropriately. It is important to avoid using strong purging medicinals because of the underlining deficiency.

3. Modern research have proven some medicinals to be effective against liver cancer, making the formula more pertinent. The use of the following medicinals need to be considered when treating liver cancer: *bái huā shé shé cǎo* (Herba Hedyotis Diffusae), *bàn zhī lián* (Herba Scutellariae Barbatae), *bàn biān lián* (Herba Lobeliae Chinensis), *quán shēn* (Rhizoma Bistortae), *shé méi* (Herba Duchesneae Indicae), *mǎ biān cǎo* (Herba Verbenae), *fèng wěi cǎo* (Herba Petridis Multifidae), *zǐ cǎo* (Radix Arnebiae), *kǔ shēn* (Radix Sophorae Flavescentis), *pú gōng yīng* (Herba Taraxaci), *chóng lóu* (Rhizoma Paridis), *yě jú huā* (Flos Chrysanthemi Indici), *zhǒng jié fēng* (Herba Sarcandrae) and *xià kū cǎo* (Spica Prunellae). The following medicinals have strong invigorating blood and dissolving stasis functions and can also be considered in treating liver cancer with stubborn mass: *dà jì* (Herba Cirsii Japonici), *bá qiā* (Rhizoma Smilacis Chinae), *guǐ jiàn yǔ* (Ramulus Euonymi), *dì biē chóng* (Eupolyphaga seu Steleophaga), *hǔ zhàng* (Rhizoma Polygoni Cuspidati), *dān shēn* (Radix et Rhizoma

Salviae Miltiorrhizae), *sān léng* (Rhizoma Sparganii), *shuǐ hóng huā zǐ* (Fructus Polygoni Orientalis) and *shuǐ zhì* (Hirudo). The following medicinals are effective to soften hardness and dissipate masses: *hǎi zǎo* (Sargassum), *xià kū cǎo* (Spica Prunellae) and *mǔ lì* (Concha Ostreae).

4. The practitioner needs to pay close attention when the patient is in the advanced stage of liver cancer demonstrating with tympanites presenting a bulgy abdomen, pale yellow complexion, and exposed veins. This demonstrates a poor prognosis and the combination of western and Chinese medicine can be combined for more effective results.

BRIEF SUMMARY

Liver cancer is a common malignant tumor that progresses rapidly. The disease location is in the liver, but the disease also has a close relation to the gallbladder, spleen, stomach, and kidney. The basic pathomechanism is the liver failing in governing the free flow of qi and the nature of disease causing stasis of blood, dampness, heat and toxins. The disease differentiation is mainly an excess in the branch and a deficiency of qi and blood at the root. The main treatment principle is to soothe the liver, move the qi, activate blood circulation and remove stasis, clear heat and drain dampness, remove toxins and stop pain.

COMPREHENSION QUESTIONS

1. What is the brief etiopathology of liver cancer?

2. How can we differentiate the liver cancer and gallbladder distention in clinical practice?

3. What are the principles of treatment for the liver cancer?

4. Multiple choice question:

1) Mrs. Zhang, 38 years old. The patient suddenly felt severe stabbing pain in the right hypochondriac area aggravated in the evening radiating to the shoulder and back. There was a large hard lump in the right ribs which refused pressure and other lumps would come and go below the left ribs. Other symptoms were sallow yellow and dull facial complexion, fatigue, lack of strength, abdominal distension and fullness and enlarged abdomen, yellowish skin, exposed veins, poor appetite, alternating constipated or loose stools, irregular menstruation, dark purple tongue with static spots and macules, and wiry and choppy pulse. The recommended formula is:

A. *Yī Guàn Jiān* (Effective Integration Decoction)
B. *Shēng Huà Tāng* (Engendering and Transforming Decoction)
C. *Yīn Chén Tāng* (Virgate Wormwood Decoction)
D. *Fù Yuán Huó Xuè Tāng* (Original Qi-Restoring and Blood-Moving Decoction)

E. *Chái Hú Shū Gān Săn* (Bupleurum Liver-Soothing Powder)

2) Mr. Qi, 45 years old. The patient suffered from hypochondriac pain with a rigid mass below the ribs that refused pressure. Other clinical manifestations were vexing heat in the five centers (chest, palms and soles), tidal fever, night sweats, dizziness, poor appetite, abdominal distension and enlargement, haematemesis, hemafecia and subcutaneous bleeding, red tongue, a scanty coating and a thready and rapid pulse. The therapeutic methods are:

A. Nourish blood and soften liver, cool blood and resolve toxins
B. Clear heat and promote gallbladder function, drain fire and resolve toxins
C. Soothe liver and strengthen spleen, invigorate blood and dissolve stasis
D. Move qi to invigorate blood, dissolve stasis and disperse accumulation
E. Enrich yin and soothe the liver, boost qi to harmonize the collaterals

Answers

1. Liver cancer is caused by the stagnation of qi, blood, dampness, heat, stasis, and toxin, which causes a mass in the liver and is mainly resulted from deficiency of qi, blood and *zang-fu* organs combined with the internal damage from the excessive seven emotions or depression.

2. Liver cancer is characterized by rigid increasing mass refusing pressure in the right hypochondriac area with persistent pain, emaciated body, lack of strength, poor appetite, and sometimes accompanied with icteric eyes, body skin, dark urine, and/or coma. The condition of the patient is in a dangerous and critical state which worsens very quickly.

Gallbladder distension is mainly marked by right hypochondriac distending pain refusing pressure usually triggered by alcohol or greasy food accompanied by abdominal distension and fullness, bitter taste in the mouth, frequent sighing, and belching. Gallbladder distension is sometimes due to the presence of gallstones.

3. Treatment principles of liver cancer is to dredge the excessive pathogenic factors while supplementing the deficiency. The general treatment principles will move qi and blood, remove stasis and dredge toxins, strengthen the spleen and drain dampness, nourish original qi and liver blood, warm yang and nourish yin. However, the treatment should be determined according to the disease course and the condition of the patient. The practitioners also need to supplement the healthy qi deficiency while removing the pathogenic factors.

4. 1) D, 2) A.

Part IV

Spleen & Stomach Conditions

4.1 Abdominal Pain

Abdominal pain is mainly characterized by pain in the area of the upper and lower abdomen reaching from the stomach below the ribs to the lower abdomen and pubic hair. It is a very commonly seen symptom in clinic and it covers many various types of diseases of the stomach, small intestines, large intestines, uterus and bladder including irritable bowel syndrome, dyspepsia, acute and chronic pancreatitis, gastrointestinal spasms, incomplete bowel obstruction, intestinal adhesion, urinary bladder or kidney stones and intestinal parasites.

In Chinese medicine, abdominal pain is divided in upper abdominal and lower abdominal pain and bloating. These symptoms can be due to multiple types of pathogens such as food damage, cold, heat, dampness, phlegm, blood stasis, internal rheum retention, qi stagnation due to emotional disorder. These symptoms might also be due to internal damage such as yin, yang, qi and blood depletion. Pain is general known to be caused by qi and blood stagnation; however, differentiating the cause of this stagnation will bring light on the type of treatment necessary to treat the disease pattern. The treatment itself will modify the pattern and close attention needs to be taken to modify the treatment approach according to the new patterns.

Analysing the pattern according to the eight guiding principles, we can evaluate if the pattern is an excess or deficient type, a cold or heat pattern, and a yin or yang pattern. Here is a list of the most commonly seen patterns with their recommended treatment principles, acupuncture points and formulas.

CLINICAL PATTERNS DIFFERENTIATION AND TREATMENTS

1. Internal Cold Retention

Symptoms: Sudden and acute abdominal cramping which is aggravated by cold and alleviated by heat, no thirst, loose or normal stools, clear and profuse urination, a normal or pale tongue body with a white and greasy coating and a deep and tight pulse.

Treatment Principle:

- Warm the abdominal area and middle *jiao*
- Disperse cold and stop pain

Main Acupuncture Points:

- RN 12 (*zhōng wǎn*): To harmonize spleen and stomach, warm middle *jiao* and regulate qi
- RN 8 (*shén què*): Moxibustion indirectly or on salt to warm the yang and regulate fluid passages
- ST 36 (*zú sān lǐ*): To invigorate the spleen, tonify qi and stop pain
- SP 4 (*gōng sūn*): To invigorate spleen, harmonize middle *jiao* and regulate qi
- ST 25 (*tiān shū*): To invigorate spleen and stomach, regulate qi

Supporting Points:

- RN 4 (*guān yuán*): Front-*mu* point of the small intestine to regulate original qi
- EX-CA 3 (*sān jiǎo jiǔ*): To stop diarrhea, regulate qi and stop pain

Recommended Formula: *Liáng Fù Wán* (良附丸, Lesser Galangal and Cyperus Pill) from the *A Collection of Fine Formulas from Various Sources* (*Liáng Fāng Jí Yè*, 良方集腋) plus *Zhèng Qì Tiān Xiāng Sǎn* (正气天香散, Qi-Correcting Lindera and Cyperus Powder) from the *Compendium of Medicine* (*Yī Xué Gāng Mù*, 医学纲目)

Substitute Formula: *Hòu Pò Wēn Zhōng Tāng* (厚朴温中汤, Officinal Magnolia Bark Center-Warming Decoction)

Patent Formula: *Liáng Fù Wán* (良附丸, Lesser Galangal and Cyperus Pill)

2. Accumulation of Damp-Heat

Symptoms: Abdominal pain which dislikes pressure, chest stuffiness and discomfort, constipation or loose stools with a sensation of incomplete evacuation, restlessness, thirst with a desire to drink, sweating, dark-yellow urine, red tongue with a yellow, greasy coating and a slippery and rapid pulse.

Treatment Principle:

- Clear heat and resolve dampness
- Move stools and unblock large intestine qi

Main Acupuncture Points:

- RN 12 (*zhōng wǎn*): To harmonize spleen and stomach and regulate qi
- ST 36 (*zú sān lǐ*): To invigorate spleen, tonify qi and stop pain
- ST 39 (*xià jù xū*): Lower *he*-sea point of the small intestine to clear intestinal damp-heat, resolve stagnation and stop abdominal pain
- ST 44 (*nèi tíng*): To clear damp-heat and harmonize intestines
- LI 11 (*qū chí*): *He*-sea point of the large intestine to drain dampness, regulate qi and stop abdominal pain
- LV 13 (*zhāng mén*): Front-*mu* point of the spleen to invigorate spleen, regulate stomach and stop abdominal pain

Supporting Points:

- BL 27 (*xiǎo cháng shù*): To expel damp-heat, treat dysentery, stop abdominal pain and regulate intestines
- LI 4 (*hé gǔ*): To clear heat, treat headaches and fever

Recommended Formula: *Dà Chéng Qì Tāng* (大承气汤, Major Purgative Decoction) from the *Treatise on Cold Damage* (*Shāng Hán Lùn*, 伤寒论)

Substitute Formulas:

- *Xiǎo Chéng Qì Tāng* (小承气汤, Minor Purgative Decoction)
- *Hòu Pò Sān Wù Tāng* (厚朴三物汤, Officinal Magnolia Bark Three Substances Decoction)

3. Food Retention

Symptoms: Abdominal fullness, distension and pain which dislikes pressure and is alleviated after passing stools, poor appetite, aversion to food, nausea, vomiting, acid reflux, belching, halitosis, constipation or loose stools containing undigested food, greasy tongue coating, slippery and excessive pulse.

Treatment Principle:

- Resolve food retention and move stools
- Regulate qi and stop pain

Main Acupuncture Points:

- ST 25 (*tiān shū*): To invigorate spleen and stomach, regulate qi
- RN 12 (*zhōng wǎn*): To harmonize spleen and stomach, warm middle *jiao* and regulate qi
- ST 36 (*zú sān lǐ*): To invigorate spleen, tonify qi and stop pain
- ST 44 (*nèi tíng*): To clear damp-heat and harmonize intestines
- RN 10 (*xià wǎn*): To regulate qi, dispel food stagnation and stop abdominal pain
- BL 21 (*wèi shù*): Back-*shu* point of the stomach to invigorate spleen and harmonize stomach, resolve dampness and promote digestion

Supporting Points:

- DU 5 (*xuán shū*): To treat diarrhea with undigested food, stop abdominal pain and benefit lumbar region
- GB 25 (*jīng mén*): To resolve belching, acid reflux and abdominal pain

Recommended Formula: *Zhǐ Shí Dǎo Zhì Wán* (枳实导滞丸, Immature Bitter Orange Stagnation-Moving Pill) from the *Clarifying Doubts about Damage from Internal and External Causes* (*Nèi Wài Shāng Biàn Huò Lùn*, 内外伤辨惑论)

Substitute and Patent Formula: *Bǎo Hé Wán* (保和丸, Harmony-Preserving Pill)

4. Liver Qi Stagnation

Symptoms: Distending and migrating abdominal pain, radiating to the hypochondriac and rib-sides which is alleviated by belching or flatulence and aggravated by anger, a slightly red tongue with a thin white coating and a wiry pulse.

Treatment Principle:

- Soothe the liver and regulate qi
- Relax the intestine and stop pain

Main Acupuncture Points:

- LV 3 (*tài chōng*): *Yuan* point of the liver to spread liver qi, soothe emotions and stop pain
- RN 17 (*dàn zhōng*): Sea of qi to regulate qi, unbind the chest and soothe emotions
- PC 6 (*nèi guān*): To regulate qi, unbind the chest and stop abdominal pain
- GB 34 (*yáng líng quán*): To spread liver qi and stop hypochondriac pain
- RN 10 (*xià wǎn*): To regulate qi, harmonize the middle and stop abdominal pain

Supporting Points:

- GB 24 (*rì yuè*): Front-*mu* point of the gallbladder to resolve hypochondriac pain, spread liver qi and harmonize intestines
- LV 2 (*xíng jiān*): To treat qi stagnation transforming to fire

Recommended Formula: *Chái Hú Shū Gān Sǎn* (柴胡疏肝散, Bupleurum Liver-Soothing Powder) from *The Complete Works of [Zhang] Jing-yue* (*Jǐng Yuè Quán Shū*, 景岳全书)

Substitute Formula: *Xiāo Yáo Sǎn* (逍遥散, Free Wanderer Powder)

Patent Formula: *Chái Hú Shū Gān Wán* (柴胡舒肝丸, Bupleurum Liver-Soothing Pill)

5. Internal Retention of Blood Stasis

Symptoms: Persistent, severe, stabbing and fixed abdominal pain, dry mouth, painful menstrual cycle, dark stools, a purple tongue and a thin and choppy pulse.

Treatment Principle:

- Invigorate blood and resolve stasis
- Harmonize the collaterals and stop pain
- Move the stool and dredge the intestines

Main Acupuncture Points:

- RN 12 (*zhōng wǎn*): To harmonize spleen and stomach, regulate middle qi and stop abdominal pain
- RN 6 (*qì hǎi*): To invigorate spleen and harmonize blood, promote circulation and treat gynecological disorders
- ST 36 (*zú sān lǐ*): To circulate qi and blood, invigorate spleen and stop pain
- SP 10 (*xuè hǎi*): To promote blood circulation and resolve stasis, harmonize menstruation and cool blood
- BL 17 (*gé shù*): Influential point of the blood to promote blood circulation and resolve stasis, harmonize blood and stop abdominal pain

Supporting Points:

- LV 3 (*tài chōng*): *Yuan* point of the liver to soothe emotions, circulate qi and blood, stop abdominal pain

- ST 29 (*guī lái*): To treat menstrual disorders

Recommended Formula: *Shào Fŭ Zhú Yū Tāng* (少腹逐瘀汤, Lower Abdominal Stasis Expelling Decoction) from the *Correction of Errors in Medical Works* (*Yī Lín Găi Cuò*, 医林改错)

Substitute Formula: *Gé Xià Zhú Yū Tāng* (膈下逐瘀汤, Expelling Stasis Below the Diaphragm Decoction)

Patent Formula: *Shào Fŭ Zhú Yū Wán* (少腹逐瘀丸, Lower Abdominal Stasis Expelling Pill)

6. Deficient Cold of the Middle *Jiao*

Symptoms: Dull, intermittent abdominal pain which is alleviated by warmth and pressure, eating or resting but is aggravated by cold, hunger or fatigue, poor appetite, a pale complexion, loose stools, mental fatigue, shortness of breath, aversion to cold, cold extremities, pale and swollen tongue with a white and moist coating, deep, weak and slow pulse.

Treatment Principle:

- Warm the middle *jiao* and tonify spleen
- Relieve spasms and stop pain

Main Acupuncture Points:

- BL 20 (*pí shù*): Back-*shu* point of the spleen to regulate middle *jiao* qi, invigorate spleen and stop abdominal pain
- BL 21 (*wèi shù*): Back-*shu* point of the stomach to invigorate spleen and harmonize stomach, resolve dampness and promote digestion
- ST 36 (*zú sān lĭ*): To invigorate spleen, supplement the healthy qi and stop pain
- LV 13 (*zhāng mén*): Front-*mu* point of the spleen to invigorate spleen, regulate stomach and stop abdominal pain
- RN 12 (*zhōng wăn*): To harmonize spleen and stomach, warm middle *jiao* and regulate qi
- RN 8 (*shén què*): Apply indirect moxa or moxa on salt to warm the yang and regulate fluid passages

Supporting Points:

- BL 23 (*shèn shù*): Back-*shu* point of the kidney to fortify yang and benefit original qi
- EX-CA 5 (*wèi shàng*): To tonify and raise the middle qi
- RN 4 (*guān yuán*): Front-*mu* point of the small intestine to benefit the uterus, tonify original qi, supplement deficiencies and regulate menstruation

Recommended Formula: *Xiăo Jiàn Zhōng Tāng* (小建中汤, Minor Center-Fortifying Decoction) from the *Treatise on Cold Damage* (*Shāng Hán Lùn*, 伤寒论)

Substitute Formula: *Fù Zĭ Lĭ Zhōng Wán* (附子理中丸, Aconite Center-Regulating Pill)

Patent Formula: *Xiăo Jiàn Zhōng Jiāo Náng* (小建中胶囊, Minor Center-Fortifying Capsule)

Summary Chart for Abdominal Pain

Patterns	Main Points	Supporting Points	Formulae
Internal Cold Retention	RN 12, RN 8, ST 36, SP 4, ST 25	RN 4 for irregular menstruation EX-CA 3 for diarrhea	*Liáng Fù Wán* plus *Zhèng Qì Tiān Xiāng Sǎn* or *Hòu Pò Wēn Zhōng Tāng*
Accumulation of Damp-Heat	RN 12, ST 36, ST 39, ST 44, LI 11, LV 13	BL 27 for dysentery LI 4 for headaches and fever	*Dà Chéng Qì Tāng* or *Xiǎo Chéng Qì Tāng* or *Hòu Pò Sān Wù Tāng*
Food Retention	ST 25, RN 12, ST 36, ST 44, RN 10, BL 21	DU 5 for diarrhea with undigested food GB 25 for acid reflux and belching	*Zhǐ Shí Dǎo Zhì Wán* or *Bǎo Hé Wán*
Liver Qi Stagnation	LV 3, RN 17, PC 6, GB 34, RN 10	GB 24 for thoracic pain and intestinal disorders LV 2 for qi stagnation transforming into fire	*Chái Hú Shū Gān Sǎn* or *Xiāo Yáo Sǎn*
Internal Retention of Blood Stasis	RN 12, RN 6, ST 36, SP 10, BL 17	LV 3 for emotional outbursts ST 29 for irregular menstruation	*Shào Fǔ Zhú Yū Tāng* or *Gé Xià Zhú Yū Tāng*
Deficient Cold of the Middle *Jiao*	BL 20, BL 21, ST 36, LV 13, RN 12, RN 8	BL 23 for kidney yang deficiency EX-CA 3 for middle qi sinking RN 4 for uterine cold and irregular menstruation	*Xiǎo Jiàn Zhōng Tāng* or *Fù Zǐ Lǐ Zhōng Wán*

CASE STUDY 1: Acute Abdominal Pain

Mr. Li, 35 years old.

Main Complaint: Abdominal pain refusing pressure for half a day.

Medical History: The patient was irritated yesterday and drank a cup of wine. At 5 o'clock this morning, he began to have serious abdominal pain, distension and stuffiness with borborygmus.

Presenting Symptoms: Abdominal pain refusing pressure, chest and rib-side fullness, bitter taste in the mouth, dry throat, dizziness, vexation, vomiting, constipation, scanty and dark urine, a pale red tongue with a yellow, thick and greasy coating and a wiry and tight pulse.

Physical Examination: Temperature: 37.8 ℃, pulse: 85 bpm, respiration: 20 bpm, blood pressure: 130/80 mmHg. The patient looked uncomfortable and groaned from the severe pain with very coarse breathing. His abdomen was slightly depressed and there was obvious tenderness and mild rebound tenderness in the middle and upper abdomen. The abdominal muscles were tensed. Laboratory examination showed a serum amylase at 128 U and urine amylase at 1024 U.

Pattern Differentiation

Anger causes qi counterflow with pathogenic fire to affect the local and upper area. In this case, the pathogenic factors accumulate in the spleen and stomach in combination with the pathogenic heat of the alcohol. Therefore, symptoms such as acute abdominal pain refusing pressure accompanied by distension and stuffiness, nausea and vomiting occured. Heat stagnation in the abdominal area and intestines causes the stagnation of qi in the *fu*-organs and leads to pain and constipation. The symptoms of bitter taste in the mouth, dizziness, chest and rib-side distress and fullness are resulted from the excessive anger impairing the liver and the liver failing to flow freely ascending with the gallbladder fire. Scanty and dark urine, yellow, thick and greasy coating, and wiry and tight pulse are signs of excess heat.

Diagnosis

TCM Diagnosis: Abdominal pain due to excess heat in the spleen with liver qi stagnation

Western Medicine Diagnosis: Abdominal pain

Treatment

The main pathomechanism of this case is liver qi stagnation with the retention of excessive heat in the spleen and stomach causing the healthy qi movement disorder in the middle *jiao* causing the abdominal pain.

Principles:

- Clear heat and remove toxins
- Unblock the interior by purging the intestines
- Move qi and relieve pain

Formula: Modified *Qīng Yí Tāng* (Pancreas-Clearing Decoction) combined with *Dà Chéng Qì Tāng* (Major Purgative Decoction)

Ingredients:

柴胡	*chái hú*	15 g	Radix Bupleuri
黄芩	*huáng qín*	9 g	Radix Scutellariae
白芍	*bái sháo*	12 g	Radix Paeoniae Alba
牡蛎	*mŭ lì*	12 g	Concha Ostreae
厚朴	*hòu pò*	9 g	Cortex Magnoliae Officinalis
川楝子	*chuān liàn zĭ*	9 g	Fructus Toosendan
枳实	*zhĭ shí*	9 g	Fructus Aurantii Immaturus
延胡索	*yán hú suŏ*	9 g	Rhizoma Corydalis

葛花	gé huā	9 g	Flos Puerariae Lobatae
防风	fáng fēng	9 g	Radix Saposhnikoviae
胡黄连	hú huáng lián	6 g	Rhizoma Picrorhizae
大黄	dà huáng	9 g	Radix et Rhizoma Rhei (added later)
芒硝	máng xiāo	9 g	Natrii Sulfas (infused)

Formula Analysis

This formula is composed of *Qīng Yí Tāng* (Pancreas-Clearing Decoction) with *Dà Chéng Qì Tāng* (Major Purgative Decoction) and other medicinals.

The former formula contains *chái hú, huáng qín, hú huáng lián, bái sháo, yán hú suǒ, dà huáng* and *máng xiāo*. In this formula, *chái hú* acts to soothe the liver and resolve constraint. *Huáng qín* and *hú huáng lián* are used to clear heat and purge fire. *Bái sháo* and *yán hú suǒ* move qi and relieve pain. *Dà huáng* and *máng xiāo* unblock the bowels and discharge heat.

When combined with the latter formula, the combination of *hòu pò* and *zhǐ shí* with *dà huáng* and *máng xiāo* strengthens the effect of purgation and resolves binding heat. *Mǔ lì* is added to soften hardness and relax bowels, *gé huā* to alleviate alcohol effect, and *fáng fēng* to resolve constraint and relieve pain.

The Chinese patent of *Qīng Yí Tāng Chōng Jì* (Pancreas-Clearing Infusion Granules) was taken orally twice a day and the patient was advised to eat only light food by avoiding cold or greasy food.

Follow-up Consultations

In the evening of the 1st day, the patient's blood pressure reduced to 94/60 mmHg. On the 2nd day, his fever reached 38.4 ℃ and it went back to normal 3 days later. His amylase resumed to normal on the 2nd day, the muscle tension disappeared on the 3rd day, and the abdominal pain remitted totally on the 4thday. On the 10th day, the patient had no more symptoms and was discharged from the hospital.

CASE STUDY 2: Acute Abdominal Pain
By Dr. Xing Xi-bo

Ms. Chu, 24 years old.

Main Complaint: Abdominal pain for 2 weeks.

Presenting Symptoms: The patient suffered from severe abdominal pain for 2 weeks accompanied with nausea, vomiting, anorexia, vexation, constipation, intolerable epigastric pain, chest distension and oppression. She was lying curled up with her knees close to her chest unable to lie on her back. The tongue was red with a yellow and greasy coating and the pulse was thin and rapid.

Physical Examination: Temperature: 37.5 ℃. The sclera was non-icteric, but she refused pressure on the abdomen and there was obvious tenderness below the xiphoid process. Laboratory tests showed WBC 10050 /mm^3, hemodiastase of 1024 U (Wintrobe), urinary amylase of 512 U.

Diagnosis

TCM Diagnosis: Abdominal pain due to liver qi stagnation with damp-heat retention

Western Medicine Diagnosis: Abdominal pain

Treatment

The pathogenesis of this case is mainly spleen deficiency failing to transport and inhibited qi flow due to damp-heat constraint in the intestines causing the qi to stagnate.

Principles:

- Clear heat and drain dampness
- Soothe the liver and strengthen spleen qi
- Promote blood circulation to stop pain

Ingredients:

银花	*yín huā*	15 g	Flos Lonicerae Japonicae
连翘	*lián qiào*	15 g	Fructus Forsythiae
重楼	*chóng lóu*	15 g	Rhizoma Paridis
白芍	*bái sháo*	15 g	Radix Paeoniae Alba
木香	*mù xiāng*	9 g	Radix Aucklandiae
香附	*xiāng fù*	9 g	Rhizoma Cyperi
乳香	*rǔ xiāng*	9 g	Olibanum
没药	*mò yào*	9 g	Myrrha
五灵脂	*wǔ líng zhī*	9 g	Faeces Trogopterori
枳壳	*zhǐ qiào*	9 g	Fructus Aurantii
栀子	*zhī zǐ*	9 g	Fructus Gardeniae
桃仁	*táo rén*	9 g	Semen Persicae
红花	*hóng huā*	9 g	Flos Carthami
黄连	*huáng lián*	9 g	Rhizoma Coptidis

Follow-up Consultations

After 2 doses of the formula, the abdominal pain was slightly alleviated but there was some increasing back pain. The patient had experienced 4 months without menses. The patient also experienced epigastric distension, fullness and an occasional dull pain. Her pulse was deep, thready and rapid and the tongue was red with a thin and white coating. These symptoms clearly demonstrate a pattern of liver qi constraint with the failure of spleen to transport. The formula was modified to fit the new pattern.

银花	*yín huā*	15 g	Flos Lonicerae Japonicae
白芍	*bái sháo*	15 g	Radix Paeoniae Alba
代赭石	*dài zhě shí*	12 g	Haematitum
陈皮	*chén pí*	9 g	Pericarpium Citri Reticulatae
连翘	*lián qiào*	9 g	Fructus Forsythiae
半夏	*bàn xià*	9 g	Rhizoma Pinelliae
乳香	*rǔ xiāng*	9 g	Olibanum
白术	*bái zhú*	9 g	Rhizoma Atractylodis Macrocephalae
川楝子	*chuān liàn zǐ*	9 g	Fructus Toosendan
厚朴	*hòu pò*	6 g	Cortex Magnoliae Officinalis
木香	*mù xiāng*	6 g	Radix Aucklandiae
高丽参	*gāo lì shēn*	4.5 g	Radix et Rhizoma Ginseng
甘草	*gān cǎo*	4.5 g	Radix et Rhizoma Glycyrrhizae

After taking 7 doses of the formula, the appetite improved greatly and the abdominal pain resolved. Recent laboratory tests showed WBC had been decreased to 5000 /mm^3, and the serum amylase was 32 U. Her pulse was deep, thin, and powerful. Afterwards, the patient was given a new formula to reinforce qi and strengthen the spleen, while clearing heat and removing dampness, regulating qi and activating blood.

Clinical Analysis

In this case, damp-heat constraint in the body caused the liver qi to stagnate and assault the spleen and stomach resulting in sudden abdominal pain and chest oppression. In the formula, *yín huā, lián qiào, zhī zǐ* and *chóng lóu* are used to clear heat and remove toxins. *Huáng lián* can clear heat and dry dampness. *Chuān liàn zǐ, mù xiāng, xiāng fù* and *zhǐ qiào* can soothe the liver and rectify qi, resolve constraint and relieve pain. *Táo rén, hóng huā, rǔ xiāng* and *mò yào* can stop pain by activating blood and removing stasis. *Bái sháo* nourishes yin, softens the liver and stops pain. After the pain diminished, *gāo lì shēn* and *bái zhú* are added to reinforce qi and strengthen the spleen.

CASE STUDY 3: Abdominal Cold Pain
By Dr. Pu Ying-lu

Ms. Xie, a teacher. 1st consultation on August 2nd, 1963.

Main Complaint: Abdominal cold pain for more than 3 months.

Presenting Symptoms: The patient suffered from cold pain in the abdominal area for over 3 months which was mild during the day and severe in the evening. She took some medications without any effective results. Therefore, she sought acupuncture and moxibustion treatment for a cure.

Presenting Symptoms: Abdominal cold pain which prefers pressure, in favor of hot drinks, poor sleep, low appetite, dizziness and heaviness of the head, and aversion to cold. The urine and stool were normal, the tongue was light pink with a white coating and a deep and slow pulse.

Physical Examination: The patient was alert with a fluent speech and a white complexion.

Diagnosis

TCM Diagnosis: Abdominal pain due to deficiency cold

Western Medicine Diagnosis: Abdominal pain

Treatment

Principles:

- Warm the interior and disperse cold
- Move qi and relieve pain
- Strengthen the spleen and harmonize the stomach

Acupuncture Point Combination: ST 25 (*tiān shū*), SP 6 (*sān yīn jiāo*), RN 24 (*chéng jiāng*), RN 4 (*guān yuán*), ST 36 (*zú sān lǐ*).

Manipulations: Apply even supplementation and drainage method to ST 25, SP 6 and RN 24 and retain the needles for 40 minutes. Apply moxibustion to RN 4 and ST 36 for 10 minutes. This treatment was given once a day every day.

After the 1st acupuncture treatment, the abdominal pain slightly relieved and 3 more treatments resolved the pain completely. The patient was asked to apply moxibustion to RN 4 and ST 36 to consolidate the treatment. A follow-up one week later showed there was no more abdominal pain.

Clinical Analysis

According to the pathogenic factors and disease pattern perceived within the symptoms and signs of the patient, this case of abdominal pain is due to a deficient cold pattern. As the qi of the *ying* and *wei* levels are deficient, the pathogenic cold enters the channels and vessels, leading to obstruction of yang qi and abdominal pain. The pulse was tight indicating coldness while it was also slow denoting deficiency. Therefore, there are symptoms of mild pain during the day and severe at night but relieved with pressure. The patient favoured hot drinks with an aversion to cold which demonstrated a deficient cold pattern. *The Spiritual Pivot* (*Líng Shū*, 灵枢) records: "For abdominal pain, apply acupuncture treatment around the navel. The pain can be relieved immediately after the treatment." ST 25 is located 2 *cun* lateral to the navel and is the front-*mu* point of the large intestine, which can be used to unblock qi and relieve pain. RN4, SP 6 and ST 36 are combined to invigorate qi. The moxibustion is applied to treat deficient cold by restoring yang of the stomach and kidney. RN 24 is an empirical point for pain around the navel, as it is mentioned in the *Practical Records of Chinese Medicine Vol. 3: Verses of Practical Acupuncture and Moxibustion* (*Zhōng Yī Shí Yàn Lù Juàn Sān: Zhēn Jiǔ Shí Yàn Gē Jué*, 中医实验录卷三・针灸实验歌诀): "Select LU 5 and SP 6 for abdominal pain and RN 24 for pain around the navel."

CASE STUDY 4: Epigastric Dull Pain

Mr. Liu, age 52, a worker.

Main Complaint: Epigastric discomfort and dull pain for half a year and aggravation for a month.

Medical History: The patient complained of epigastric discomfort and dull pain, heartburn, poor appetite, without acid reflux and belching for half a year. The onset began after drinking alcohol. These symptoms aggravated one month ago, accompanied by dry mouth, feverish sensation in the palms, soles and chest, vexation, dry stool, insomnia and dreaminess. The patient had a history of drinking and smoking for many years and was fond of pungent foods.

Presenting Symptoms: Epigastric discomfort and dull pain with feverish sensation, dry mouth, hot sensation of the palms, soles and chest, vexation, dry stool, insomnia, dreaminess, poor appetite, no acid regurgitation and belching, red tongue with cracks without coating and a deep and thin pulse.

Physical Examination: There was normal body temperature, heart beat, respiration and blood pressure. The patient was thin with no abnormal findings of his heart and lung, but there was mild tenderness in the epigastric region, but no muscular tone and rebound pain. The liver and spleen were not palpated. The blood test, urine test, and stool test were all normal.

Pattern Differentiation

This patient has a history of smoking and drinking for many years and favors pungent foods. Cigarettes, alcohol and pungent foods are hot in property and easily cause fluid consumption. Prolonged heat constraint impairs yin which causes a malnourishment of the stomach and results in dull pain of the epigastric area. As the body fluids are deficient they fail to nourish the orifices causing the symptom of dry mouth and constipation. The red tongue without coating and the deep thin pulse are also signs of body fluid deficiency.

Diagnosis

TCM Diagnosis: Stomachache due to stomach yin and body fluid deficiency
Western Medicine Diagnosis: Epigastric pain

Treatment

Pungent products like alcohol can easily consume yin fluid and impair the spleen and stomach, leading to failure of transportation and transformation. In addition, heat constraint impairs both yin and stomach membrane which result in fluid deficiency and lack of nourishment to the stomach. If this condition lingers for years, it often causes diseases. Accordingly, the treatment principle is to enrich yin and boost stomach. The formula is a modified *Yì Wèi Tāng* (Stomach-Boosting Decoction) together with *Yī Guàn Jiān* (Effective Integration Decoction).

Principles:

- Nourish yin and tonify stomach
- Strengthen the spleen and nourish body fluids

Formula: Modified *Yì Wèi Tāng* (Stomach-Boosting Decoction) combined with *Yī Guàn Jiān* (Effective Integration Decoction).

Ingredients:

北沙参	*běi shā shēn*	15 g	Radix Glehniae
麦冬	*mài dōng*	15 g	Radix Ophiopogonis
生地	*shēng dì*	15 g	Radix Rehmanniae
玉竹	*yù zhú*	10 g	Rhizoma Polygonati Odorati
石斛	*shí hú*	10 g	Caulis Dendrobii
枸杞子	*gǒu qǐ zǐ*	10 g	Fructus Lycii
当归	*dāng guī*	12 g	Radix Angelicae Sinensis
川楝子	*chuān liàn zǐ*	9 g	Fructus Toosendan
白芍	*bái sháo*	15 g	Radix Paeoniae Alba
甘草	*gān cǎo*	5 g	Radix et Rhizoma Glycyrrhizae

Formula Analysis

In this formula, *běi shā shēn* and *mài dōng* harmonize the stomach and nourish yin. *Shēng dì, yù zhú, shí hú* and *gǒu qǐ zǐ* nourish liver yin and stomach fluids. *Dāng guī* nourishes the liver and invigorates blood. *Chuān liàn zǐ* soothes the liver and rectifies qi. *Bái sháo* and *gān cǎo* relieve pain by harmonizing *ying*. Moreover, *xiāng yuán* (Fructus Citri), *fó shǒu* (Fructus Citri Sarcodactylis) and other medicinals can be added depending on the presenting symptoms.

If there is the presence of epigastric burning pain with acid regurgitation, *Zuǒ Jīn Wán* (Left Metal Pill) can be taken with this formula.

The Chinese patent formula *Yīn Xū Wèi Tòng Piàn* (Yin Deficiency and Stomach Pain Tablets) was also given orally (6 tablets each dose) 3 times a day.

Follow-up Consultations

After 20 doses of the formula, the epigastric pain and discomfort were completely resolved.

KEY CLINICAL POINTS

Generally speaking, clinical practice should be based on the presenting patterns according to the eight guiding principles to discern the severity of cold or heat, deficiency or excess, and condition of qi and blood. The treatment principle for abdominal pain is to unblock the qi constraint by treating excess with purgation, treating deficiency with supplementation, treating heat with cold medicinals and treating cold patterns with warming medicinals. We also need to take these clinical key points into account:

1. Use warming and unblocking treatment principles to treat abdominal pain due to congealed cold.

Warming and dredging medicinals are mainly pungent-warm or pungent-hot in quality. They are often combined with blood moving and pain relieving medicinals. They are usually used to warm and activate qi, purge interior cold, promote the smooth flow of qi and blood, dry dampness and unblock the collaterals. However, purely using acrid hot medicinals, such as *Sì Nì Tāng* (Frigid Extremities Decoction), can only restore yang to rescue from counterflow, which has little effect on warming and unblocking to relieve pain. Therefore, warming and unblocking methods must be combined with other medicinals. The first category is qi moving medicinals, such as *gāo liáng jiāng* and *xiāng fù* in the formula *Liáng Fù Wán* (Lesser Galangal and Cyperus Pill). The second category is blood cooling and supplementing medicinals, such as simultaneous application of *guì zhī, xì xīn, dāng guī* and *bái sháo* in the formula *Dāng Guī Sì Nì Tāng* (Chinese Angelica Frigid Extremities Decoction). The third category is blood activating and stasis removing medicinals, such as *Shào Fù Zhú Yū Tāng* (Lower Abdominal Stasis-Expelling Decoction). The fourth category is sweet medicinals to relax muscles and stop pain by nourishing, such as *gān cǎo, dà zǎo* and *yí táng*.

2. Apply heat clearing and bowel unblocking method to treat acute abdominal pain of heat pattern.

This method mainly applies heat clearing and toxin removing medicinals, such as *yín huā* and *huáng lián*, and bowel unblocking ingredients, such as *dà huáng* and *máng xiāo* to relieve pain by unblocking stools. Nowadays, it is used to treat chronic or acute pancreatitis with favourable curative effect. As for intestinal obstruction, modified *Tiáo Wèi Chéng Qì Tāng* (Stomach-Regulating and Purgative Decoction) together with qi rectifying ingredients like *mù xiāng* and *bīng láng* can be prescribed to rectify qi and unblock the bowels. It is important to notice, that these formulas have strong purging effect and when used incorrectly or over a long period of time can injure the stomach qi. It is then contraindicated to apply this purging method after the pattern has changed. Additionally, avoid using this formula on pattern of abdominal pain due to deficiency.

3. Pay attention to abdominal pain due to worm accumulation.

Many intestinal parasites such as roundworm, tapeworm, and hookworm can cause abdominal pain. For abdominal pain due to parasites, it requires to begin by calming the worms and then we use medicinals to expel them. If the abdominal pain lingers after expelling the worms, it is because there are still worms in the intestines and the method needs to be applied again.

In case of prolonged worm accumulation, the patient will also suffer from qi and blood deficiency and spleen and stomach depletion. In these cases, we also need to strengthen healthy qi while expelling pathogens. Formulas such as *Huà Chóng Wán* (Worm-Expelling Pill) and *Wū Méi Wán* (Mume Pill) with modification can be selected to expel these worms. The treatment is ultimately to kill and expel worms with assistance of purgative medicinals to discharge worms while warming the middle *jiao*.

COMPREHENSION QUESTIONS

1. What are the key points to diagnose the abdominal pain?
2. What are the key differences between abdominal pain and the *Pǐ* syndrome?
3. Multiple choice questions:

1) Mr. Zhou, 18 years old. The patient suffered from abdominal distension and fullness, belching with putrid smell, acid reflux and inhibited bowel movements which followed overeating two days ago. His tongue coating was thick and greasy. The doctor prescribed *Bǎo Hé Wán* (Harmony-Preserving Pill) without any alleviating effect. We need to combine *Bǎo Hé Wán* with:

A. *Xiǎo Chéng Qì Tāng* (Minor Purgative Decoction)
B. *Dà Chéng Qì Tāng* (Major Purgative Decoction)
C. *Zhǐ Shí Dǎo Zhì Wán* (Immature Bitter Orange Stagnation-Moving Pill)
D. *Xiǎo Xiàn Xiōng Tāng* (Minor Chest-Draining Decoction)
E. *Lǐ Zhōng Tāng* (Center-Regulating Decoction)

2) Mr. Zhang, 27 years old. After a dinner party, the patient suffered from a stomachache with distension and a dull pain with palpation, belching with putrid smell, acid reflux, vomiting with smelly undigested food, pain relieved by vomiting, no appetite, unsatisfying defecation that is relieved by passing stools, a thick and greasy tongue coating and a slippery pulse. The recommended formula is:

A. *Dà Chéng Qì Tāng* (Major Purgative Decoction)
B. *Xiǎo Chéng Qì Tāng* (Minor Purgative Decoction)
C. *Huò Xiāng Zhèng Qì Wán* (Agastache Qi-Correcting Pill)
D. *Bàn Xià Xiè Xīn Tāng* (Pinellia Heart-Draining Decoction)
E. *Bǎo Hé Wán* (Harmony-Preserving Pill)

3) A 29-year-old male was suffering from wandering epigastric distension and pain, frequent belching, inhibited defecation, a thin and white tongue coating and a wiry pulse.

3.1) The differentiation pattern of this case is:
A. Liver qi invading the stomach
B. Stagnation of blood stasis
C. Heat constraint of the liver and stomach
D. Food stagnation
E. Pathogenic cold invading the stomach

3.2) The optimal treatment principle is to:
A. Soothe the liver and rectify qi
B. Harmonize the spleen and stomach
C. Rectify qi and harmonize the stomach
D. Rectify qi and invigorate blood
E. Boost qi and strengthen the spleen

3.3) The recommended formula is:
A. *Xiāo Yáo Săn* (Free Wanderer Powder)
B. *Huà Gān Jiān* (Liver Resolving Decoction)
C. *Chái Hú Shū Gān Săn* (Bupleurum Liver-Soothing Powder)
D. *Dà Chái Hú Tāng* (Major Bupleurum Decoction)
E. None of the above

4) Mr. Qian, 16 years old. The patient was suffering from epigastric distension, fullness and pain, belching with putrid smell, acid regurgitation, constipation, a thick and greasy tongue coating and a slippery pulse.
4.1) The differentiation pattern for this case is:
A. Liver qi constraint that transforms fire
B. Liver qi constraint with qi stagnation and blood stasis
C. Food stagnation and inhibited bowels
D. External wind cold and internal food stagnation
E. None of the above

4.2) The optimal treatment principle is to:
A. Soothe the liver and rectify qi, clear heat and drain fire
B. Soothe the liver, rectify qi, and invigorate the blood
C. Promote digestion and guide out food stagnation by purging the intestines
D. Scatter wind cold, promote digestion and purge food stagnation
E. None of the above

4.3) The doctor prescribed *Băo Hé Wán* (Harmony-Preserving Pill) without any effect. At present, the recommended formula is:
A. *Dà Chéng Qì Tāng* (Major Purgative Decoction)

B. *Lǐ Zhōng Tāng* (Center-Regulating Decoction)
C. *Bǎo Hé Wán* (Harmony-Preserving Pill)
D. *Dà Chái Hú Tāng* (Major Bupleurum Decoction)
E. *Liáng Gé Sǎn* (Diaphragm-Cooling Powder)

5) Mr. Zhang, 40 years old. The patient suffered from epigastric distension, fullness and pain that were triggered by emotional stress, the pain radiates to the hypochondriac area with frequent belching, inhibited bowel movements, a thin and white tongue coating and a wiry pulse.

5.1) The differentiation pattern of this case is:
A. Liver qi invading the stomach
B. Pathogenic heat retention in the liver and stomach
C. Stagnation of blood stasis
D. Food stagnation
E. None of the above

5.2) If the patient does not improve after the treatment and there are symptoms of epigastric urgent burning pain, irritability, acid regurgitation, dry mouth with a bitter taste, a red tongue with a yellow tongue coating and a wiry and rapid pulse. The recommended formula is:
A. *Chái Hú Shū Gān Sǎn* (Bupleurum Liver-Soothing Powder)
B. *Dà Chái Hú Tāng* (Major Bupleurum Decoction)
C. *Xiāo Yáo Sǎn* (Free Wanderer Powder)
D. *Yǎng Wèi Tāng* (Stomach Boosting Decoction)
E. *Huà Gān Jiān* (Liver Resolving Decoction)

5.3) If the condition remains without improvement after further treatment and the manifestations are hematemesis, flushed face, red tongue, vexation, constipation, and a wiry, rapid and forceful pulse. The recommended formula is:
A. *Huáng Tǔ Tāng* (Yellow Earth Decoction)
B. *Guī Pí Tāng* (Spleen-Restoring Decoction)
C. *Xiè Xīn Tāng* (Heart-Draining Decoction)
D. *Bàn Xià Xiè Xīn Tāng* (Pinellia Heart-Draining Decoction)

5.4) If the symptoms are relieved after treatment, but there are still epigastric dull pain, dry mouth and throat, dry and constipated stool, a red tongue with a lack of fluids and a thin and rapid pulse. The recommended formula is:
A. *Yǎng Wèi Tāng* (Stomach Boosting Decoction)
B. *Lǐ Zhōng Tāng* (Center-Regulating Decoction)
C. *Huà Gān Jiān* (Liver Resolving Decoction)
D. *Yī Guàn Jiān* (Effective Integration Decoction) combined with *Sháo Yào Gān Cǎo*

Tāng (Peony and Licorice Decoction)

Answers

1. All sorts of pain in the area from below the stomach to above the pubic area fall into the realm of abdominal pain. The possible types of abdominal pain include cold pain, burning pain, dull pain, distending pain, stabbing pain, pulling pain and so on. The clinical manifestations of abdominal pain are different according to which organs are affected and by which pathogenic factors. If the intestines are involved, there will be symptoms of lower abdominal cramping pain and bloating, diarrhea or constipation. If the urinary bladder is affected by damp-heat, there will be burning lower abdominal pain radiating to the external genitalia with continuous, dribbling and burning urination. If the pain is due to roundworms, there will be severe abdominal pain which worsens with cold and eating accompanied by vomiting. There are various pathological causes for abdominal pain, clearly identifying the pattern is the only effective way to offer a cure.

2. Both abdominal pain and *pǐ* syndrome share the same location of disease presenting in the epigastric area below the heart. However, the *pǐ* syndrome is a symptom characterized as blockage sensation occurring only below the heart accompanied by chest fullness and oppression. As we just mentioned abdominal pain refers to a larger area and various types of pain including the area affected by the *pǐ* syndrome. When the abdominal pain shares the same symptom presentation of the *pǐ* syndrome we classify it and treat it as a *pǐ* syndrome.

3. 1) A, 2) E, 3.1) A, 3.2) A, 3.3) C, 4.1) C, 4.2) C, 4.3) A, 5.1) A, 5.2) E, 5.3) C, 5.4) D.

4.2 *Pǐ* Syndrome

The *pǐ* syndrome is characterized by subjective stuffiness or obstruction sensation in the area below the heart region accompanied by chest distension and fullness without any palpable lumps. It can be classified into two different syndromes according to the affected area: chest *pǐ* and epigastric *pǐ*. These syndromes are very commonly seen and have various excessive and deficiency patterns with a fairly high level of relapse which make them difficult to be treated. The description of the *pǐ* syndrome is often seen in disease conditions such as chronic gastritis, functional dyspepsia, gastric neurosis and gastroptosis, heart conditions and so on. Their treatment principles remain according to their Chinese medicine differentiation.

The *pǐ* syndrome is closely related to the condition of the stomach and is also affected by the liver and spleen. Its occurrence involves the condition of the flow of qi in the middle *jiao* and the failure of the spleen and stomach in their corresponding ascending and descending functions often caused by food damage, liver qi stagnation, phlegm retention, dampness and heat stagnation or weakness in the spleen and stomach. In the initial stage, an excess pattern is commonly seen due to the accumulation of pathogenic factors. However, in chronic or reoccurring cases we often see a pattern related to the spleen failing to raise the clear yang and the stomach unable to lower turbid yin creating the sensation of blockage in the epigastric area below the heart. If the excessive pattern lasts for a long time without effective treatment, the condition of the healthy qi will weaken and will gradually impair the stomach and spleen leading to a deficiency pattern. Prolonged pathogenic damp-heat retention or heat stagnation in the liver and stomach will also cause a deficient *pǐ* syndrome due to stomach yin depletion.

CLINICAL PATTERNS DIFFERENTIATION AND TREATMENTS

1. Internal Retention of Pathogenic Heat

Symptoms: Heartburn, a subjective sensation of obstruction and heat in the epigastric area, halitosis, mouth and tongue ulcers, aversion to heat, restlessness, irritability, flushed face, red eyes, dry mouth, insomnia, dark yellow urine, dry stools or constipation, a red tongue with yellow coating and a rapid pulse.

Treatment Principle:
- Clear heat and nourish body fluids
- Regulate stomach and relieve fullness

Main Acupuncture Points:
- RN 12 (*zhōng wǎn*): Front-*mu* point of the stomach to regulate middle qi, harmonize spleen and stomach
- BL 21 (*wèi shù*): Back-*shu* point of the stomach to harmonize middle *jiao* and promote digestion
- ST 36 (*zú sān lǐ*): To invigorate spleen, tonify qi and stop pain
- PC 6 (*nèi guān*): To regulate middle qi, clear heat, regulate stomach and calm the spirit
- HT 5 (*tōng lǐ*): *Luo*-connecting point of the heart to clear heart heat, treat mouth ulcers and calm the spirit
- ST 25 (*tiān shū*): Front-*mu* point of the large intestine to invigorate stomach and intestines, regulate qi, improve digestion and resolve stagnation

Supporting Points:
- ST 44 (*nèi tíng*): To clear damp-heat and harmonize intestines
- RN 10 (*xià wǎn*): To regulate qi, dispel food stagnation and treat abdominal distention

Recommended Formula: *Dà Huáng Huáng Lián Xiè Xīn Tāng* (大黄黄连泻心汤, Rhubarb and Coptis Heart-Draining Decoction) from the *Treatise on Cold Damage* (*Shāng Hán Lùn*, 伤寒论)

Substitute Formula: *Zhǐ Shí Dǎo Zhì Wán* (枳实导滞丸, Immature Bitter Orange Stagnation-Moving Pill)

Patent Formula: *Qīng Wèi Huáng Lián Wán* (清胃黄连丸, Stomach-Clearing Coptis Pill)

2. Food Retention

Symptoms: Belching, a subjective sensation of obstruction and heaviness in the epigastric area, acid reflux, nausea, vomiting of undigested food, diarrhea, halitosis, borborygmus with abdominal pain and fullness, poor appetite, fatigue, sweating after exertion, a thick and greasy tongue coating and a slippery pulse.

Treatment Principle:
- Promote digestion and activate the middle *jiao*
- Invigorate qi to relieve fullness

Main Acupuncture Points:
- ST 24 (*huá ròu mén*): To harmonize stomach, transform stagnation and calm the spirit
- RN 10 (*xià wǎn*): To regulate qi, dispel food stagnation and stop abdominal pain
- RN 12 (*zhōng wǎn*): Front-*mu* point of the stomach to regulate middle qi, harmonize spleen and stomach

- ST 36 (*zú sān lǐ*): To invigorate spleen, tonify qi and promote circulation
- BL 21 (*wèi shù*): Back-*shu* point of the stomach to invigorate spleen and harmonize stomach, promote digestion
- PC 6 (*nèi guān*): To regulate middle qi, clear heat, regulate stomach and calm the spirit

Supporting Points:

- DU 5 (*xuán shū*): To treat diarrhea with undigested food, stop abdominal pain and benefit lumbar region
- GB 25 (*jīng mén*): To resolve belching and acid reflux

Recommended Formula: *Bǎo Hé Wán* (保和丸, Harmony-Preserving Pill) from the *Teachings of [Zhu] Dan-xi* (*Dān Xī Xīn Fǎ*, 丹溪心法)

Substitute Formula: *Jiàn Pí Wán* (健脾丸, Spleen-Fortifying Pill)

Patent Formula: *Bǎo Hé Wán* (保和丸, Harmony-Preserving Pill)

3. Internal Retention of Turbid Phlegm

Symptoms: A subjective sensation of obstruction and heaviness in the epigastric area, edema in the limbs, poor appetite, nausea, headaches which are aggravated in damp weather, chest and epigastric fullness, fatigue, heaviness of the body, excessive salivation, vomiting, loose stools, a greasy tongue coating and a slippery pulse.

Treatment Principle:

- Strengthen the spleen and resolve dampness
- Regulate qi and remove obstruction

Main Acupuncture Points:

- SP 9 (*yīn líng quán*): To expel damp-heat, harmonize middle *jiao* and regulate fluid passages
- SP 8 (*dì jī*): *Xi*-cleft point of the spleen to resolve dampness and regulate spleen, improve digestion and benefit appetite
- ST 40 (*fēng lóng*): To expel phlegm and dampness, clear phlegm from the chest area
- ST 36 (*zú sān lǐ*): To expel dampness, invigorate spleen, tonify qi and promote circulation
- RN 11 (*jiàn lǐ*): To invigorate spleen and stomach, regulate fluid passages and treat edema
- BL 21 (*wèi shù*): Back-*shu* point of the stomach to invigorate spleen and harmonize stomach, resolve dampness and promote digestion

Supporting Points:

- ST 25 (*tiān shū*): Front-*mu* point of the large intestine to resolve dizziness due to damp- heat, regulate qi and resolve stagnation
- GB 24 (*rì yuè*): Front-*mu* point of the gallbladder to resolve hypochondriac pain, expel damp-heat and benefit the gallbladder

Recommended Formula: *Píng Wèi Sǎn* (平胃散, Stomach-Calming Powder) combined with *Èr Chén Tāng* (二陈汤, Two Matured Substances Decoction). Both formulas are from the *Beneficial Formulas from the Taiping Imperial Pharmacy* (*Tài Píng Huì Mín Hé Jì Jú Fāng*, 太平惠民和剂局方)

Substitute Formula: *Xiāng Shā Liù Jūn Zǐ Tāng* (香砂六君子汤, Costusroot and Amomum Six Gentlemen Decoction)

Patent Formula:

- *Xiāng Shā Píng Wèi Wán* (香砂平胃丸, Costusroot and Amomum Stomach-Calming Pill)
- *Xiāng Shā Liù Jūn Zǐ Wán* (香砂六君子丸, Costusroot and Amomum Six Gentlemen Pill)

4. Liver Qi Stagnation Affecting the Stomach

Symptoms: A subjective sensation of obstruction and pain in the epigastric area, restlessness, irritability, belching, diarrhea, bitter taste, frequent sighing, hypochondriac pain, poor appetite or indigestion, abdominal distention, dysmenorrhea, a thin tongue coating and a wiry pulse.

Treatment Principle:

- Soothe the liver and invigorate qi
- Relieve fullness and nourish the stomach

Main Acupuncture Points:

- BL 18 (*gān shù*): Back-*shu* point of the liver to spread liver qi, regulate emotions and promote circulation
- BL 21 (*wèi shù*): Back-*shu* point of the stomach to invigorate spleen and harmonize stomach, promote digestion and stop hypochondriac pain
- LV 3 (*tài chōng*): *Yuan*-source point of the liver to soothe liver, regulate menstruation, stop vomiting and calm the spirit
- LV 14 (*qī mén*): Front-*mu* point of the liver to spread liver qi, harmonize liver and stomach
- ST 36 (*zú sān lǐ*): To invigorate spleen, support the healthy qi and promote circulation
- RN 12 (*zhōng wǎn*): Front-*mu* point of the stomach to regulate middle qi, harmonize spleen and stomach

Supporting Points:

- GB 24 (*rì yuè*): Front-*mu* point of the gallbladder to resolve hypochondriac pain and benefit the gallbladder
- LV 8 (*qū quán*): To spread liver qi and invigorate blood

Recommended Formula: *Sì Nì Sǎn* (四逆散, Frigid Extremities Powder) from the *Treatise on Cold Damage* (*Shāng Hán Lùn*, 伤寒论) combined with *Yuè Jú Wán* (越鞠丸, Constraint-Resolving Pill) from the *Teachings of [Zhu] Dan-xi* (*Dān Xī Xīn Fǎ*, 丹溪心法)

Substitute Formula: *Chái Hú Shū Gān Sǎn* (柴胡疏肝散, Bupleurum Liver-Soothing Powder)

Patent Formula:

- *Chái Hú Shū Gān Wán* (柴胡舒肝丸, Bupleurum Liver-Soothing Pill)
- *Yuè Jú Wán* (越鞠丸, Constraint-Resolving Pill)

5. Deficiency of the Spleen and Stomach

Symptoms: A subjective sensation of obstruction and emptiness in the epigastric area, lassitude, reluctance to speak, poor appetite, sloppy stools or stools with undigested food, abdominal distension, edema, spontaneous sweating, irregular menstrual cycle, spotting, a light red tongue body with thin color and a thready and weak pulse.

Treatment Principle:

- Supplement qi and warm the middle *jiao*
- Strengthen spleen and regulate stomach

Main Acupuncture Points:

- BL 20 (*pí shù*): Back-*shu* point of the spleen to invigorate spleen, tonify qi, harmonize middle *jiao* and stop vomiting
- BL 21 (*wèi shù*): Back-*shu* point of the stomach to invigorate spleen and harmonize stomach, resolve dampness and promote digestion
- RN 6 (*qì hăi*): To invigorate spleen and harmonize blood, promote circulation and treat gynecological disorders
- SP 9 (*yīn líng quán*): To harmonize middle *jiao*, expel dampness, regulate menstruation and benefit lower *jiao*
- ST 36 (*zú sān lǐ*): To invigorate spleen and harmonize stomach, nourish the original qi, resolve edema and regulate menstruation

Supporting Points:

- ST 40 (*fēng lóng*): To expel phlegm and dampness, nourish spleen, harmonize stomach and intestines
- RN 12 (*zhōng wăn*): To warm middle *jiao*, harmonize spleen and stomach, regulate qi and stop abdominal pain

Recommended Formula: *Bŭ Zhōng Yì Qì Tāng* (补中益气汤, Center-Supplementing and Qi-Boosting Decoction) from the *Treatise on the Spleen and Stomach* (*Pí Wèi Lùn*, 脾胃论)

Substitute Formula: *Shēn Líng Bái Zhú Săn* (参苓白术散, Ginseng, Poria and Atractylodes Macrocephalae Powder)

Patent Formula: *Bŭ Zhōng Yì Qì Wán* (补中益气丸, Center-Supplementing and Qi-Boosting Pill)

Summary Chart for *Pǐ* Syndrome

Patterns	Main Points	Supporting Points	Formulae
Internal Retention of Pathogenic Heat	RN 12, BL 21, ST 36, PC 6, HT 5, ST 25	ST 44 for intestinal damp-heat RN 10 for food stagnation	*Dà Huáng Huáng Lián Xiè Xīn Tāng* or *Zhǐ Shí Dăo Zhì Wán*

Continued

Patterns	Main Points	Supporting Points	Formulae
Food Retention	ST 24, RN 10, RN 12, ST 36, BL 21, PC 6	DU 5 for diarrhea with undigested food and lumbar pain GB 25 for belching and acid reflux	*Bǎo Hé Wán* or *Jiàn Pí Wán*
Internal Retention of Turbid Phlegm	SP 9, SP 8, ST 40, ST 36, RN 11, BL 21	ST 25 for dizziness due to stagnated damp-heat GB 24 for coastal pain	*Píng Wèi Sǎn* plus *Èr Chén Tāng* or *Xiāng Shā Liù Jūn Zǐ Tāng*
Liver Qi Stagnation Affecting the Stomach	BL 18, BL 21, LV 3, LV 14, ST 36, RN 12	GB 24 for coastal pain LV 8 for blood stasis due to qi stagnation	*Sì Nì Sǎn* plus *Yuè Jú Wán* or *Chái Hú Shū Gān Sǎn*
Deficiency of the Spleen and Stomach	BL 20, BL 21, RN 6, SP 9, ST 36	ST 40 for dampness accumulation RN 12 for middle *jiao* cold	*Bǔ Zhōng Yì Qì Tāng* or *Shēn Líng Bái Zhú Sǎn*

CASE STUDY 1: Chronic Epigastric Fullness

Mr. Li, 28 years old.

Main Complaint: Epigastric distention and fullness for 5 years with aggravation for 2 weeks.

Medical History: Five years ago, the patient had his appendix removed since he experienced a lower appetite and discomfort in the upper abdominal area. Two weeks ago, after improper food intake, the patient experienced repeated epigastric distension, fullness and pain which was aggravated by eating. The patient experienced frequent belching and the fullness was relieved by passing gas. An abdominal ultrasound showed no abnormal findings and there were no abnormal findings of the stomach mucus membrane. The patient was diagnosed with functional dyspepsia. Motilium and other drugs were administrated, but had no curative effect. Therefore, he consulted with Chinese medicine.

Presenting Symptoms: Epigastric distention and fullness, poor appetite and digestion, frequent belching, mental fatigue, lack of strength, lusterless complexion, normal sleep, normal urination, slightly dry stool, a pale red tongue with a thin white coating and a deep and weak pulse.

Physical Examination: Temperature: 36.9 ℃, pulse: 80 bpm, respiration: 20 bpm, blood pressure: 120/75 mmHg. The patient was aware with a sallow yellow complexion. His abdomen was soft and symmetric without apparent mass or depression. There was a tenderness in the upper abdomen with palpation. The bowel sounds were normal and the liver and spleen are not palpable. There was no tenderness in the hepatic region and a gastroscopy showed no abnormal findings.

Pattern Differentiation

With a disease history of 5 years, his spleen and stomach are weak. Together with improper diet, his middle *jiao* qi was insufficient, lacking strength to receive and transport food. Therefore, there were manifestations of abdominal distension and pain, poor appetite and digestion, and frequent belching. Mental fatigue, lack of strength, lusterless complexion, and deep and weak pulse were all signs of spleen and stomach weakness. The disease location was in the spleen and stomach and it was a deficiency pattern.

Diagnosis

TCM Diagnosis: Deficiency *pǐ* syndrome due to depletion of the spleen and stomach

Western Medicine Diagnosis: Functional dyspepsia

Treatment

The pathomechanism of this case is mainly spleen qi deficiency where the spleen fails to transport the food and nutrients appropriately leading to the epigastric distension and fullness as well as the poor appetite and digestion.

Principles:

- Supplement the center and tonify qi
- Strengthen the spleen and harmonize the stomach

Formula: Modified *Bǔ Zhōng Yì Qì Tāng* (Center-Supplementing and Qi-Boosting Decoction)

Ingredients:

黄芪	*huáng qí*	30 g	Radix Astragali
党参	*dǎng shēn*	20 g	Radix Codonopsis
白术	*bái zhú*	15 g	Rhizoma Atractylodis Macrocephalae
陈皮	*chén pí*	6 g	Pericarpium Citri Reticulatae
升麻	*shēng má*	10 g	Rhizoma Cimicifugae
柴胡	*chái hú*	10 g	Radix Bupleuri
当归	*dāng guī*	10 g	Radix Angelicae Sinensis
山楂	*shān zhā*	30 g	Fructus Crataegi
麦芽	*mài yá*	30 g	Fructus Hordei Germinatus (dry-fried)
谷芽	*gǔ yá*	30 g	Fructus Setariae Germinatus (dry-fried)
鸡内金	*jī nèi jīn*	10 g	Endothelium Corneum Gigeriae Galli (dry-fried)
甘草	*gān cǎo*	3 g	Radix et Rhizoma Glycyrrhizae

Formula Analysis

In the formula, *huáng qí* is the chief ingredient which supplements the middle *jiao* and fortifies qi. *Dǎng shēn* and *bái zhú* supplement qi and fortify the spleen. *Dāng guī* nourishes the blood and harmonizes the *ying* level, as well as assists *huáng qí* and *dǎng shēn* to supplement qi. *Chén pí* can rectify qi and harmonize the stomach. *Shēng má* and *chái hú* raise yang and lift the sunken. *Gān cǎo* relieves spasm and pain, and also harmonizes the other ingredients. In addition, *shān zhā, gǔ yá, mài yá* and *jī nèi jīn* are combined to promote digestion, relieve food accumulation and fortify the stomach. The combination of these ingredients is able to boost the middle *jiao,* fortify the spleen and promote transportation. The Chinese medicinal patent *Jiàn Pí Wán* (Spleen-Fortifying Pill) was also given to the patient at the dosage of 9 g twice a day. The patient was also asked to avoid acrid, spicy, fatty and oily food.

Follow-up Consultations

After 7 doses of the formula, the abdominal distension and fullness was relieved, the appetite improved and the patient felt more energized. The formula was given for 8 more weeks with the addition of ginseng to further strengthen the middle *jiao* and treat the *pǐ* syndrome and all symptoms alleviated.

CASE STUDY 2: Chronic Epigastric *Pǐ* Syndrome
By Dr. Li Shou-shan

Mr. Chi, 66 years old. First consultation on November 2nd, 1986.

Main Complaint: Epigastric *pǐ* syndrome with fullness for over 10 years with recent aggravation.

Medical History: The patient suffered from stomach diseases for over 10 years with symptoms of abdominal fullness and discomfort which aggravated on an empty stomach and was slightly relieved after eating, though the discomfort resumed soon afterwards. The patient was only able to eat about 150 to 200 g a day and was becoming gradually thinner. A gastroscopy showed chronic atrophic gastritis with severe intestinal metaplasia. The patient had been prescribed some Chinese and Western medicines, such as Hericium Erinaceus Tablet and Vatacoenayme without any obvious effect.

Presenting Symptoms: Epigastric fullness and discomfort, poor appetite and digestion, fatigue, lack of strength, loose stool, belching, frequent flatulence, a pale red tongue with a white slippery coating and a deep wiry pulse.

Physical Examination: The patient was very thin but aware. His facial complexion was slightly yellow and lusterless. There were petechiae on the tongue and the sublingual veins were thick and long in a light purple colour and with several nodules. His abdomen was soft without any lumps or mass. There was slight tenderness in the upper abdominal area upon pressure. A routine blood test showed: RBC 3.5 $\times 10^{12}$/L, Hb 90 g/L. His body weight was 55 kg.

Diagnosis

TCM Diagnosis: Stomach *pǐ* syndrome (spleen and stomach weakness, qi stagnation and blood stasis)

Western Medicine Diagnosis: Chronic atrophic gastritis with severe intestinal metaplasia

Treatment

The root of this condition is the depletion of the spleen and stomach qi with some qi stagnation as an excess in the branch.

Principles:

- Supplement the middle *jiao* and dissipate *pǐ* syndrome
- Rectify qi and remove blood stasis

Formula: Modified *Zhǐ Zhú Wán* (Immature Bitter Orange and Atractylodes Macrocephala Pill)

Ingredients:

黄芪	*huáng qí*	25 g	Radix Astragali
党参	*dǎng shēn*	15 g	Radix Codonopsis
丹参	*dān shēn*	15 g	Radix et Rhizoma Salviae Miltiorrhizae
白术	*bái zhú*	15 g	Rhizoma Atractylodis Macrocephalae
白芍	*bái sháo*	15 g	Radix Paeoniae Alba
香橼	*xiāng yuán*	15 g	Fructus Citri (peel)
广木香	*guǎng mù xiāng*	3 g	Radix Aucklandiae
砂仁	*shā rén*	3 g	Fructus Amomi
鸡内金	*jī nèi jīn*	20 g	Endothelium Corneum Gigeriae Galli
姜半夏	*jiāng bàn xià*	7.5 g	Rhizoma Pinelliae Praeparatum
陈皮	*chén pí*	10 g	Pericarpium Citri Reticulatae
桂枝	*guì zhī*	10 g	Ramulus Cinnamomi
炙甘草	*zhì gān cǎo*	10 g	Radix et Rhizoma Glycyrrhizae Praeparata cum Melle

Follow-up Consultations

After taking this modified formula for over 2 months, the symptoms of the *pǐ* syndrome resolved, his appetite resumed, urination and defecation became normal, his body weight increased by 7 kg, and his facial complexion was pinkish. The patient had a red tongue with a thin white coating, the sublingual vessels were pale red, thin and short, and the pulse was weak and slippery. He was treated for 3 months altogether and then was re-examined with a gastroscopy and biopsy which showed a superficial gastritis without any trace of intestinal metaplasia. The blood test was also back to normal. The patient stopped taking the medication and his condition did not relapse within the following two years.

Clinical Analysis

The type of chronic atrophic gastritis lies in the stomach and is characterized by gastric distension, pain and fullness which is directly related to the *pǐ* syndrome in Chinese medicine. Since this case is mainly a deficiency turning into excess causing the epigastric *pǐ* symptoms, the priority of the treatment needs to tend to the deficient root by reinforcing the healthy qi and strengthening the middle *jiao*. Since this case also involves cancerous metaplasia, the pathogenic accumulation also needs to be addressed in the treatment principle of rectifying qi and moving blood stasis.

It is important to notice that Dr. Li Shou-shan always inspected sublingual vein, because he believed that the pale purple and long sublingual vein with or without nodules are often indicators of intestinal metaplasia. In these cases, he would often supplement the formula with the medicinals *jī nèi jīn, dān shēn, bái huā shé shé cǎo* and so on.

CASE STUDY 3: Acute Dull Epigastric Pain
By Dr. Xi Yong-jiang

Mr. Xu, 36 years old.

Main Complaint: Dull pain in the upper abdomen for over one month.

Medical History: The patient ate a large amount of food very quickly due to the stress at work last month.

Presenting Symptoms: Since then, he felt a dull pain in his upper abdomen after having meals, accompanied with belching, acid reflux, slightly loose stools once to twice a day, sometimes insomnia and occasional foul breath, a pale tongue with whitish greasy coating and a thready pulse.

Physical Examination: The patient was conscious with a fluent speech, slightly emaciated with a slightly yellow complexion. His abdomen was flat, symmetric and soft with a slight tenderness in the upper abdomen but no rebound tenderness. The liver and spleen were impalpable. There were no abnormal findings from the gastroscopy.

Diagnosis

TCM Diagnosis: *Pǐ* syndrome with fullness due to spleen and stomach depletion

Western Medicine Diagnosis: Dull epigastric pain

Principles:

- Soothe the liver and invigorate the spleen
- Remove obstruction and stop pain

Acupuncture Point Combinations:

1. Back side of the body: DU 11 (*shén dào*), DU 9 (*zhì yáng*), BL 17 (*gé shù*), BL 18 (*gān shù*), BL 20 (*pí shù*), BL 21 (*wèi shù*), BL 22 (*sān jiāo shù*), SP 6 (*sān yīn jiāo*).

2. Front side of the body: RN 12 (*zhōng wǎn*), RN 10 (*xià wǎn*), LI 10 (*shǒu sān lǐ*), ST 36 (*zú sān lǐ*), ST 40 (*fēng lóng*), LV 3 (*tài chōng*), SP 8 (*dì jī*), SP 5 (*shāng qiū*).

3. Moxa therapy: RN 17 (*dàn zhōng*), RN 11 (*jiàn lǐ*), RN 8 (*shén què*), LI 10 (*shǒu sān lǐ*), ST 36 (*zú sān lǐ*).

Apply needling tonifying method to back-*shu* points and even method to points on limbs. Apply two moxa cones on medicinal ginger slices on RN 17, RN 11 and RN 8 the size of a half ginkgo.

Follow-up Consultations

These acupuncture and moxibustion treatments were given twice a week and ten treatments made one course. After one course of treatments, the patient confirmed that the upper abdominal distending pain was resolved, the foul breath improved, but there was still a slight distension in the epigastric area.

After three months of treatment, the abdominal pain and distension pain were completely resolved and the patient gained a bit of weight and felt stronger with a healthy spirit.

Clinical Analysis

RN 12 is the front-*mu* point of the stomach channel, and the influential point of the *fu*-organs, which can fortify and activate the middle *jiao* while regulating the qi. ST 36 rectifies the *fu*-organs and is the *he*-sea point of the stomach channel and the earth point within the earth channel. They can both supplement deficiencies and drain excesses to regulate the stomach and intestinal qi, harmonize stomach and relieve pain. Therefore, these two points are the optimal points for treating stomach and abdomen diseases. When giving acupuncture or moxibusiton treatment to these two points, some patients experience some flatulence and instant release from the fullness and bloating. If the needles are inserted to the depth about 1 to 1.5 *cun*, many sensitive patients can feel gastrointestinal peristalsis and borborygmus. Some patients may continue to have belching even two days after acupuncture treatment, but the abdominal distension and fullness will vanish and the appetite will improve, indicating significant effect on gastrointestinal peristalsis.

KEY CLINICAL POINTS

In the initial stage, the condition of *pǐ* syndrome is mostly an excess pattern, but if it lasts for a long time, it will become a deficiency pattern as the qi of the middle *jiao* is consumed and the body fluids are damaged. Clinically, it is commonly seen as a deficient root and excess branch. The fundamental principles are harmonizing and fortifying the spleen and stomach, rectifying qi and dissipating nodule. In addition, the following clinical points need to be taken into account.

1. Even if the condition of *pǐ* syndrome and fullness is located in the stomach,

it is closely related to the function of the spleen. The spleen and stomach are both located in the middle *jiao* and easily affect each other. Chronic conditions of the stomach will always involve the spleen function resulting in spleen yang impairment, transportation and transformation disorder, clear qi failing to ascend and turbid qi failing to descend. In this sense, there will be ascending and descending disorder in the middle *jiao* leading to the epigastric *pǐ* syndorme. Therefore, the treatment principle is to nourish and strengthen the spleen qi and warm the middle *jiao* yang qi to remove stasis.

2. Chronic *pǐ* syndrome usually presents a complex of deficiency-excess pattern where both deficient cold and stagnant heat create the fullness and pain which need to be treated simultaneously with acrid and bitter medicinals. Generally, we also need to add warm, sweet and acrid medicinals to treat the *pǐ* syndrome to warm and supplement the deficient cold pattern. However, the chronic *pǐ* syndrome due to heat constraint in the upper and cold in the lower with symptoms of gastric distension and fullness, fatigue, anorexia, bitter taste and dryness in the mouth, a pale tongue with a slightly yellowish greasy coating should be treated with one of Zhang Zhong-jing's *Xiè Xīn Tāng* (Heart-Draining Decoction) formulas with *huáng qín* and *huáng lián* to warm the middle and lower while clearing empty heat in the upper.

3. The *pǐ* syndrome due to damp-heat retention or long standing liver qi stagnation turning into heat will injure the body fluid and yin. Therefore, we need to be careful when using acrid and drying medicinals, such as *shā rén, hòu pò, chén pí* and *fǎ bàn xià,* since they might further damage the fluids. In the course of rectifying qi and dissipating *pǐ*, we need to apply light natured medicinal to properly nourish stomach yin, such as *zhǐ qiào, fó shǒu, zhú rú,* and *hòu pò huā.* Similarly, the chosen medicinals to nourish stomach yin, should not be too greasy since they might hinder the qi movement.

COMPREHENSION QUESTIONS

1. Illustrate the diagnostic criteria of *pǐ* syndrome.
2. What are the treatment principles for the *pǐ* syndrome?
3. Multiple choice questions:

1) Mr. Zhang, 36 years old. The patient suffered from epigastric stuffiness, fullness and discomfort, nausea, vomiting, dry mouth without desire for drinking, poor appetite and digestion. His tongue was red with yellow greasy coating. Which *pǐ* syndrome is this?

A. Disharmony of the liver and stomach
B. Food stagnation
C. Insufficiency of stomach yin
D. Turbid phlegm accumulation in the middle *jiao*
E. Damp-heat accumulation in the stomach

2) Mr. Li, 43 years old. The patient suffered from epigastric pain, stuffiness and fullness, hunger without any desire to eat, nausea, belching, dry mouth and throat, constipation, a red tongue with scanty coating and a thin and rapid pulse. Which *pǐ* syndrome is this?

A. Spleen and stomach weakness
B. Disharmony of the liver and stomach
C. Insufficiency of stomach yin
D. Food stagnation
E. Damp-heat accumulation in the stomach

Answers

1. *Pǐ* syndrome is characterized by a subjective sensation of epigastric stuffiness, distension and fullness with softness and painlessness upon pressure and without any visible mass and nodule. It can present as an acute or a chronic case but it is often a reoccurring remitting condition. It is usually induced or triggered by irregular diet, emotional stress, poor living styles and season changes.

2. The fundamental treatment principles are to rectify the function of the spleen and stomach in the ascending and descending movement of qi and nutrients to disperse the *pǐ* syndrome and fullness. In this condition, we usually have to purge the excess by moving qi, dissipate stagnation, stop pain while supplementing deficiency.

3. 1) E, 2) C.

4.3 Vomiting

Vomiting is a syndrome due to the failure of the stomach qi to harmonize and descend causing the ascending of qi, food and fluids. Usually vomiting with sound and without stomach contents is called dry vomiting. Clinically, it is present in the courses of many diseases such as nervous vomiting, acute gastritis, cardiogenic vomiting, prolapse of stomach mucosa, intestinal obstruction, acute pancreatitis and so on.

The pathological manifestations of this disease are due to excess and deficiency patterns. Excess syndromes are caused by the pathogenic factors, such as external pathogenic factors, food stagnation, phlegm retention, and liver qi invading the stomach resulting in the obstruction of the stomach qi to ascend and cause vomiting. Deficiency syndromes are caused by qi and yin deficiency of the spleen and stomach, leading to disorder of transportation and transformation, and stomach qi failing to harmonize and descend. Generally, initial stage of vomiting belongs to the excess syndrome. If vomiting lasts for a long time, the spleen and stomach may be injured and become weak, and lead to a deficiency syndrome. If weakness of the spleen and stomach is further damaged by food, a deficiency and excess complex syndrome will occur.

CLINICAL PATTERNS DIFFERENTIATION AND TREATMENTS

1. Pathogenic Factors Attacking the Stomach

Symptoms: Sudden and violent vomiting of all contents in the stomach, chills and fever, body aches, chest and gastric fullness and discomfort, a white and greasy tongue coating and a soft and moderate pulse.

Treatment Principle:

- Remove pathogenic factors and release the exterior
- Resolve turbidity and harmonize the middle *jiao*

Main Acupuncture Points:

- RN 12 (*zhōng wǎn*): Front-*mu* point of the stomach to regulate spleen and stomach, harmonize middle *jiao* and descend rebellious qi
- ST 36 (*zú sān lǐ*): To expel dampness, strengthen healthy qi, invigorate spleen and promote circulation
- PC 6 (*nèi guān*): To alleviate nausea and vomiting, descend rebellious qi, regulate

stomach and unbind the chest

- SP 4 (*gōng sūn*): To resolve dampness, alleviate vomiting, regulate *chong* and *ren mai*, invigorate spleen and harmonize middle *jiao*
- SJ 5 (*wài guān*): To release the exterior and clear heat

Supporting Points:

- LI 4 (*hé gŭ*): To release the exterior, clear *yang ming* heat and stop toothache
- ST 25 (*tiān shū*): To invigorate spleen and stomach, clear damp-heat, alleviate vomiting and resolve stagnation

Recommended Formula: *Huò Xiāng Zhèng Qì Săn* (藿香正气散, Agastache Qi-Correcting Powder) from the *Beneficial Formulas from the Taiping Imperial Pharmacy* (*Tài Píng Huì Mín Hé Jì Jú Fāng*, 太平惠民和剂局方)

Substitute Formula: *Xīn Jiā Xiāng Rú Yĭn* (新加香薷饮, Newly Supplemented Mosla Beverage)

Patent Formula: *Huò Xiāng Zhèng Qì Ruăn Jiāo Náng* (藿香正气软胶囊, Agastache Qi-Correcting Soft Capsule)

2. Food Retention

Symptoms: Foul-smelling vomiting, halitosis, gastric or abdominal distension and fullness, belching, poor appetite, symptoms aggravate after eating and alleviate after vomiting, foul-smelling loose stools or constipation, a thick and greasy tongue coating and a slippery and excessive pulse.

Treatment Principle:

- Promote digestion and strengthen spleen qi
- Harmonize the stomach and descend stomach qi

Main Acupuncture Points:

- PC 6 (*nèi guān*): To alleviate nausea and vomiting, descend rebellious qi, regulate stomach
- RN 12 (*zhōng wăn*): Front-*mu* point of the stomach to regulate spleen and stomach, harmonize middle *jiao* and regulate qi
- ST 36 (*zú sān lĭ*): To invigorate spleen, support the healthy qi, stop pain and promote circulation
- RN 10 (*xià wăn*): To regulate qi, dispel food stagnation and stop abdominal pain
- ST 21 (*liáng mén*): To harmonize middle *jiao*, transform stagnation, raise qi and alleviate vomiting
- BL 21 (*wèi shù*): Back-*shu* point of the stomach, to invigorate spleen and harmonize stomach, and promote digestion

Supporting Points:

- LI 9 (*tài yuān*): To treat vomiting, headaches and dizziness due to *yang ming* fire
- SJ 6 (*zhī gōu*): To redirect the rebellious stomach qi downward, clear heat and resolve constipation

Recommended Formula: *Băo Hé Wán* (保和丸, Harmony-Preserving Pill) from the

Teachings of [Zhu] Dan-xi (*Dān Xī Xīn Fǎ*, 丹溪心法)

Substitute Formula: *Zhǐ Shí Dǎo Zhì Wán* (枳实导滞丸, Immature Bitter Orange Stagnation-Moving Pill)

Patent Formula: *Bǎo Hé Wán* (保和丸, Harmony-Preserving Pill)

3. Internal Obstruction of Phlegm

Symptoms: Vomiting of clear fluids or saliva, gastric discomfort, poor appetite, dizziness, blurry vision, palpitations, a white and greasy tongue coating and a slippery pulse.

Treatment Principle:

- Warm the spleen and resolve phlegm
- Harmonize the stomach and descend stomach qi

Main Acupuncture Points:

- PC 6 (*nèi guān*): To alleviate nausea and vomiting, descend rebellious qi and regulate stomach
- RN 12 (*zhōng wǎn*): Front-*mu* point of the stomach to harmonize spleen and stomach, warm middle *jiao* and regulate qi
- ST 36 (*zú sān lǐ*): To invigorate spleen, support the correct qi, stop pain and promote circulation
- ST 40 (*fēng lóng*): To expel phlegm and dampness from the lung, heart and chest
- SP 9 (*yīn líng quán*): To harmonize middle *jiao*, expel dampness and resolve edema
- SP 4 (*gōng sūn*): To resolve dampness, alleviate vomiting, regulate *chong* and *ren mai*, invigorate spleen and harmonize middle *jiao*

Supporting Points:

- LV 3 (*tài chōng*): *Yuan*-source point of the liver to clear liver and gallbladder damp-heat, alleviate vomiting, clear head and eyes, unbind the chest and stop pain
- SP 8 (*dì jī*): *Xi*-cleft point of the spleen to resolve dampness and regulate spleen, improve digestion and benefit appetite

Recommended Formula: *Líng Guì Zhú Gān Tāng* (苓桂术甘汤, Poria, Cinnamon, Bighead Atractylodes and Licorice Decoction) combined with *Xiǎo Bàn Xià Tāng* (小半夏汤, Minor Pinellia Decoction) from the *Essentials from the Golden Cabinet* (*Jīn Guì Yào Lüè*, 金匮要略)

Substitute Formula: *Wēn Dǎn Tāng* (温胆汤, Gallbladder-Warming Decoction)

4. Liver Qi Stagnation Affecting the Stomach

Symptoms: Vomiting with acid reflux, frequent belching, hypochondriac pain, a red tongue around the edges with a thin greasy coating and a wiry pulse.

Treatment Principle:

- Soothe the liver and regulate qi
- Harmonize the stomach and descend stomach qi

Main Acupuncture Points:

- PC 6 (*nèi guān*): To alleviate nausea and vomiting, descend rebellious qi and regulate stomach
- BL 18 (*gān shù*): Back-*shu* point of the liver to spread liver qi, clear liver and gallbladder heat, unbind the chest and promote circulation
- RN 12 (*zhōng wǎn*): Front-*mu* point of the stomach to harmonize spleen and stomach, warm middle *jiao* and regulate qi
- ST 36 (*zú sān lǐ*): To invigorate spleen, support the correct qi, stop pain and promote circulation
- LV 3 (*tài chōng*): *Yuan*-source point of the liver to spread liver qi, subdue liver yang, unbind the chest and stop pain
- GB 34 (*yáng líng quán*): To spread liver and gallbladder qi, clear damp-heat and stop pain

Supporting Points:

- GB 25 (*jīng mén*): To resolve belching and acid reflux
- SP 11 (*jī mén*): To clear damp-heat and open and regulate lower *jiao*

Recommended Formula: *Chái Hú Shū Gān Săn* (柴胡疏肝散, Bupleurum Liver-Soothing Powder) from *The Complete Works of [Zhang] Jing-yue* (*Jĭng Yuè Quán Shū*, 景岳全书)

Substitute Formula: *Yuè Jú Wán* (越鞠丸, Constraint-Resolving Pill)

Patent Formula: *Chái Hú Shū Gān Wán* (柴胡舒肝丸, Bupleurum Liver-Soothing Pill)

5. Deficient Cold in the Spleen and Stomach

Symptoms: Intermittent vomiting, pale complexion, fatigue, dry mouth with no desire to drink, aversion to cold, cold limbs, loose stools, a pale and swollen tongue with thin white and moist coating and a deep, weak and slow pulse.

Treatment Principle:

- Warm the middle *jiao* and strengthen the spleen
- Harmonize the stomach and descend stomach-qi

Main Acupuncture Points:

- BL 20 (*pí shù*): Back-*shu* point of the spleen to regulate middle *jiao* qi, invigorate spleen, alleviate vomiting and stop abdominal pain
- BL 21 (*wèi shù*): Back-*shu* point of the stomach to invigorate spleen and harmonize stomach, alleviate nausea and vomiting, promote digestion and stop hypochondriac pain
- ST 36 (*zú sān lǐ*): To invigorate spleen, nourish original qi, alleviate vomiting and promote circulation
- RN 12 (*zhōng wǎn*): Front-*mu* point of the stomach to harmonize spleen and stomach, warm middle *jiao* and regulate qi
- RN 4 (*guān yuán*): Front-*mu* point of the small intestine to tonify original qi, supplement deficiencies, regulate *chong* and *ren mai*

- RN 8 (*shén què*): Apply moxibustion to warm the yang and resolve edema

Supporting Points:

- BL 30 (*bái huán shù*): To warm the uterus and lower *jiao*, treat leukorrhea and seminal emission
- SP 14 (*fù jié*): To invigorate spleen and warm middle *jiao*, descend rebellious qi and umbilical pain

Recommended Formula: *Lǐ Zhōng Wán* (理中丸, Center-Regulating Pill) from the *Treatise on Cold Damage* (*Shāng Hán Lùn*, 伤寒论)

Substitute Formula: *Fù Zǐ Lǐ Zhōng Wán* (附子理中丸, Aconite Center-Regulating Pill)

Patent Formula: *Lǐ Zhōng Wán* (理中丸, Center-Regulating Pill)

6. Stomach Yin Deficiency

Symptoms: Frequent vomiting, dry retching, dry mouth, dry throat, hunger with no desire to eat, a dry and red tongue and a thready and rapid pulse.

Treatment Principle:

- Nourish stomach yin and supplement body fluids
- Descend rebellious qi and relieve vomiting

Main Acupuncture Points:

- BL 20 (*pí shù*): Back-*shu* point of the spleen to regulate middle *jiao* qi, invigorate spleen, alleviate vomiting and stop abdominal pain
- BL 21 (*wèi shù*): Back-*shu* point of the stomach to invigorate spleen and harmonize stomach, alleviate nausea and vomiting, promote digestion and stop hypochondriac pain
- PC 8 (*láo gōng*): To tonify stomach yin, clear middle *jiao* heat and resolve halitosis
- RN 12 (*zhōng wǎn*): Front-*mu* point of the stomach to regulate spleen and stomach, harmonize middle *jiao* and descend rebellious qi
- KI 6 (*zhào hǎi*): To nourish yin and clear deficient heat
- SP 6 (*sān yīn jiāo*): To invigorate spleen and nourish yin, harmonize the lower *jiao*, regulate menstruation, alleviate vomiting and improve digestion

Supporting Points:

- LV 3 (*tài chōng*): *Yuan*-source point of the liver to nourish liver yin and blood, treat irregular menstruation
- LU 10 (*yú jì*): To descend rebellious qi, harmonize stomach and heart, moisten dry throat and clear lung heat

Recommended Formula: *Mài Mén Dōng Tāng* (麦门冬汤, Ophiopogon Decoction) from the *Essentials from the Golden Cabinet* (*Jīn Guì Yào Lüè*, 金匮要略)

Substitute Formula: *Yì Wèi Tāng* (益胃汤, Stomach-Boosting Decoction)

Patent Formula: *Yǎng Wèi Shū Jiāo Náng* (养胃舒胶囊, Stomach-Nourishing Capsule)

Summary Chart for Vomiting

Patterns	Main Points	Supporting Points	Formulae
Pathogenic Factors Attacking the Stomach	RN 12, ST 36, PC 6, SP 4, SJ 5	LI 4 for toothache due to *yang ming* heat ST 25 for damp-heat affliction	*Huò Xiāng Zhèng Qì Sǎn* or *Xīn Jiā Xiāng Rú Yǐn*
Food Retention	PC 6, RN 12, ST 36, RN 10, ST 21, BL 21	LI 9 for headaches and dizziness due to *yang ming* fire SJ 6 for constipation	*Bǎo Hé Wán* or *Zhǐ Shí Dǎo Zhì Wán*
Internal Obstruction of Phlegm-rheum	PC 6, RN 12, ST 36, ST 40, SP 9, SP 4	LV 3 for liver and gallbladder damp-heat SP 8 for indigestion and poor appetite	*Líng Guì Zhú Gān Tāng* plus *Xiǎo Bàn Xià Tāng* or *Wēn Dǎn Tāng*
Liver Qi Invading the Stomach	PC 6, BL 18, RN 12, ST 36, LV 3, GB 34	GB 25 for acid reflux SP 11 for lower *jiao* accumulation	*Chái Hú Shū Gān Sǎn* or *Yuè Jú Wán*
Deficient Cold in the Spleen and Stomach	BL 20, BL 21, ST 36, RN 12, RN 4, RN 8	BL 30, for uterine cold, irregular menstruation and seminal emission SP 14 for umbilical pain due to middle *jiao* cold	*Lǐ Zhōng Wán* or *Fù Zǐ Lǐ Zhōng Wán*
Stomach Yin Deficiency	BL 20, BL 21, PC 8, RN 12, KI 6, SP 6	LV 3 for stomach and liver yin deficiency LU 10 for dry and painful throat	*Mài Mén Dōng Tāng* or *Yì Wèi Tāng*

CASE STUDY 1: Vomiting with Constipation

Mr. Sun, 46 years old. 1st consultation on May 30th, 1997.

Main Complaint: Dry mouth and vomiting for a month.

Medical History: The patient suffered from gastritis 6 years ago. He took Chinese and Western medications intermittently. Most of the Chinese medicinals taken were warm, hot, aromatic and dry in quality. His condition was sometimes mild and sometimes severe. In the recent month, he had symptoms of dry mouth and throat without any appetite and later on he also suffered from constipation. He received western medical treatment which was ineffective. The patient had a history of drinking alcohol and smoking.

Presenting Symptoms: Vomiting saliva, no appetite, dry mouth and throat, constipation, slightly yellow urine, a red tongue without coating and a thin pulse.

Physical Examination: Temperature: 36.8 ℃, pulse: 90 bpm, respiration: 20 bpm, blood pressure: 120/70 mmHg. The patient was conscious with a red face and a hoarse voice. His chest was symmetric and the respiratory sounds were normal without any dry or moist rales. There was tenderness in the epigastric region and his abdomen was flat. A fibergastroscope test showed atrophic gastritis.

Pattern Differentiation

The patient has suffered from pain in the stomach area for a long time and often takes aromatic and dry medicinals which easily consume qi and damage yin. This damage combined with the inability for the stomach to descend the qi and harmonize, lack of appetite, nausea and vomiting of saliva will result. Extensive vomiting and anorexia cause body fluid deficiency seen in the symptoms of dry throat, mouth and constipation. The signs of red tongue without coating and thin pulse are also signs of lack of body fluids.

Diagnosis

TCM Diagnosis: Vomiting due to stomach qi and yin deficiency
Western Medicine Diagnosis: Vomiting with constipation

Treatment

The chief pathomechanisms of this case are mainly the lack of body fluids and stomach qi deficiency with the inability to harmonize and descend causing symptoms of belching, vomiting and dry mouth and throat.

Principles:

- Nourish yin and supplement body fluids
- Strengthen the stomach qi and stop vomiting

Formula: Modified *Mài Mén Dōng Tāng* (Ophiopogon Decoction)

Ingredients:

党参	*dǎng shēn*	15 g	Radix Codonopsis
沙参	*shā shēn*	15 g	Radix Adenophorae seu Glehniae
麦冬	*mài dōng*	15 g	Radix Ophiopogonis
石斛	*shí hú*	15 g	Caulis Dendrobii
半夏	*bàn xià*	15 g	Rhizoma Pinelliae
旋覆花	*xuán fù huā*	10 g	Flos Inulae
竹茹	*zhú rú*	10 g	Caulis Bambusae in Taenia
葛根	*gé gēn*	15 g	Radix Puerariae Lobatae
火麻仁	*huǒ má rén*	15 g	Fructus Cannabis
生姜	*shēng jiāng*	10 g	Rhizoma Zingiberis Recens
香橼	*xiāng yuán*	12 g	Fructus Citri
山药	*shān yào*	15 g	Rhizoma Dioscoreae
甘草	*gān cǎo*	6 g	Radix et Rhizoma Glycyrrhizae

Formula Analysis

The medicinals *dǎng shēn, shān yào, shā shēn, gé gēn, shí hú* and *mài dōng* are in the formula to fortify the spleen, tonify the stomach and enrich fluids. *Bàn xià, xuán fù huā, zhú rú* and *shēng jiāng* serve to redirect the counterflow of qi and stop vomiting. *Xiāng yuán* moves qi and disinhibits the stagnation of qi and *huǒ má rén* moistens the intestines to unblock the stools. An addition dose of 9 g of *Mài Dōng Dì Huáng Wán* (Ophiopogon and Rehmannia Pill) was taken twice a day and the patient was advised to avoid raw, cold, oily, greasy and dry food.

Follow-up Consultations

After three doses of the formula, the symptoms of nausea and vomiting were resolved, his mouth was not as dry and there was a normal amount of saliva. The patient continued to take 3 more doses, he was able to pass stools and his appetite was normal. The patient was advised to avoid aromatic and dry food to prevent from a relapse.

CASE STUDY 2: Acute Vomiting
By Dr. Li Jie-ming

Ms. Zou, 24 years old. 1st consultation on December 11th, 1991.

Main Complaint: Nausea and vomiting for over a month.

Medical History: A month ago, the patient suffered from nausea and vomiting especially after meals, accompanied by belching, anorexia and epigastric pain. She was given metoclopramide, aluzyme and other orally administered medication from the school nurse but symptoms remained the same and she was sent to a hospital for treatment. A gastroscopy and a test of the liver function showed no abnormal findings and the patient was diagnosed as "gastric neurosis".

Presenting Symptoms: Nausea, vomiting, chest and epigastric stuffiness and distress, frequent belching, poor appetite, dry mouth without desire to drink, loose stools once or twice per day, a pale tongue with a slightly greasy coating and a thin pulse.

Diagnosis

TCM Diagnosis: Vomiting due to internal obstruction of phlegm and fluid retention

Western Medicine Diagnosis: Vomiting

Treatment

The pathomechanism of this case is mainly deficiency of the spleen and stomach with retention of phlegm, and failure of the stomach qi to harmonize and descend causing vomiting.

Principles:

- Direct qi downward and stop vomiting
- Strengthen the spleen and harmonize the stomach

Formula: Modified *Xuán Fù Dài Zhě Tāng* (Inula and Hematite Decoction)

Ingredients:

旋覆花	*xuán fù huā*	12 g	Flos Inulae (wrapped)
代赭石	*dài zhě shí*	15 g	Haematitum (decocted first)
陈皮	*chén pí*	12 g	Pericarpium Citri Reticulatae
半夏	*bàn xià*	10 g	Rhizoma Pinelliae
党参	*dǎng shēn*	15 g	Radix Codonopsis
苏梗	*sū gěng*	12 g	Caulis Perillae
藿香	*huò xiāng*	10 g	Herba Agastachis (added later)
佩兰	*pèi lán*	10 g	Herba Eupatorii
鸡内金	*jī nèi jīn*	10 g	Endothelium Corneum Gigeriae Galli
谷芽	*gǔ yá*	15 g	Fructus Setariae Germinatus
麦芽	*mài yá*	15 g	Fructus Hordei Germinatus
生姜	*shēng jiāng*	6 g	Rhizoma Zingiberis Recens
砂仁	*shā rén*	6 g	Fructus Amomi (cracked)
木香	*mù xiāng*	12 g	Radix Aucklandiae
白术	*bái zhú*	12 g	Rhizoma Atractylodis Macrocephalae (dry-fried)
大枣	*dà zǎo*	20 g	Fructus Jujubae

Follow-up Consultations

After 3 doses of the formula, the symptoms of chest and epigastric fullness and distress, belching, nausea, and vomiting were significantly relieved and her appetite improved. After 7 more doses, all symptoms were mostly resolved and the tongue was pale red with a white coating and the pulse was thin. At this time, *mù xiāng* was removed from the formula and the patient took another 3 doses to consolidate the treatment.

Clinical Analysis

The symptom of vomiting is classified into four patterns: cold, hot, deficiency and excess, but the main pathogenesis is the counterflow of stomach qi moving upward causing the vomiting. Therefore, the common treatment principle in all patterns is to harmonize the stomach and redirect the stomach qi downwards. A formula commonly used by Dr. Li is *Xuán Fù Dài Zhě Tāng* (Inula and Hematite Decoction). The medicinal *xuán fù huā* can redirect the stomach qi downwards and stop vomiting, dissolve phlegm and promote urination. *Bàn xià* can redirect the counterflow downwards and eliminate phlegm. *Shēng jiāng* serves to warm the middle, harmonize the stomach, redirect the counterflow downwards, stop vomiting and eliminate phlegm. *Dài zhě shí* is strong at redirecting the counterflow downwards. *Dǎng shēn, gān cǎo* and *dà zǎo* can tonify qi, harmonize the middle *jiao* and supplement deficiency. This formula is greatly efficient while its ingredients are fairly simple. Modification of this formula is also possible to treat the pattern causing the vomiting.

In this case of vomiting, aside from deficiency of spleen and phlegm stagnation, there is food retention for which Dr. Li added the aromatics medicinals *huò xiāng* and *pèi lán* to remove turbidity, awaken the spleen and reinforce the stomach. *Jī nèi jīn, gǔ yá* and *mài yá* can promote digestion and remove food stagnation. *Chén pí, mù xiāng, shā rén, bái zhú,* and *sū gěng* can move qi and fortify the spleen. All the ingredients of this formula can restore the transportation function of the middle *jiao*, remove phlegm and dampness, promote digestion and stop vomiting.

CASE STUDY 3: Nervous Vomiting
By Dr. Chen Shao-long

Mr. Cheng, 16 years old. 1st consultation on May 18th, 1997.

Main Complaint: Paroxysmal vomiting for three years with aggravation for two days.

Medical History: Three years ago, the patient vomited before and after having examinations at school. Intravenous dripping of metoclopramide was slightly effective in the past but had not proven effective in the last two days. No organic lesions were found by examination. It was diagnosed as "nervous vomiting".

Presenting Symptoms: Restlessness, hypochondriac and epigastric fullness, distension and discomfort, mild aversion to wind and cold, occasional nausea, belching, paroxysmal vomiting of yellowish-green watery liquid which relieved part of his symptoms. The tongue was pale with thick and slightly greasy coating and the pulse was wiry and thready.

Physical Examination: The patient was conscious with a pale complexion. His abdomen was distended without any tenderness. The liver and gallbladder were not palpable below the costal region.

Diagnosis

TCM Diagnosis: Vomiting due to liver qi stagnation attacking the stomach
Western Medicine Diagnosis: Nervous vomiting

Treatment

Principles:

- Calm the heart and tranquilize the mind
- Regulate qi and smooth the liver
- Harmonize the stomach and redirect counterflow downward

Main Acupuncture Points: DU 20 (*bǎi huì*), PC 7 (*dà líng*), ST 36 (*zú sān lǐ*), SP 4 (*gōng sūn*), LV 3 (*tài chōng*).

Manipulations: Apply 90 small moxa cones of moxibustion on DU 20 and needle ST 36, SP 4, LV 3 and PC 7 by applying the supplementation method at first and then follow with the drainage method while retaining the needles for 30 minutes after obtaining qi.

Follow-up Consultations

One treatment later, his vomiting stopped instantly, but there were still nausea, distension and fullness in the epigastrium and rib-side regions. Three treatments later, all symptoms resolved. Another two treatments were given to consolidate the effect. There was no relapse in the following year.

Clinical Analysis

This disease is due to the failure of the stomach qi to descend which creates a counterflow of qi and causes vomiting. This case of vomiting is caused by the stress during the examination causing liver qi stagnation affecting the stomach. The *du mai* is the sea of all yang channels which governs all the yang of the body. The DU 20 is at the top of the head, being the confluent point of all the yang channels and is also the key point of the *du mai*. Therefore, moxibustion on this point can invigorate yang qi of the whole body, harmonize qi movement, and balance yin and yang. PC 7 is on the pericardium channel of hand *jue yin* which mainly treats disorders of the heart, mind and spleen. The combination of DU 20 and PC 7 serves to calm the heart and tranquilize the mind, redirect qi downwards and harmonize the stomach. As the *The Yellow Emperor's Inner Classic* (*Huáng Dì Nèi Jīng*, 黄帝内经) states: "*He*-sea point can treat the diseases of *fu*-organs." This explains choosing ST 36, the *he*-sea point of foot *yang ming* channel to regulate the function of the stomach and intestines. SP 4 and LV 3 are combined to fortify the spleen and boost qi, as well as to purge the stagnation of liver qi.

KEY CLINICAL POINTS

The treatment principle of vomiting is to harmonize the stomach and redirect the counterflow downwards, but we must also treat the pattern cause to have timely results. Generally speaking, excessive patterns are usually easier to treat and deficient and complex patterns are more difficult to treat and are more prone to relapses. Hence, treating chronic cases will need a longer course of treatment with a longer observation period after the symptoms have receded. Meanwhile, these additional key points are also worth noticing.

1. *Bàn Xià* is a strong medicinal to treat vomiting. In the medical classical text *Essentials from the Golden Cabinet* (*Jīn Guì Yào Lüè*, 金匮要略), the major and minor *Bàn*

Xià Tāng (Pinellia Decoction) formulas are noted to treat vomiting. Zhu Liang-chun, a famous TCM doctor, believes "only raw *bàn xià* has significant curative effect to stop vomiting". However, raw *bàn xià* is toxic, so it should be decocted 30 minutes before adding other ingredients until the toxicity is reduced. If *bàn xià* is smashed with fresh ginger before decocting, the efficacy on treating vomiting increases. In addition, *shān yào* (Rhizoma Dioscoreae) porridge can be taken as its sticky quality retains the medicinal effect in the stomach. Since *shān yào* can supplement the lung, promote fluid production in the upper, boost the kidney and inhibit surging of the *chong mai* in the lower, it is especially appropriate to combine with *bàn xià* to treat severe vomiting.

2. *Dà huáng* and *gān cǎo* can also treat vomiting, especially when the regular methods and medicinals have shown no effect. These two medicinals can treat vomiting immediately after food or when suffering from uremia. In the *Essentials from the Golden Cabinet (Jīn Guì Yào Lüè,* 金匮要略), it states: "for vomiting immediately after having food, *Dà Huáng Gān Cǎo Tāng* (Rhubarb and Licorice Decoction) governs." This formula contains only two ingredients, *dà huáng* 9 g and *gān cǎo* 6 g, but its curative effect is usually quite immediate. In clinical practice, we should mainly consider these medicinals when vomiting happens soon after eating rather than in other patterns. As *dà huáng* is bitter and cold, and able to relax the bowels, promote urination, regulate the center, promote digestion, and harmonize five *zang*-organs, it is taken as a chief ingredient. *Gān cǎo*, the deputy ingredient, acts to revive the center, thus making the clear qi ascend and the turbidity descend. Therefore, the stomach qi becomes smooth and the vomiting is cured spontaneously.

3. Besides the acupuncture points already mentioned, ear acupuncture can also be used to treat vomiting such as the areas of the *wèi* (stomach), *gān* (liver), *jiāo gǎn* (sympathetic), *pí zhì xià* (subcortex) and *shén mén* (*shen men*).

4. Prolonged vomiting will produce a severe body fluid and original qi deficiency which will cause a series of other severe symptoms which also must be addressed in the treatment approach.

BRIEF SUMMARY

The basic pathogenesis of vomiting is the failure of the stomach qi to descend and harmonize. It involves many pathogenic factors with deficiency and excess patterns but they all cause the counterflow of stomach qi upward presenting as the symptom of vomiting. The deficiency syndrome is due to the deficiency of stomach causing the failure of the stomach qi to descend and harmonize, while the excess syndrome due to pathogenic factors such as six excesses, improper diet, phlegm, retained fluid, qi stagnation, and static blood attacking the stomach and resulting in counterflow of stomach qi. The location of vomiting lies in the stomach and it is also related to the spleen and liver. The deficiency syndrome mostly involves the spleen, while the excess syndrome implicates the liver. Therefore, the treatment principles are rectifying the spleen and stomach, redirecting the qi counterflow and relieving vomiting. The primary selection of acupuncture points are the front-*mu* and back-*shu* points of the stomach, respectively RN 12 (*zhōng wǎn*) and BL 21 (*wèi shù*) to harmonize the stomach and stop vomiting. PC 6 (*nèi guān*) can rectify the chest and stomach qi and redirect qi counterflow downwards, making it one of the primary points to treat vomiting.

COMPREHENSION QUESTIONS

1. What are the disease causes and pathomechanism of vomiting?
2. What are the differentiating patterns and associated treatment for vomiting?
3. Multiple choice questions:

1) The patient suffered from vomiting after eating improper food with intermittent occurrence and remission, poor appetite, bright pale complexion, fatigue, lack of strength, preferred warmth, aversion of cold, cool extremities, thirst without desire to drink, loose stools, a pale tongue with a thin and white coating and a soggy and weak pulse. Select the most appropriate formula:

A. Modified *Lǐ Zhōng Tāng* (Center-Regulating Decoction)
B. Modified *Yī Guàn Jiān* (Effective Integration Decoction) combined with *Sháo Yào Gān Cǎo Tāng* (Peony and Licorice Decoction)
C. Modified *Sì Qī Tāng* (Four for Seven Decoction)
D. Modified *Xiǎo Bàn Xià Tāng* (Minor Pinellia Decoction) combined with *Líng Guì Zhú Gān Tāng* (Poria, Cinnamon Twig, Atractylodes Macrocephala and Licorice Decoction)
E. Modified *Huò Xiāng Zhèng Qì Sǎn* (Agastache Qi-Correcting Powder)

2) Female, 42 years old. The patient suffered from nausea and vomiting for 3 months with accompanied symptoms of poor appetite, indigestion, epigastric stuffiness and distress, difficult stools, a white and slippery tongue coating and a deficient and wiry pulse. The disease pattern is:

A. Exogenous pathogens attacking the stomach
B. Internal food stagnation
C. Internal obstruction of phlegm and fluid retention
D. Liver qi attacking the stomach
E. Spleen and stomach qi deficiency

Answers

1. The general pathomechanism of vomiting is the failure of the stomach qi to harmonize and descend causing the counterflow of stomach qi presenting as vomiting. There are various causes for this syndrome. Exogenous pathogens include the six excesses and turbidity such as cold, heat, dampness, phlegm, wind and qi and

blood stasis. This syndrome might also be due to improper diet such as excessive food intake, having too much cold, raw, acrid, spicy, sweet, fatty and insanitary food, excessive drinking of alcohol, all of which harm the stomach and spleen, causing the counterflow of stomach qi. Emotional, physical and mental stress or over exhaustion can also impair the spleen and stomach qi resulting in vomiting.

2. These are the clinical patterns and their treatment approaches:

• For pathogenic factors attacking the stomach, the recommended formula is: *Huò Xiāng Zhèng Qì Săn* (Agastache Qi-Correcting Powder) or *Xīn Jiā Xiāng Rú Yĭn* (Newly Supplemented Mosla Beverage)

• For food retention, the recommended formula is: *Băo Hé Wán* (Harmony-Preserving Pill) or *Zhĭ Shí Dăo Zhì Wán* (Immature Bitter Orange Stagnation-Moving Pill)

• For internal obstruction of turbid phlegm, the recommended formula is: *Líng Guì Zhú Gān Tāng* (Poria, Cinnamon, Bighead Atractylodes and Licorice Decoction) combined with *Xiăo Bàn Xià Tāng* (Minor Pinellia Decoction), or *Wēn Dăn Tāng* (Gallbladder-Warming Decoction)

• Liver qi stagnation affecting the stomach, the recommended formula is: *Chái Hú Shū Gān Săn* (Bupleurum Liver-Soothing Powder) or *Yuè Jú Wán* (Constraint-Resolving Pill)

• Deficient cold of the spleen and stomach, the recommended formula is: *Lĭ Zhōng Wán* (Center-Regulating Pill) or *Fù Zĭ Lĭ Zhōng Wán* (Aconite Center-Regulating Pill)

3. 1) A, 2) E.

4.4 Constipation

Constipation is a common functional gastrointestinal disease characterized by the decreased frequency of defecation, difficult of defecation, incomplete defecation, dry and scant constipated stool without any organic diseases causing the symptoms.

There are various pathomecanisms leading to constipation. Some are deficiency patterns including qi deficiency, blood and body fluid deficiency, some are due to overwork and exhaustion, some are due to poor life styles such as irregular diet, emotional and mental stress, aging and so on. Other patterns are excess patterns such as heat accumulation in the stomach and intestines, cold accumulation, phlegm retention and blood stasis. The disease location lies in the large intestine, but it is also closely related to the functions of the spleen, stomach, lung, liver and kidney. The spleen and stomach are the sea of transformation and transportation. The spleen governs transformation and transportation, while the stomach harmonizes and descends the qi to the intestines. In the understanding of digestion of Chinese medicine, every organ has an important function to fulfill. The food is eaten through the mouth and received and digested by the stomach and then transformed, transported and distributed by the spleen. The stomach qi descends the nutrient to the intestine so the nutrients are absorbed and the turbid fluid and qi are expelled. The liver regulates the smooth flow of qi to assure the proper functions of all organs accordingly. The kidney and spleen have warming and nourishing functions and the lung has descending and purification functions. If any of these organs are attacked by pathogenic factors or are deficient and can not function properly it might cause constipation. If there is liver qi stagnation, the *fu* organs will be blocked and the stools will not move out freely. If the kidney qi is deficient, the large intestine will be too weak to expel the stools. If the lung qi does not descend properly, the stomach and large intestine of the *yang ming* channels will also be inhibited. Furthermore, constipation can manifest as a cold, heat, deficiency and excess pattern. Identifying the correct pattern and treating it accordingly will bring about clinical success.

CLINICAL PATTERNS DIFFERENTIATION AND TREATMENTS

1. Excess Heat Accumulation in the Intestines

Symptoms: Dry stools, difficult and infrequent defecation, scanty, yellow or reddish colored urine, flushed face, fever, abdominal distension and pain, dry mouth, halitosis, a red tongue with a dry yellow coating and a slippery and rapid pulse.

Treatment Principle:

- Clear heat and resolve stagnation
- Moisten the large intestine and resolve constipation

Main Acupuncture Points:

- BL 25 (*dà cháng shù*): Back-*shu* point of the large intestine to regulate intestinal qi and resolve stagnation
- ST 25 (*tiān shū*): Front-*mu* point of the large intestine to invigorate stomach and intestines, regulate qi, stop pain, clear heat and resolve stagnation
- SJ 6 (*zhī gōu*): To downbear rebellious qi, clear heat and resolve constipation
- LI 4 (*hé gǔ*): *Yuan*-source point of the large intestine to active the intestines, regulate qi, stop pain and resolve constipation
- ST 37 (*shàng jù xū*) and LI 11 (*qū chí*): upper and lower *he*-sea points of the large intestine, to regulate intestines, resolve stagnation, clear heat and stop pain
- ST 44 (*nèi tíng*): To clear intestinal heat and harmonize intestines

Supporting Points:

- KI 6 (*zhào hǎi*): To nourish yin and clear deficient heat
- LI 9 (*shàng lián*): To treat vomiting, headaches and dizziness due to *yang ming* fire

Recommended Formula: *Má Zǐ Rén Wán* (麻子仁丸, Cannabis Fruit Pill) from the *Treatise on Cold Damage* (*Shāng Hán Lùn*, 伤寒论)

Substitute Formula:

- *Rùn Cháng Wán* (润肠丸, Intestines-Moistening Pill)
- *Dà Chéng Qì Tāng* (大承气汤, Major Purgative Decoction)

Patent Formula:

- *Dāng Guī Lóng Huì Wán* (当归龙荟丸, Chinese Angelica, Gentian, and Aloe Pill)
- *Má Rén Ruǎn Jiāo Náng* (麻仁软胶囊, Cannabis Fruit Soft Capsule)

2. Qi Stagnation in the Intestines

Symptoms: Difficult or incomplete defecation, belching, flatulence, borborygmus, chest and hypochondrium fullness and discomfort, abdominal distension and pain, poor appetite, emaciation, all symptoms aggravated by emotional and mental stress, a pale red tongue with a thin white greasy coating and a wiry pulse.

Treatment Principle:

- Regulate qi and resolve stasis
- Soothe the intestines and resolve constipation

Main Acupuncture Points:

- ST 25 (*tiān shū*): Front-*mu* point of the large intestine to invigorate stomach and intestines, regulate qi, improve digestion and resolve stagnation
- ST 28 (*shuǐ dào*): To regulate lower *jiao* qi and resolve constipation
- LV 3 (*tài chōng*): *Yuan*-source point of the liver to spread liver qi, soothe emotions, unbind the chest and stop pain

- RN 12 (*zhōng wăn*): To harmonize spleen and stomach, warm middle *jiao* and regulate qi
- BL 25 (*dà cháng shù*): Back-*shu* point of the large intestine to regulate intestinal qi and resolve stagnation
- SJ 6 (*zhī gōu*): To treat chest and hypochondriac pain and regulate qi

Supporting Points:

- GB 24 (*rì yuè*): Front-*mu* point of the gallbladder to resolve hypochondriac pain, spread liver qi and harmonize intestines
- PC 6 (*nèi guān*): To regulate qi, unbind the chest and stop abdominal pain

Recommended Formula: *Liù Mó Tāng* (六磨汤, Six Milled Ingredients Decoction) from the *Standards for Diagnosis and Treatment* (*Zhèng Zhì Zhŭn Shéng*, 证治准绳)

Substitute Formula:

- *Chái Hú Shū Gān Săn* (柴胡疏肝散, Bupleurum Liver-Soothing Powder)
- *Sì Mò Tāng* (四磨汤, Four Milled Ingredients Decoction)

Patent Formula:

- *Chái Hú Shū Gān Wán* (柴胡舒肝丸, Bupleurum Liver-Soothing Pill)
- *Mù Xiāng Shùn Qì Wán* (木香顺气丸, Costus Root Qi-Balancing Pill)

3. Spleen Qi Deficiency

Symptoms: Constipation with borborygmus, unable to complete defecation because of lack of strength, defecation followed by sweating and shortness of breath, pale complexion, lassitude, fatigue, reluctance to speak, a pale and tender tongue with thin white coating and a weak pulse.

Treatment Principle:

- Invigorate spleen to supplement qi
- Warm the lower *jiao* and moisten the intestines

Main Acupuncture Points:

- BL 20 (*pí shù*): Back-*shu* point of the spleen to regulate middle *jiao* qi, invigorate spleen and stop abdominal pain
- BL 25 (*dà cháng shù*): Back-*shu* point of the large intestine to regulate intestinal qi and resolve stagnation
- ST 25 (*tiān shū*): Front-*mu* point of the large intestine to invigorate stomach and intestines, regulate qi, improve digestion and resolve stagnation
- ST 37 (*shàng jù xū*): Lower *he*-sea point of the large intestine to regulate intestines, resolve stagnation, clear heat and stop pain
- RN 6 (*qì hăi*): To invigorate spleen and tonify original qi, promote circulation resolve fatigue
- SJ 6 (*zhī gōu*): To unbind the chest, descend rebellious qi and resolve constipation

Supporting Points:

- SP 8 (*dì jī*): *Xi*-cleft point of the spleen to resolve dampness and regulate spleen, improve digestion and benefit appetite

- ST 36 (*zú sān lǐ*): To expel dampness, invigorate spleen, tonify qi and promote circulation

Recommended Formula: *Huáng Qí Tāng* (黄芪汤, Astragalus Decoction) from the *Appendices to the 'Essentials from the Golden Cabinet'* (*Jīn Guì Yì*, 金匮翼)

Substitute Formula: *Bǔ Zhōng Yì Qì Tāng* (补中益气汤, Center-Supplementing and Qi-Boosting Decoction)

Patent Formula: *Biàn Mì Tōng Kǒu Fú Yè* (便秘通口服液, Constipation-Relieving Oral Liquid)

4. Yin Deficiency and Intestinal Dryness

Symptoms: Extremely dry stools, dizziness, tinnitus, soreness and weakness of the lumbus and knees, emaciation, malar flush, restlessness, insomnia, tidal fever, night sweats, a red tongue with a scanty coating and a thready and rapid pulse.

Treatment Principle:

- Nourish yin and supplement body fluids
- Moisten the intestines and resolve constipation

Main Acupuncture Points:

- ST 25 (*tiān shū*): Front-*mu* point of the large intestine to invigorate stomach and intestines, regulate qi, improve digestion and resolve stagnation
- BL 25 (*dà cháng shù*): Back-*shu* point of the large intestine to regulate intestinal qi and resolve stagnation
- ST 28 (*shuǐ dào*): To regulate lower *jiao* qi and resolve constipation
- ST 36 (*zú sān lǐ*): To invigorate spleen, support the correct qi and promote circulation
- SP 6 (*sān yīn jiāo*): To invigorate spleen and nourish yin, harmonize the lower *jiao*
- KI 6 (*zhào hǎi*): To nourish yin, clear deficient heat and resolve constipation

Supporting Points:

- RN 4 (*guān yuán*): Front-*mu* point of the small intestine to tonify original qi, supplement deficiency and regulate small intestine
- LV 3 (*tài chōng*): *Yuan*-source point of the liver to nourish liver yin and blood, treat irregular menstruation

Recommended Formula: *Zēng Yè Tāng* (增液汤, Humor-Increasing Decoction) from the *Systematic Differentiation of Warm Diseases* (*Wēn Bìng Tiáo Biàn*, 温病条辨)

Substitute Formula:

- *Liù Wèi Dì Huáng Wán* (六味地黄丸, Six Ingredients Rehmannia Pill)
- *Yì Wèi Tāng* (益胃汤, Stomach-Boosting Decoction)

Patent Formula: *Wǔ Rén Rùn Cháng Wán* (五仁润肠丸, Five-Seed Intestines-Moistening Pill)

5. Spleen and Kidney Yang Deficiency

Symptoms: Fatigue, difficult defecation, clear profuse urination, pale complexion, cold limbs, abdominal pain and coldness, soreness in lumbus and knees, a pale tongue with teeth marks and a white moist coating and a deep, weak and slow pulse.

Treatment Principle:

- Warm yang and strengthen spleen
- Tonify the kidney qi and warm the *mingmen*
- Promote bowel movement and resolve constipation

Main Acupuncture Points:

- ST 25 (*tiān shū*): Front-*mu* point of the large intestine to invigorate stomach and intestines, regulate qi, improve digestion and resolve stagnation
- BL 25 (*dà cháng shù*): Back-*shu* point of the large intestine to regulate intestinal qi and resolve stagnation
- BL 20 (*pí shù*): Back-*shu* point of the spleen to regulate middle *jiao* qi, invigorate spleen and stop abdominal pain
- RN 8 (*shén què*): Apply moxibustion to warm the yang and resolve edema
- RN 4 (*guān yuán*): Front-*mu* point of the small intestine to tonify original qi, supplement deficiency and regulate small intestine
- DU 3 (*yāo yáng guān*): To tonify original qi, benefit lumbus and lower limbs, dispel dampness and regulate menstruation

Supporting Points:

- BL 23 (*shèn shù*): Back-*shu* point of the kidney to tonify kidney and fortify yang, strengthen qi, strengthen lumbar region, benefit urination and menstruation
- RN 12 (*zhōng wǎn*): To harmonize spleen and stomach, warm middle *jiao* and regulate qi

Recommended Formula: *Jì Chuān Jiān* (济川煎, Fluid-Replenishing Decoction) from *The Complete Works of [Zhang] Jing-yue* (*Jǐng Yuè Quán Shū*, 景岳全书)

Substitute Formula:

- *Wēn Pí Tāng* (温脾汤, Spleen-Warming Decoction)
- *Jì Shēng Shèn Qì Wán* (济生肾气丸, Life-Saving Kidney Qi Pill)

Patent Formula:

- *Bàn Liú Wán* (半硫丸, Pinellia and Sulfur Pill)
- *Jì Shēng Shèn Qì Wán* (济生肾气丸, Life-Saving Kidney Qi Pill)

Summary Chart for Constipation

Patterns	Main Points	Supporting Points	Formulae
Excess Heat Accumulation in the Intestines	BL 25, ST 25, SJ 6, LI 4, ST 37, LI 11, ST 44	KI 6 for yin deficiency causing deficient heat LI 9 for vomiting, headaches and dizziness due to *yangming* fire	*Má Zǐ Rén Wán* or *Rùn Cháng Wán* or *Dà Chéng Qì Tāng*
Qi Stagnation in the Intestines	ST 25, ST 28, LV 3, RN 12, BL 25, SJ 6	GB 24 for hypochondriac pain due to qi stagnation PC 6 for abdominal pain due to qi stagnation	*Liù Mò Tāng* or *Chái Hú Shū Gān Sǎn* or *Sì Mò Tāng*

Continued

Patterns	Main Points	Supporting Points	Formulae
Spleen Qi Deficiency	BL 20, BL 25, ST 25, ST 37, RN 6, SJ 6	SP 8 for indigestion due to dampness ST 36 for dampness accumulation	*Huáng Qí Tāng* or *Bǔ Zhōng Yì Qì Tāng*
Yin Deficiency and Intestinal Dryness	ST 25, BL 25, ST 28, ST 36, SP 6, KI 6	RN 4 for intestinal deficiency LV 3 for liver yin deficiency and dysmenorrhea	*Zēng Yè Tāng* or *Liù Wèi Dì Huáng Wán* or *Yì Wèi Tāng*
Spleen and Kidney Yang Deficiency	ST 25, BL 25, BL 20, RN 8, RN 4, DU 3	BL 23 for spleen and kidney yang deficiency RN 12 for middle *jiao* cold	*Jì Chuān Jiān* or *Wēn Pí Tāng* or *Jì Shēng Shèn Qì Wán*

CASE STUDY: Chronic Constipation

Ms. Wang, 36 years old.

Main Complaint: Difficult defecation for over half a year.

Medical History: The patient suffered from difficult defecation for over half a year. It often took the patient over one hour to pass stool and she often self medicated with *niú huáng jiě dú piàn* (Bovine Bezoar Toxins Removing Tablets), *dà huáng piàn* (Rhubarb Tablets), and glycerine enema for relief. However, soon after the constipation would return and was gradually worsening.

Presenting Symptoms: Bloating and distension in the lower abdomen with the desire to defecate without being able to pass stool, lack of strength and profuse sweating after defecation, pale complexion, mental fatigue, poor appetite, a pale red tongue with teeth marks and a thin and white coating and a thin and weak pulse.

Physical Examination: Temperature: 36.5 ℃, pulse: 80 bpm, respiration: 20 bpm, blood pressure: 120/70 mmHg. The patient was conscious and cooperative. Her skin and sclera were non-icteric and there were no enlarged lymph nodes, liver or spleen. Respiratory sounds were clear and the heart was regular without heart murmurs. Her abdomen wall was soft with no tenderness, or rebound tenderness. The routine urine and blood tests showed no abnormal findings. Colonoscopy indicated no abnormal findings.

Pattern Differentiation

As the spleen governs the functions of transportation and transformation, when the spleen is deficient, there is impaired transportation and transformation of the food and it causes dampness stagnation. When this deficiency is combined with large intestines qi deficiency, it is too weak to expel toxins and dampness through the stools resulting in constipation. In these conditions, the purgation method should be

avoided. In the *Teachings of Dan-xi* (*Dān Xī Xīn Fǎ*, 丹溪心法), it states: "If we apply strong medicinals to purge, it will consume the body fluids, qi and blood. Though the bowels are unblocked temporary, the constipation will soon resume." This is a case of spleen and lung qi deficiency with body fluid deficiency. The patient regularly used strong bitter and cold medicinals to purge the stool for temporary relief, but it would further damage the qi and fluids and the constipation eventually worsened. The lung and large intestine have an interior and exterior relationship. When the lung qi is deficient combined with a spleen qi deficiency pattern, there will be a weakness to defecate. In this case the pale complexion, mental fatigue, poor appetite, abdominal distension and discomfort which aggravates after meals, a pale red tongue with teeth marks and a thin and weak pulse indicate spleen qi deficiency.

Diagnosis

TCM Diagnosis: Constipation due to spleen and lung qi deficiency with body fluid depletion

Western Medicine Diagnosis: Constipation

Treatment

The main pathomechanism of this case is spleen and lung qi deficiency, with body fluid deficiency.

Principles:

- Supplement qi and fortify the spleen
- Moisten the intestines to promote defecation

Formula: Modified *Huáng Qí Tāng* (Astragalus Decoction)

Ingredients:

黄芪	*huáng qí*	20 g	raw Radix Astragali
党参	*dǎng shēn*	10 g	Radix Codonopsis
白术	*bái zhú*	10 g	raw Rhizoma Atractylodis Macrocephalae
枳壳	*zhǐ qiào*	10 g	Fructus Aurantii
桔梗	*jié gěng*	10 g	Radix Platycodonis
郁李仁	*yù lǐ rén*	15 g	Semen Pruni
山楂	*shān zhā*	15 g	Fructus Crataegi

Formula Analysis

In this formula, *huáng qí* strongly supplements the lung and spleen qi. *Dǎng shēn* and *jié gěng* assist *huáng qí* to tonify qi. *Yù lǐ rén* smoothens the intestines and relaxes the bowels. *Zhǐ qiào* breaks stagnant qi and leads qi downwards, and when combined with *jié gěng* they harmonize the middle *jiao* qi as one medicinal descends and the other ascends. Scorch fried *shān zhā* serves to promote digestion. Raw *bái zhú* strengthens the spleen and moistens the intestines to resolve constipation.

Ear Acupuncture Point Combination:

sympathetic (*jiāo gǎn*)	rectum (*zhí cháng*)	large intestine (*dà cháng*)
liver (*gān*)	spleen (*pí*)	subcortex (*pí zhì xià*)
endocrine (*nèi fēn mì*)	*sanjiao* (*sān jiāo*)	

The patient can also receive ear acupuncture or ear seeds to stimulate the bowel movements. Use adhesive tape to fasten *wáng bù liú xíng* on the selected ear points and tender points on the ear. Apply on each ear alternatively and change every two days. The patient should press the ear points for about 10 minutes until the area is hot, distending, and painful about 5 times a day. Usually 30 days make one course of period.

Follow-up Consultations

After a week of the formula, her bowels were slightly easier to pass. After 20 more doses, the patient passed stool without any difficulty.

KEY CLINICAL POINTS

Constipation is a fairly commonly seen symptom in clinic and there are various differentiations and causes which vary greatly. Simply purging the stools is often not efficient or only brings temporary relief. Only treating the deeper cause of the constipation will bring lasting results.

Educating the patient suffering from habitual constipation is very important since there is often the harmful habit of regularly taking purgative medicine which further harms the body fluids and qi. Advise the patient to avoid using such medicine and to develop healthy eating habits according to their condition. When the patient is suffering from constipation due to qi deficiency, advise them to eat food which nourish qi and promote the bowels such as finer and root vegetables. When the patient suffers from constipation due to cold stagnation, advise them to avoid all cold foods and increase their intake of warming food such as porridge, soups and so on. When the patient is suffering from heat stagnation constipation, advise them to avoid hot, spicy and greasy food and add more fruits and vegetable to their diet such as apples, bananas, pineapples. These changes in diet can be combined with the medicinals to fully relieve the syndrome. Also the patient can develop a healthy exercise program of walking over 30 minutes in the evening after dinner, swimming or slight jogging. Excessive sweating should also be avoided to prevent from harming the body fluid any further. Avoiding mental and emotional stress should also be taken into account and maintaining a calm and healthy attitude is recommended.

BRIEF SUMMARY

The disease location of constipation is in the intestines, but this condition is also affected by disorders of the spleen, stomach, lung, liver and kidney. Both external pathogenic factors such as cold and heat, dampness and phlegm and internal damage from irregular or improper diet and excessive emotions can cause constipation. Organ disorders such as deficiency of yin, yang, qi and blood can all cause intestinal obstruction due to the lack of intestines warmth and body fluid leading to dry and difficult stools. The main treatment principles are to unblock and rectify the bowel movement and moisten the intestines to promote defecation.

COMPREHENSION QUESTIONS

1. What are the differentiation patterns and recommended formulas for constipation?

2. How can we differentiate from the cold, heat, deficiency and excess patterns causing constipation?

3. What are the key clinical points for constipation?

4. Multiple choice questions:

1) Male, 70 years old. The patient suffered from forceless defecation, shortness of breath, spontaneous sweating, weakness after defecation, dry stools, a pale tongue with thin coating and a weak pulse. The treatment principle is to:

A. Boost kidney yang
B. Warm yang and tonify qi
C. Tonify qi and moisten the intestines
D. Nourish blood and moisten the intestines
E. Nourish yin and relax bowels

2) A patient has dry constipated stool with difficult defecation for months. The accompanying symptoms include feverish sensation, vexation, abdominal distension, fullness and pain, dry mouth with bad breath, scanty and dark brown urine, a red tongue with yellow and dry coating and a slippery and rapid pulse. The recommended formula is:

A. *Má Zǐ Rén Wán* (Cannabis Fruit Pill)
B. *Gēng Yī Wán* (Toilette Pill)
C. *Dà Chéng Qì Tāng* (Major Purgative Decoction)
D. *Zēng Yè Tāng* (Humor-Increasing Decoction)
E. *Dà Chái Hú Tāng* (Major Bupleurum Decoction)

3) Mr. Li, 75 years old. The patient suffered from constipation with dry stools,

lusterless complexion, vertigo, blurry vision, palpitations, insomnia, pale nails, pale lips and tongue and a thin pulse. The pattern differentiation is:

A. Constipation due to blood deficiency
B. Constipation due to qi deficiency
C. Constipation due to yang deficiency
D. Constipation due to both qi and blood deficiency
E. Constipation due to qi stagnation

4) Mr. Zhang, 28 years old. The patient has a strong constitution with a good appetite but has just recovered from a cold. His stool is relatively dry and has only one defecation every several days, accompanied by abdominal distension and fullness, red complexion and vexing heat, dry mouth with bad breath, dark red lips, a red tongue with yellow coating and a slippery and rapid pulse. The pattern differentiation is:

A. Yin and body fluid deficiency and dryness of the intestines
B. Heat accumulation in the stomach and intestines with fluids consumption
C. Blood and body fluid deficiency causing constipation
D. Heat binding and qi stagnation and excess in the stomach and intestines
E. Heat binding and food stagnation in the stomach and intestines

5) Mr. Zhang, 80 years old. The patient has suffered from constipation over a long period of time and had no favorable effect from taking *fān xiè yè*. His main complaint is weakness during defecation causing constipation followed by excessive sweating, mental fatigue, weakness, a pale tongue with a thin coating and a deficient and weak pulse. The treatment principle is to:

A. Tonify qi and moisten the intestines
B. Warm yang to promote defecation
C. Move qi and remove food stagnation
D. Nourish blood and moisten the intestines
E. Tonify qi and nourish blood, moisten the intestines to promote defecation

6) Mr. Liu, 39 years old. The patient suffered from constipation for a long period of time and was highly susceptible to depression. The accompanied symptoms were chest and hypochondriac fullness and distension, upper and lower abdominal distension and distress which aggravate after meals, frequent belching, a slightly greasy tongue coating and a wiry pulse. The recommended formula is:

A. *Chái Hú Shū Gān Săn* (Bupleurum Liver-Soothing Powder)
B. *Sì Nì Săn* (Frigid Extremities Powder)
C. *Liù Mò Tāng* (Six Milled Ingredients Decoction)
D. *Dà Chéng Qì Tāng* (Major Purgative Decoction)
E. *Mù Xiāng Shùn Qì Wán* (Costus Root Qi-Balancing Pill)

Answers

1. The common pattern differentiation for constipation and recommended formulas are the following:

- Excessive heat stagnated in the intestines, the recommended formula is: *Má Zǐ Rén Wán* (Cannabis Fruit Pill), *Rùn Cháng Wán* (Intestines-Moistening Pill) or *Dà Chéng Qì Tāng* (Major Purgative Decoction)
- Qi stagnation in the intestines, the recommended formula is: *Liù Mò Tāng* (Six Milled Ingredients Decoction), *Chái Hú Shū Gān Săn* (Bupleurum Liver-Soothing Powder) or *Sì Mò Tāng* (Four Milled Ingredients Decoction)
- Spleen qi deficiency, the recommended formula is: *Huáng Qí Tāng* (Astragalus Decoction) or *Bŭ Zhōng Yì Qì Tāng* (Center-Supplementing and Qi-Boosting Decoction)
- Yin deficiency with intestinal dryness, the recommended formula is: *Zēng Yè Tāng* (Humor-Increasing Decoction), *Liù Wèi Dì Huáng Wán* (Six Ingredients Rehmannia Pill) or *Yì Wèi Tāng* (Stomach-Boosting Decoction)
- Spleen and kidney yang deficiency, the recommended formula is: *Jì Chuān Jiān* (Fluid-Replenishing Decoction), *Wēn Pí Tāng* (Spleen-Warming Decoction) or *Jì Shēng Shèn Qì Wán* (Life-Saving Kidney Qi Pill)
- Cold stagnation, the recommended formula is: *Dà Huáng Fù Zǐ Tāng* (Rhubarb and Aconite Decoction)
- Food stagnation, the recommended formula is: *Zhĭ Shí Dăo Zhì Wán* (Immature Bitter Orange Stagnation-Moving Pill)
- Phlegm rheum retention, the recommended formula is: *Dăo Tán Tāng* (Phlegm-Expelling Decoction)
- Blood deficiency, the recommended formula is: *Rùn Cháng Tāng* (Intestine Moistening Decoction).

2. The pattern differentiation for constipation is based on the presenting symptoms and signs that whether the pattern is excessive or deficient, due to heat or cold, and which organs are affected. The symptoms of dryness of the mouth and throat, headache, tinnitus, red tongue with a yellow coating and a rapid and slippery pulse indicate an excessive heat pattern. If the constipation increases with cold food and cold weather and is accompanied with sharp and sudden spasms of the lower abdomen with low appetite, it is due to cold excess in the intestines. If the constipation is due to the lack of strength to expel the stool accompanied by shortness of breath and spontaneous sweating, soft and deep pulse, the pattern is due to qi deficiency. If there is dryness of the mouth and eye, dry stools, pale tongue with a thin and deep pulse, the constipation is due to body fluid and blood deficiency.

3. The key clinical points to advice your patients are to avoid using purging medicine and to develop healthy eating habits according to their condition. When the patient is suffering from constipation due to qi deficiency, advise them to eat food which nourish qi and promote the bowels such as fine and root vegetables. When

the patient suffers from constipation due to cold stagnation, advise them to avoid all cold foods and increase their intake of warming food such as porridge, soups and so on. When the patient is suffering from heat stagnation constipation, advise them to avoid hot, spicy and greasy food and add more fruits and vegetable to their diet such as apples, bananas, pineapples. These changes of diet can be combined with the medicinals to fully relieve the syndrome. Also the patient can develop a healthy exercise program of walking over 30 minutes in the evening after dinner, swimming or slight jogging. Excessive sweating should also be avoided to prevent from harming the body fluid any further. Avoid mental and emotional stress should also be taken into account and maintaining a calm and healthy attitude is recommended.

4. 1) C, 2) A, 3) A, 4) B, 5) A, 6) C.

4.5 Diarrhea

Diarrhea is characterized by frequent loose stool, undigested food in the stool, or in some cases frequent watery stool. In ancient times, this symptom was classified into two separate kinds of syndrome. One type of diarrhea was defined by frequent loose stool without urgency and the other was defined by urgent explosive watery stools. The symptoms of diarrhea are clearly differentiated by excessive and deficiency patterns, cold or heat patterns. It can be mild or severe and can occur at any age. In some younger patients or in the weak and elderly, diarrhea can be life threatening and need our immediate attention.

In western medicine, the symptoms of diarrhea is often seen in diseases such as acute enteritis, irritable bowel syndrome, intestinal tumor, intestinal tuberculosis and many others.

The location of this symptom is in the intestine and it is closely related to the function of the spleen, liver and kidney. Similar to constipation, diarrhea can result from both external and internal pathogenic factors. External contraction of pathogenic cold, heat and dampness, as well as the internal damage of food accumulation and excessive emotions, and visceral deficiency can cause diarrhea. There are both deficiency and excess, and diarrhea can be acute, moderate or chronic and life threatening. Here are the most commonly seen patterns in clinic with their recommended treatment principles, acupuncture points and formulas.

CLINICAL PATTERNS DIFFERENTIATION AND TREATMENTS

1. Cold Dampness Attacking the Spleen

Symptoms: Clear, loose and watery stools, abdominal pain and fullness which worsen with cold food or cold weather, borborygmus, poor appetite, nausea, vomiting, no thirst, aversion to cold, fever, nasal congestion, headache, body aches, heaviness of the limbs, a pale tongue with a white and greasy coating and a soft and slow pulse.

Treatment Principle:

- Release the exterior and dispel cold
- Warm the interior and transform dampness

Main Acupuncture Points:

- RN 12 (*zhōng wǎn*): Front-*mu* point of the stomach to harmonize spleen and stomach, warm middle *jiao* and regulate qi

- ST 25 (*tiān shū*): To invigorate spleen and stomach, clear dampness, alleviate vomiting and resolve stagnation
- ST 36 (*zú sān lǐ*): To expel dampness, strengthen the stomach qi, invigorate spleen, alleviate diarrhea and vomiting, promote circulation
- ST 37 (*shàng jù xū*): Lower *he*-sea point of the large intestine to resolve stagnation, expel dampness, alleviate diarrhea and stop pain
- SP 9 (*yīn líng quán*): To harmonize middle *jiao*, expel dampness and resolve edema
- RN 8 (*shén què*): Apply moxa to warm the yang and resolve edema

Supporting Points:

- BL 30 (*bái huán shù*): To warm the uterus, regulate menstruation, leucorrhea and seminal emission
- SP 14 (*fù jié*): To invigorate spleen and warm middle *jiao*, descend rebellious qi and umbilical pain

Recommended Formula: *Huò Xiāng Zhèng Qì Săn* (藿香正气散, Agastache Qi-Correcting Powder) from the *Beneficial Formulas from the Taiping Imperial Pharmacy* (*Tài Píng Huì Mín Hé Jì Jú Fāng*, 太平惠民和剂局方)

Substitute Formula: *Wèi Líng Tāng* (胃苓汤, Stomach-Calming Poria Decoction)

Patent Formula: *Huò Xiāng Zhèng Qì Ruăn Jiāo Náng* (藿香正气软胶囊, Agastache Qi-Correcting Soft Capsule)

2. Food Stagnation in the Stomach and Intestines

Symptoms: Abdominal pain which is aggravated after eating, borborygmus, foul smelling stools with undigested food, sporadic eating binges of cold, sweet or greasy food, gastric or abdominal fullness, halitosis, poor appetite, a red tongue with thick and greasy coating and a slippery and large pulse.

Treatment Principle:

- Promote digestion and expel accumulation
- Descend and harmonize the stomach qi

Main Acupuncture Points:

- BL 20 (*pí shù*): Back-*shu* point of the spleen to regulate middle *jiao* qi, invigorate spleen, alleviate diarrhea and stop abdominal pain
- BL 21 (*wèi shù*): Back-*shu* point of the stomach to invigorate spleen and harmonize stomach, alleviate diarrhea, promote digestion and stop hypochondriac pain
- ST 25 (*tiān shū*): Front-*mu* point of the large intestine to invigorate stomach and intestines, regulate qi, improve digestion and resolve stagnation
- ST 36 (*zú sān lǐ*): To expel dampness, strengthen stomach qi, invigorate spleen, alleviate diarrhea and promote circulation
- ST 37 (*shàng jù xū*): Lower *he*-sea point of the large intestine to resolve

stagnation, expel dampness, alleviate diarrhea and stop pain

• RN 10 (*xià wǎn*): To regulate qi, dispel food stagnation and stop abdominal pain

Supporting Points:

• DU 5 (*xuán shū*): To treat diarrhea with undigested food, stop abdominal pain and benefit lumbar region

• BL 35 (*huì yáng*): To clear dampness, treat hemorrhoids, alleviate diarrhea and separate clear from turbid

Recommended Formula: *Bǎo Hé Wán* (保和丸, Harmony-Preserving Pill) from the *Teachings of [Zhu] Dan-xi* (*Dān Xī Xīn Fǎ,* 丹溪心法)

Substitute Formula: *Zhǐ Shí Dǎo Zhì Wán* (枳实导滞丸, Immature Bitter Orange Stagnation-Moving Pill)

Patent Formula:

• *Bǎo Hé Wán* (保和丸, Harmony-Preserving Pill)

• *Jiàn Wèi Xiāo Shí Piàn* (健胃消食片, Stomach-Strengthening Digestive Tablet)

3. Damp-Heat Stagnation in the Intestines

Symptoms: Abdominal pain, urgent and loose defecation with foul smell and a feeling of incomplete evacuation, a burning sensation around the anus, headaches, restlessness, fever, thirst and scanty yellow urine, a red tongue with a yellow and greasy coating and a rapid and slippery pulse.

Treatment Principle:

• Clear heat and expel dampness

• Harmonize the stomach and intestines and resolve diarrhea

Main Acupuncture Points:

• ST 25 (*tiān shū*): Front-*mu* point of the large intestine to invigorate stomach and intestines, regulate qi, improve digestion and resolve stagnation

• ST 37 (*shàng jù xū*) and LI 11 (*qū chí*): Upper and lower *he*-sea points of the large intestine, to resolve stagnation, expel dampness, alleviate diarrhea and stop pain

• ST 44 (*nèi tíng*): To clear intestinal heat and harmonize intestines

• SP 9 (*yīn líng quán*): To harmonize middle *jiao*, expel dampness and resolve edema

• RN 9 (*shuǐ fēn*): To regulate fluid passages, expel edema, invigorate middle *jiao,* alleviate diarrhea, treat abdominal distension and pain

• ST 40 (*fēng lóng*): To expel phlegm and dampness from the lungs, heart and chest

Supporting Points:

• LV 13 (*zhāng mén*): Front-*mu* point of the spleen to invigorate spleen, regulate stomach and stop abdominal pain

• BL 27 (*xiǎo cháng shù*): To expel damp-heat, morbid leucorrhea, alleviate diarrhea, stop abdominal pain and regulate intestines

Recommended Formula: *Gé Gēn Huáng Qín Huáng Lián Tāng* (葛根黄芩黄连汤,

Pueraria, Scutellaria, and Coptis Decoction) from the *Treatise on Cold Damage* (*Shāng Hán Lùn*, 伤寒论)

Substitute Formula: *Xīn Jiā Xiāng Rú Yǐn* (新加香薷饮, Newly Supplemented Mosla Beverage) with *Liù Yī Sǎn* (六一散, Six-to-One Powder)

Patent Formula: *Xiāng Lián Zhǐ Xiè Piàn* (香连止泻片, Aucklandia and Coptis Anti-diarrhea Tablet)

4. Spleen and Stomach Qi Deficiency

Symptoms: Recurring loose stools with increased frequency especially after eating greasy food, poor appetite, aversion to greasy food, gastric or abdominal distension and pain, pale complexion, lassitude, a pale tongue with a thin white coating and a weak and thready pulse.

Treatment Principle:

- Strengthen the spleen and supplement qi
- Transform dampness and resolve diarrhea

Main Acupuncture Points:

- ST 25 (*tiān shū*): Front-*mu* point of the large intestine to invigorate stomach and intestines, regulate qi, improve digestion and resolve stagnation
- ST 36 (*zú sān lǐ*): To expel dampness, strengthen stomach qi, invigorate spleen, alleviate diarrhea and promote circulation
- ST 37 (*shàng jù xū*): Lower *he*-sea point of the large intestine to resolve stagnation, expel dampness, alleviate diarrhea and stop pain
- SP 9 (*yīn líng quán*): To harmonize middle *jiao*, expel dampness and resolve edema
- SP 3 (*tài bái*): *Yuan*-source point of spleen to invigorate spleen, expel dampness, harmonize spleen and stomach, treat abdominal distension and irregular menstruation
- RN 9 (*shuǐ fēn*): To regulate fluid passages, expel edema, invigorate middle *jiao*, alleviate diarrhea, treat abdominal distension and pain

Supporting Points:

- SP 8 (*dì jī*): *Xi*-cleft point of the spleen to resolve dampness and regulate spleen, improve digestion and benefit appetite
- RN 6 (*qì hǎi*): To invigorate spleen and harmonize blood, promote circulation and treat gynecological disorders

Recommended Formula: *Shēn Líng Bái Zhú Sǎn* (参苓白术散, Ginseng, Poria and Atractylodes Macrocephalae Powder) from the *Beneficial Formulas from the Taiping Imperial Pharmacy* (*Tài Píng Huì Mín Hé Jì Jú Fāng*, 太平惠民和剂局方)

Substitute Formula: *Bǔ Pí Yì Cháng Wán* (补脾益肠丸, Spleen-Tonifying and Intestines-Replenishing Pill)

Patent Formula:

- *Bǔ Pí Yì Cháng Wán* (补脾益肠丸, Spleen-Tonifying and Intestines-Replenishing Pill)

• *Xiāng Shā Liù Jūn Zǐ Wán* (香砂六君子丸, Costusroot and Amomum Six Gentlemen Pill)

5. Liver Depression and Spleen Deficiency

Symptoms: Abdominal pain and diarrhea which often occur due to excessive emotions or stress, borborygmus, flatulence, chest or hypochondriac distension and fullness in the regions, belching, poor appetite, a pale tongue with a thin white coating and a wiry pulse.

Treatment Principle:

• Soothe the liver and fortify the spleen

• Calm the mind and harmonize intestines

Main Acupuncture Points:

• ST 25 (*tiān shū*): Front-*mu* point of the large intestine to invigorate stomach and intestines, regulate qi, improve digestion and resolve stagnation

• GB 34 (*yáng líng quán*): To spread liver and gallbladder qi, unbind the chest and stop pain

• SP 9 (*yīn líng quán*): To harmonize middle *jiao*, regulate menstruation and resolve edema

• LV 13 (*zhāng mén*): Front-*mu* point of the spleen to harmonize liver and spleen, regulate stomach and alleviate diarrhea

• LV 3 (*tài chōng*): *Yuan*-source point of the liver to spread liver qi, soothe emotional outbursts, alleviate diarrhea, clear head and eyes, unbind the chest and stop pain

• DU 4 (*mìng mén*): To alleviate diarrhea, strengthen the lumbus and regulate *du mai*

Supporting Points:

• GB 24 (*rì yuè*): Front-*mu* point of the gallbladder to spread liver qi and resolve hypochondriac pain

• LV 2 (*xíng jiān*): To treat qi stagnation transforming to fire

Recommended Formula: *Tòng Xiè Yào Fāng* (痛泻药方, Important Formula for Painful Diarrhea) from *The Complete Works of [Zhang] Jing-yue* (*Jǐng Yuè Quán Shū*, 景岳全书)

Substitute Formula: *Sì Nì Sǎn* (四逆散, Frigid Extremities Powder)

Patent Formula: *Xiāo Yáo Wán* (逍遥丸, Free Wanderer Pill)

6. Kidney Yang Deficiency

Symptoms: Clear and thin stools, stool incontinence or diarrhea (which often occurs in the early morning), coupled with abdominal pain which is relieved by passing stools, borborygmus, poor appetite, cold limbs, aversion to cold, soreness and weakness in the lower back and knees, a pale tongue with a thin, white and moist coating and a deep and thready or deep, weak and slow pulse.

Treatment Principle:

- Warm the kidney and strengthen the spleen
- Harmonize and resolve diarrhea

Main Acupuncture Points:

- BL 20 (*pí shù*): Back-*shu* point of the spleen to regulate middle *jiao* qi, invigorate spleen, alleviate diarrhea and stop abdominal pain
- BL 23 (*shèn shù*): Back-*shu* point of the kidney to tonify kidney and fortify yang, supplement qi, strengthen lumbar region, benefit urination and menstruation
- RN 8 (*shén què*): Apply moxibustion to warm the yang and resolve diarrhea
- ST 25 (*tiān shū*): Front-*mu* point of the large intestine to invigorate stomach and intestines, regulate qi, improve digestion and resolve stagnation
- KI 3 (*tài xī*): *Yuan*-source point of kidney to tonify kidney yang, invigorate spleen and strengthen lumbus
- RN 12 (*zhōng wǎn*): Front-*mu* point of the stomach to harmonize spleen and stomach, warm middle *jiao* and regulate qi

Supporting Points:

- EX-CA 5 (*wèi shàng*): To tonify and raise the middle qi
- RN 4 (*guān yuán*): Front-*mu* point of the small intestine to benefit the uterus, tonify original qi, supplement deficiency and regulate menstruation

Recommended Formula: *Sì Shén Wán* (四神丸, Four Spirits Pill) from the *Standards for Diagnosis and Treatment* (*Zhèng Zhì Zhǔn Shéng*, 证治准绳)

Substitute Formula: *Zhēn Rén Yǎng Zàng Tāng* (真人养脏汤, Enlightened Master Viscera-Nourishing Decoction)

Patent Formula: *Jīn Guì Shèn Qì Wán* (金匮肾气丸, Golden Cabinet's Kidney Qi Pill)

Summary Chart for Diarrhea

Patterns	Main Points	Supporting Points	Formulae
Cold Dampness Attacking the Spleen	RN 12, ST 25, ST 36, ST 37, SP 9, RN 8	BL 30 for uterine cold, irregular menstruation and seminal emission SP 14 for umbilical pain	*Huò Xiāng Zhèng Qì Sǎn* or *Wèi Líng Tāng*
Food Stagnation in the Stomach and Intestines	BL 20, BL 21, ST 25, ST 36, ST 37, RN 10	DU 5 for diarrhea with undigested food and lumbar weakness BL 35 for hemorrhoids	*Bǎo Hé Wán* or *Zhǐ Shí Dǎo Zhì Wán*
Damp-Heat Stagnation in the Intestines	ST 25, ST 37, ST 44, SP 9, RN 9, ST 40	LV 13 for vomiting due to liver depression and spleen weakness BL 27 for excessive leucorrhea	*Gé Gēn Huáng Qín Huáng Lián Tāng* or *Xīn Jiā Xiāng Rú Yǐn* plus *Liù Yī Sǎn*
Spleen and Stomach Qi Deficiency	ST 25, ST 36, ST 37, SP 9, SP 3, RN 9	SP 8 for indigestion RN 6 for gynecological disorders	*Shēn Líng Bái Zhú Sǎn* or *Bǔ Pí Yì Cháng Wán*

Continued

Patterns	Main Points	Supporting Points	Formulae
Liver Depression and Spleen Deficiency	ST 25, GB 34, SP 9, LV 13, LV 3, DU 4	GB 24 for hypochondriac pain and distention LV 2 for liver qi stagnation transforming into fire	*Tòng Xiè Yào Fāng* or *Sì Nì Săn*
Kidney Yang Deficiency	BL 20, BL 23, RN 8, ST 25, KI 3, RN 12	EX-CA 5 for middle qi sinking RN 4 for irregular menstruation and uterine disorders	*Sì Shén Wán* or *Zhēn Rén Yăng Zàng Tāng*

CASE STUDY 1: Chronic Dawn Diarrhea

Ms. Wang, 62 years old.

Main Complaint: Reoccurring diarrhea for 3 years.

Medical History: The patient suffered from reoccurring diarrhea for over 3 years which often happened around 4 o'clock in the morning during which there were paroxysmal abdominal pain followed by yellow loose stool 2 to 3 times. After around 7 o'clock, the abdominal pain and diarrhea resolved, but the patient also suffered from mental fatigue, lumbar soreness and weakness. There was only temporary relief from self prescribed medication. There were no abnormal findings in the blood and stool tests. The patient also suffered from chronic bronchitis which could only be relieved by antibiotics or antiasthmatic medication.

Presenting Symptoms: Paroxysmal abdominal pain and frequent borborygmus before dawn which was only relieved by defecation of loose stool sometimes with undigested food. The accompanied symptoms were emaciation, aversion to cold, cold limbs, lumbar and knee soreness and pain, lethargy, poor appetite, occasional cough and panting, a pale tongue with a thin and white coating and a deep and thin pulse.

Physical Examination: Temperature: 36.5 ℃, pulse: 90 bpm, respiration: 20 bpm, blood pressure: 125/80 mmHg. The patient was conscious and there was no tenderness and rebound pain in the abdomen. The borborygmus was normal and the liver and spleen were not palpable. An electro-enteroscopy showed mild congestion in the colon.

Pattern Differentiation

The kidney yang is the root of the body warmth and function. In this case, the kidney yang is very weak which also has affected the spleen yang which is unable to transform and transport the nutrients from the food causing diarrhea at dawn. The symptoms of cold limbs, aversion to cold, weakness, poor appetite, and indigestion are all symptoms of spleen and kidney yang deficiency.

Diagnosis

TCM Diagnosis: Chronic diarrhea due to spleen and kidney yang deficiency
Western Medicine Diagnosis: Chronic Diarrhea

Treatment

The main pathomechanism of this case is kidney yang deficiency that it fails to warm the spleen and the spleen is unable to carry out transportation and transformation normally, leading to diarrhea.

Principles:

- Supplement qi and fortify the spleen
- Fortify kidney and warm the yang
- Warm the intestine to check diarrhea

Formula: Modified *Sì Shén Wán* (Four Spirits Pill) with *Zhēn Rén Yǎng Zàng Tāng* (Enlightened Master Viscera-Nourishing Decoction)

Ingredients:

补骨脂	*bǔ gǔ zhī*	10 g	Fructus Psoraleae
吴茱萸	*wú zhū yú*	10 g	Fructus Evodiae
肉豆蔻	*ròu dòu kòu*	10 g	Semen Myristicae
五味子	*wǔ wèi zǐ*	10 g	Fructus Schisandrae Chinensis
党参	*dǎng shēn*	30 g	Radix Codonopsis
广木香	*guǎng mù xiāng*	10 g	Radix Aucklandiae
诃子	*hē zǐ*	10 g	Fructus Chebulae
白术	*bái zhú*	10 g	Rhizoma Atractylodis Macrocephalae
甘草	*gān cǎo*	6 g	Radix et Rhizoma Glycyrrhizae

Formula Analysis

In this formula, *bǔ gǔ zhī* is the chief medicinal and it is acrid, bitter and greatly warming. It can supplement the *mìng mén* fire and warm the spleen. *Ròu dòu kòu* is acrid and warm and warms the spleen and stomach, astringes the intestines, treats diarrhea and assists *bǔ gǔ zhī*. *Wǔ wèi zǐ* can fortify the spleen and supplement qi, astringe essence and treat diarrhea. *Wú zhū yú* is acrid, bitter and very hot and is able to warm the spleen and kidney to disperse cold. *Dǎng shēn, mù xiāng, hē zǐ, bái zhú* and *gān cǎo* are combined to tonify qi and fortify the spleen, astringe the intestines and treat diarrhea, warm the middle and supplement deficiency. All the ingredients are combined to warm the spleen and kidney, treat diarrhea and nourish the deficient organs.

The patient was also asked to take a Chinese patent *Jīn Guì Shèn Qì Wán* (Golden Cabinet's Kidney Qi Pill) at the dosage of 9 g, twice a day. The patient was also advised to avoid raw, cold and greasy food.

Follow-up Consultations

After 7 doses of the formula, the abdominal pain at dawn was significantly relieved and stools were slightly more formed in the last 3 days, having only one bowel movement a day. The symptoms of weakness and soreness in the lumbar, weakness, aversion to cold and cold limbs were also relieved.

After one more week of the same formula, the borborygmus and all other symptoms resolved. The patient felt relieved and stopped taking the medication. A two-year follow up confirmed no relapse of the symptoms.

CASE STUDY 2: Chronic Diarrhea with Mucus

By Dr. Xu Jing-fan

Ms Li, 40 years old. 1st consultation on April 7th, 1994.

Main Complaint: Diarrhea with white mucus for 3 years and aggravation for 3 months.

Medical History: Three years ago, the patient suffered from abdominal pain and diarrhea during the summer. It was diagnosed as acute bacillary dysentery and she had mostly recovered after treatment. Two months after the episode, she experienced diarrhea with white mucus again, passing stools twice or trice a day. There were no abdominal pain or urgency without some heaviness sensation at the anus. She was given antibiotics for several months without any change in the symptoms. In the recent 3 months, the patient had experienced a lot of stress at work which affected her mood and she was having diarrhea 2-4 times a day with a large amount of white mucus. Stool test also showed the presence of mucus without any blood cells. Stool bacteria culture showed no growth of bacteria. The patient noticed that the amount of mucus increased when eating meat so she reverted to becoming vegetarian. She was prescribed both Chinese and Western medicine without any effect.

Presenting Symptoms: lethargy, fatigue, slight distending sensation in the stomach, low appetite, a pale red tongue with a thin and white coating with a white greasy coating in the root and a thin pulse. There was no cough, no phlegm coming from the lungs and no chills or fever.

Physical Examination: The temperature was 36.8 ℃ and the facial complexion a little sallow yellow. There were no abnormal findings of her lung, heart, liver and spleen. There was no tenderness in the abdomen. The stools were loose and soft with lots of sticky white mucus.

Diagnosis

TCM Diagnosis: Diarrhea due to spleen and stomach weakness with internal retention of phlegm-damp

Western Medicine Diagnosis: Diarrhea

Treatment

The main pathomechanism of this case is the spleen failing to transport and transform the fluid and food causing a retention of dampness and phlegm in the intestines seen in the symptoms of mucus in the diarrhea.

Principles:

- Invigorate the spleen and warm the center
- Drain dampness and expel phlegm

Formula: Modified *Píng Wèi Săn* (Stomach-Calming Powder) combined with *Èr Chén Tāng* (Two Matured Substances Decoction)

Ingredients:

苍术	*cāng zhú*	10 g	Rhizoma Atractylodis (dry-fried)
白术	*bái zhú*	10 g	Rhizoma Atractylodis Macrocephalae (scorch-fried)
厚朴	*hòu pò*	10 g	Cortex Magnoliae Officinalis (prepared)
陈皮	*chén pí*	10 g	Pericarpium Citri Reticulatae (dry-fried)
法半夏	*fă bàn xià*	10 g	Rhizoma Pinelliae Praeparatum
桔梗	*jié gĕng*	10 g	Radix Platycodonis
防风	*fáng fēng*	10 g	Radix Saposhnikoviae (dry-fried)
薏苡仁	*yì yĭ rén*	30 g	Semen Coicis (dry-fried)
冬瓜子	*dōng guā zĭ*	30 g	Semen Benincasae
荷叶	*hé yè*	15 g	Folium Nelumbinis
茯苓	*fú líng*	15 g	Poria
山楂	*shān zhā*	15 g	Fructus Crataegi (scorch-fried)
神曲	*shén qū*	15 g	Massa Medicata Fermentata (scorch-fried)
炙甘草	*zhì gān căo*	5 g	Radix et Rhizoma Glycyrrhizae Praeparata cum Melle

Follow-up Consultations

After taking 10 doses of the formula, her stool was gradually formed and the amount of mucus reduced. The patient passed stool once or twice a day, the greasy tongue coating reduced and her appetite improved.

Based on the previous formula, *hòu pò* was removed and *cāng zhú* was reduced to 6 g. We also added dry-fried *dăng shēn* 10 g and dry-fried *shān yào* 15 g. After another 10 doses, the patient had more energy and the appetite became normal. She passed a bowel movement once a day without mucus and she started eating meat again. A follow-up consultation 7 months later, confirmed there was no relapse of her symptoms.

Notes

Doctor Xu diagnosed this case as phlegm diarrhea because of the reoccurring symptoms of having profuse mucus in the stools without abdominal pain or urgency or rectal heaviness. Initially, the patient suffered from acute dysentery which is usually result from internal damp-heat accumulation in the intestine that impairs the intestinal membrane and causes disharmony of the qi and blood. With timely treatment, it was cured quickly. However, bitter and cold products were used as medicine and afterwards some white mucus appeared in the stool and there was a severe increase in the amount of bowel movements. At consultation, the symptoms of white greasy tongue coating and loose stool with mucus demonstrated a spleen deficiency failing to transport producing dampness and phlegm in the intestines.

The modified *Píng Wèi Săn* (Stomach-Calming Powder) was given to invigorate the spleen and warm the center and *Èr Chén Tāng* (Two Matured Substances Decoction) was added to disperse of the dampness and phlegm. The combination of *cāng zhú* and *bái zhú* reinforces the transporting function of the spleen. *Chén pí, bàn xià, yì yĭ rén, dōng guā zĭ, jié gĕng,* and *fú líng* are all common ingredients to remove phlegm. *Fáng fēng* is added to dispel wind and remove dampness. *Hé yè* can raise the clear yang. *Shān zhā* and *shén qū* assist the spleen and stomach to transport and transform. *Gān căo* harmonizes other ingredients in the formula. We can notice that the dosage of *jié gĕng* is slightly high because of its lifting effect as well as its strong phlegm eliminating effect.

CASE STUDY 3: Chronic Diarrhea
By Dr. Lu Jing-shan

Mr. Zhao, 45 years old. 1st consultation on July 5th, 1972.

Main Complaint: Occasional loose stool and diarrhea for 8 years.

Medical History: Eight years ago, the patient experienced poor appetite, abdominal pain and diarrhea due to improper diet. After having genyamycin and saccharated yeast tablets, the symptoms resolved. However, the symptoms returned after having an improper diet again.

Presenting Symptoms: In recent a year, the patient had 4 to 5 times loose stools a day accompanied by poor appetite, fatigue, lack of strength, cold sensation in the abdomen which prefers warmth, abdominal pain and discomfort, a pale tongue with teeth marks with a thin and white coating and a thin and weak pulse especially in the *guan* and *chi* positions of the right hand.

Physical Examination: The abdominal area was flat and soft without abnormal findings.

Diagnosis

TCM Diagnosis: Diarrhea due to spleen and stomach depletion

Western Medicine Diagnosis: Chronic diarrhea

Treatment

Principles:

- Warm the middle *jiao* and dissipate cold
- Fortify the spleen and treat diarrhea

Acupuncture Point Combination: RN 11 (*jiàn lǐ*) and ST 36 (*zú sān lǐ*).

Manipulations: Insert 2 *cun* long filiform needles into the two points 1.5 *cun* deep. After the sensation of qi arrival, apply supplementing method and retain the needles for 20 minutes. Withdraw the needles and apply 3 large cones moxibustion to each point. The patient was treated everyday. After 10 days, the appetite and the mental state improved, and the stools reduced to 2 to 3 times a day. After another 10 treatments, all symptoms resolved. The patient had formed stools 1 to 2 times a day and there were no relapse noticed within the following year.

Notes

The point combination of RN 11 and ST 36 is able to treat dyspepsia, poor appetite, spontaneous sweating, fatigue, lack of strength, gastric pain, abdominal pain and diarrhea caused by spleen and stomach depletion. RN 11 can raise the clear yang and fortify the middle *jiao*, while ST 36 strengthens the spleen and stomach and lowers counterflow of turbidity. The cooperation between these two points doubles the curative effect on strengthening the spleen and stomach, supplementing middle *jiao* deficiency, improving appetite, and treating diarrhea. Even if the patient had these severe symptoms for over 8 years only two courses of acupuncture and moxibustion treatment were able to resolve all her symptoms. In cases of deficiency, we need to be patient and provide the amount of treatment needed for full recovery while preventing the reoccurrence of the syndrome. In addition, it is important to advise the patient to maintain a proper and regular diet and life style.

KEY CLINICAL POINTS

The treatment for diarrhea is generally provided by promoting the function of transportation of the spleen and dispelling dampness but tending to their corresponding patterns is essential to get the best results. It is also important to remember not to overuse bitter and cold medicinals to clear heat. Similarly, it is best not solely apply sweet and warm ingredients for deficient pattern of chronic diarrhea since they easily cause dampness retention. These additional clinical concepts are also important to notice.

1. Medicinals to strengthen the spleen should be applied with flexibility

Dampness is the main pathological factor of the symptom of diarrhea. On one hand, nourishing the spleen itself will help the body to eliminate the dampness. On the other hand, adding aromatic and drying medicinals to remove or drain the dampness will also support the spleen in its transformation and transportation functions. We need to remain flexible on which step to focus on according to the presenting symptoms. We can apply formulas to fortify the spleen and remove dampness such as *Shēn Líng Bái Zhú Săn* (Ginseng, Poria and Atractylodes Macrocephalae Powder) and *Sì Jūn Zĭ Tāng* (Four Gentlemen Decoction).

2. Do not promote urination to treat chronic diarrhea

In some cases of acute diarrhea, it is sometimes recommended to expel dampness by urination to dry the stool and treat diarrhea. However, cases of chronic diarrhea are often caused by spleen deficiency failing to transport and transform or affected by other organs which have caused an accumulation of dampness over a long period of time. In a mild case, aromatic medicinals are needed to remove dampness, while in a severe case, bitter and warm medicinals should be applied to dry dampness. If we promote urination in these cases, the healthy qi and body fluids will be damaged.

3. Be cautious of using strengthening and astringent methods.

These treatment methods can not be applied to treat acute diarrhea to avoid retaining the pathogenic factor. However, in chronic diarrhea, it is best to avoid tonifying before the pathogenic dampness, cold, food accumulation, heat and phlegm have not been totally removed. Otherwise, the pattern will worsen.

4. We must identify the appropriate pathogenic factor in a deficiency-excess pattern.

It is easy to understand that a pattern of chronic diarrhea usually leads to a deficient state. But the causes of chronic diarrhea are complex and are often accompanied by pathogenic cold, heat, phlegm, dampness, and other pathogenic factors. The practitioner should first determine the pattern, the root cause and branch manifestations. While during the treatment, we must pay attention to the priority of the manifesting symptoms between the root and branch to evaluate which treatment approach is appropriate at that moment. Such as using acrid medicinals to open orifices and bitter medicinals to descend while using the harmonizing method to balance the liver and spleen.

COMPREHENSION QUESTIONS

1. How is diarrhea differentiated from dysentery?
2. What are the treatment principles for diarrhea?
3. Multiple choice questions.

1) Signs and symptoms: abdominal pain, borborygmus, diarrhea with smelly stools which smell like rotten eggs, abdominal pain which is relieved after defecation, abdominal distension and fullness, acid and indigested food regurgitation, no appetite, a turbid or greasy and thick tongue coating and a slippery pulse.

The recommended formula is:

A. Modified *Sì Shén Wán* (Four Spirits Pill)

B. Modified *Băo Hé Wán* (Harmony-Preserving Pill)

C. Modified *Shēn Líng Bái Zhú Săn* (Ginseng, Poria and Atractylodes Macrocephalae Powder)
D. Modified *Gé Gēn Huáng Qín Huáng Lián Tāng* (Pueraria, Scutellaria, and Coptis Decoction)
E. Modified *Huò Xiāng Zhèng Qì Săn* (Agastache Qi-Correcting Powder)

2) Signs and symptoms: occasional loose stool and diarrhea for a long period of time, poor appetite, abdominal and epigastric distension and discomfort after meals, obviously increased defecation after having greasy food, a sallow yellowish and lusterless complexion, mental fatigue, a pale tongue with white coating and a thin weak pulse.

The main pathomechanism is:
A. disturbance of qi movement with the liver failing to govern smooth flow of qi
B. chronic diarrhea due to kidney yang deficiency
C. spleen and stomach weakness leading to the disorder of transportation and transformation
D. diet irregularities with internal food retention
E. damp-heat obstruction causing the disorder of transmission and transformation

Answers

1. Both of the symptoms of diarrhea and dysentery are demonstrated as increased bowel movements with loose stool. However, diarrhea is mainly characterized by increased loose stool, undigested food in the stool, or even watery stool. Its abdominal pain occurs similarly with borborygmus and relieved after defecation. Dysentery is mainly characterized by abdominal pain, tenesmus with red and white purulent blood and mucus in the stools. Its abdominal pain occurs with tenesmus at the same time and remains after defecation.

2. The basic pathomechanism of diarrhea is spleen deficiency with dampness retention. The fundamental treatment principle is to fortify the spleen and remove dampness. Acute diarrhea is mainly due to damp exuberance, so the treatment emphasis is on removing dampness assisted with promoting urination. Furthermore, according to conditions of cold-damp and damp-heat, warming and removing cold dampness or clearing and removing damp-heat can be applied respectively. If the diarrhea is complicated with exterior pathogen, apply releasing the exterior for support. For complication of summer-heat, clear the summer-heat. For complication of food damage, promote digestion. Chronic diarrhea mainly lies in the spleen deficiency, so it is key to fortify the spleen qi. For diarrhea due to liver qi over-acting the spleen, we need to smooth the liver and strengthen the spleen. For kidney yang deficiency, we need to warm the kidney and fortify the spleen. For sinking of middle *jiao* qi, we need to raise the yang qi. For lingering chronic diarrhea, using astringent medicinals is appropriate. If the case of complex pattern with both cold and heat

and deficiency-excess patterns, the treatment should be tailored to the presenting symptoms. It is worth reading, the *Required Readings from the Medical Ancestors* (*Yī Zōng Bì Dú*, 医宗必读). It is an ancient medical book which lists nine methods for treating diarrhea, including percolating with bland medicinals, lifting, clearing, draining, moderating with sweet medicinals, restraining with acid medicinals, drying the spleen, warming the kidney, and astringing discharge.

3. 1) B, 2) C.

4.6 Dysentery

Dysentery is an enteric infectious disease commonly seen in the summer and autumn mainly manifested as increased episodes of defecation, abdominal pain, abdominal urgency with rectal heaviness and stools mixed with red and white sticky mucus. In Western medicine, this syndrome is mainly associated to bacillary dysentery and amebic dysentery.

In Chinese medicine, the causes of dysentery include external contraction of seasonal pathogen such as heat dampness, cold and phlegm, toxins due to improper diet and internal damage or deficiency. The main pathomechanism is accumulation of pathogen in the intestines causing qi and blood stagnation which leave the intestines failing to transport the bowels. In an acute onset, excessive pattern is more likely where the damp-heat pattern of dysentery is more common, although the cold-damp pattern is also seen and must clearly be identified to provide the appropriate treatment. In chronic cases of dysentery, there is a complex pattern of both deficiency and excess, where the long standing pathogens have caused internal deficiency to the organs. In these cases, it is often seen as intermittent dysentery and the treatment must include both expelling the pathogens while tonifying the internal qi and blood while fortifying the organs. Within the deficiency patterns, there are the yin deficiency and yang deficiency dysentery. The deficient types of dysentery manifest with symptoms of being unable to eat or vomiting directly after eating. Patterns in the following list are the most commonly seen with their treatment principles, acupuncture points and formulas.

CLINICAL PATTERNS DIFFERENTIATION AND TREATMENTS

1. Damp-Heat Dysentery

Symptoms: Abdominal pain, tenesmus, bloody stools with white mucus, a burning sensation around the anus, scanty and dark-yellow urine, a greasy and slightly yellow tongue coating and a slippery and rapid pulse.

Treatment Principle:

- Clear heat and resolve dampness
- Remove toxin and stop pain
- Regulate qi and circulate blood

Main Acupuncture Points:

- ST 25 (*tiān shū*): Front-*mu* point of the large intestine to invigorate spleen and stomach, clear damp-heat and resolve dysentery
- SP 10 (*xuè hǎi*): To promote blood flow and dispel stasis, invigorate the spleen, resolve dampness and cool blood
- ST 36 (*zú sān lǐ*): To expel dampness, invigorate spleen, tonify qi, promote blood circulation and resolve dysentery
- ST 44 (*nèi tíng*): To clear toxic heat and dampness, regulate *yang ming* channels
- LI 11 (*qū chí*) and ST 37 (*shàng jù xū*): Upper and lower *he*-sea points of the large intestine, to resolve stagnation, expel damp-heat, cool blood, regulate qi and stop pain
- ST 40 (*fēng lóng*): Main point for expelling phlegm and dampness

Supporting Points:

- BL 27 (*xiǎo cháng shù*): To expel damp-heat, morbid leucorrhea, alleviate diarrhea, stop abdominal pain and regulate intestines
- GB 24 (*rì yuè*): Front-*mu* point of the gallbladder to resolve hypochondriac pain, expel damp-heat and benefit the gallbladder

Recommended Formula: *Sháo Yào Tāng* (芍药汤, Peony Decoction) from the *Collection of Writings on the Mechanism of Disease, Suitability of Qi, and the Safeguarding of Life as Discussed in the 'Basic Questions'* (*Sù Wèn Bìng Jī Qì Yí Bǎo Mìng Jí*, 素问病机气宜保命集)

Substitute Formula: *Huáng Qín Tāng* (黄芩汤, Scutellaria Decoction)

Patent Formula: *Xiāng Lián Piàn* (香连片, Cyperus and Coptis Tablet)

2. Toxic Heat Dysentery

Symptoms: Sudden onset of dysentery with bloody stools (with fresh or dark blood), severe abdominal pain, tenesmus, high fever with thirst, headache, restlessness, in severe cases convulsions or coma might occur, a dark-purple tongue with dry, yellow coating, slippery and a rapid pulse.

Treatment Principle:

- Clear heat and cool blood
- Relieve dysentery and clear the upper

Main Acupuncture Points:

- ST 36 (*zú sān lǐ*): To invigorate spleen, tonify qi, alleviate diarrhea, promote circulation and resolve dysentery
- ST 44 (*nèi tíng*): To clear intestinal heat and harmonize intestines
- LI 4 (*hé gǔ*): To clear *yang ming* heat, clear the head, reduce fever, alleviate dysentery and stop pain
- LI 11 (*qū chí*): *He*-sea point of the large intestine to resolve stagnation, expel dampness, alleviate diarrhea and stop pain
- LV 3 (*tài chōng*): *Yuan*-source point of the liver to spread liver qi, alleviate diarrhea, clear head and eyes, regulate blood and stop pain

• SP 10 (*xuè hǎi*): To promote blood flow and dispel stasis, invigorate the spleen and cool blood

Supporting Points:

• HT 5 (*tōng lǐ*): *Luo*-connecting point of the heart to clear intestinal heat, treat mouth ulcers and calm the spirit

• RN 10 (*xià wǎn*): To regulate qi, dispel food stagnation and treat abdominal distension

Recommended Formula: *Bái Tóu Wēng Tāng* (白头翁汤, Pulsatilla Decoction) from the *Treatise on Cold Damage* (*Shāng Hán Lùn*, 伤寒论)

Substitute Formula: *Gé Gēn Huáng Qín Huáng Lián Tāng* (葛根黄芩黄连汤, Pueraria, Scutellaria, and Coptis Decoction) combined with *Huáng Lián Jiě Dú Tāng* (黄连解毒汤, Coptis Toxin-Resolving Decoction)

Patent Formula: *Gé Gēn Qín Lián Wán* (葛根芩连丸, Pueraria, Scutellaria, and Coptis Pill)

3. Damp-Cold Dysentery

Symptoms: Stools containing profuse white and sticky mucus and blood, abdominal pain, tenesmus, poor appetite, gastric fullness, head and body heaviness, a pale tongue with a white, greasy coating and a soggy and moderate pulse.

Treatment Principle:

• Warm and tonify qi

• Expel cold and resolve dampness

• Activate qi and stop pain

Main Acupuncture Points:

• ST 25 (*tiān shū*): Front-*mu* point of the large intestine to invigorate spleen and stomach, expel dampness, regulate qi and resolve dysentery

• RN 12 (*zhōng wǎn*): Front-*mu* point of the stomach to harmonize spleen and stomach, warm middle *jiao* and regulate qi

• RN 8 (*shén què*): Apply moxibustion to warm the yang and regulate fluid passages

• ST 36 (*zú sān lǐ*): To expel dampness, strengthen immune system, invigorate spleen, tonify correct qi, alleviate diarrhea, promote circulation and regulate dysentery

• RN 6 (*qì hǎi*): To invigorate spleen, tonify original qi, fortify yang and promote circulation

• BL 20 (*pí shù*): Back-*shu* point of the spleen to regulate middle *jiao* qi, invigorate spleen, alleviate diarrhea and stop abdominal pain

Supporting Points:

• BL 30 (*bái huán shù*): To warm the uterus, regulate menstruation, leucorrhea and seminal emission

• SP 14 (*fù jié*): To invigorate spleen and warm middle *jiao*, descend rebellious qi

and umbilical pain

Recommended Formula: *Wèi Líng Tāng* (胃苓汤, Stomach-Calming Poria Decoction) from the *Teachings of [Zhu] Dan-xi* (*Dān Xī Xīn Fǎ*, 丹溪心法)

Substitute Formula: *Bú Huàn Jīn Zhèng Qì Sǎn* (不换金正气散, Priceless Qi-Righting Powder)

Patent Formula: *Huò Xiāng Zhèng Qì Ruǎn Jiāo Náng* (藿香正气软胶囊, Agastache Qi-Correcting Soft Capsule)

4. Yin Deficiency Dysentery

Symptoms: Stools containing purulent blood or viscous fresh blood, burning pain around the umbilicus, difficult bowel movements, poor appetite, restlessness, dry mouth, dry eyes, a dark-red tongue with scanty coating and a thready and rapid pulse.

Treatment Principle:

- Nourish yin and body fluids
- Harmonize *ying* and *wei* qi
- Clear the intestines and stop pain

Main Acupuncture Points:

- ST 25 (*tiān shū*): Front-*mu* point of the large intestine to invigorate spleen and stomach, regulate qi and resolve dysentery
- ST 36 (*zú sān lǐ*): To invigorate spleen, tonify qi, promote circulation and resolve dysentery
- RN 12 (*zhōng wǎn*): Front-*mu* point of the stomach to harmonize spleen and stomach, benefit middle *jiao*, regulate qi and stop abdominal pain
- KI 6 (*zhào hǎi*): To clear deficient fire and regulate yin motility vessel
- SP 6 (*sān yīn jiāo*): To invigorate spleen and nourish yin, harmonize the lower *jiao*, regulate menstruation and improve digestion
- KI 3 (*tài xī*): *Yuan*-source point of kidney to tonify kidney yin, clear deficient fire and invigorate spleen

Supporting Points:

- SP 14 (*fù jié*): To invigorate spleen, warm middle *jiao*, descend rebellious qi and relieve umbilical pain
- RN 4 (*guān yuán*): Front-*mu* point of the small intestine to tonify original qi, supplement deficiency, regulate small intestine and harmonize menstruation

Recommended Formula: *Zhù Chē Wán* (驻车丸, Carriage-Halting Pill) from the *Important Formulas Worth a Thousand Gold Pieces for Emergency* (*Bèi Jí Qiān Jīn Yào Fāng*, 备急千金要方)

Substitute Formula: *Huáng Lián Ē Jiāo Tāng* (黄连阿胶汤, Coptis and Ass-Hide Gelatin Decoction)

5. Yang Deficiency Dysentery

Symptoms: Thin, clear stools containing white mucus or incontinence, dull abdominal pain, poor appetite, mental fatigue, cold limbs, lumbar coldness and soreness, a pale tongue with thin and white coating and a deep, thready and weak pulse.

Treatment Principle:

- Warm and tonify kidney and spleen
- Strengthen the bowel holding functions

Main Acupuncture Points:

- ST 25 (*tiān shū*): Front-*mu* point of the large intestine to invigorate spleen and stomach, regulate qi and resolve dysentery
- RN 8 (*shén què*): Apply moxibustion to warm the yang and rescue from collapse
- ST 36 (*zú sān lǐ*): To invigorate spleen, tonify correct qi, alleviate diarrhea and promote circulation
- BL 20 (*pí shù*): Back-*shu* point of the spleen to regulate middle *jiao* qi, invigorate spleen, alleviate diarrhea and stop abdominal pain
- BL 23 (*shèn shù*): Back-*shu* point of the kidney to tonify kidney and fortify yang, supplement qi and strengthen lumbar region
- RN 12 (*zhōng wǎn*): Front-*mu* point of the stomach to harmonize spleen and stomach, warm middle *jiao* and regulate qi

Supporting Points:

- RN 10 (*xià wǎn*): To regulate qi, dispel food stagnation and stop abdominal pain
- BL 27 (*xiǎo cháng shù*): To treat morbid leucorrhea, treat hemorrhoid, resolve dysentery, stop abdominal pain and regulate intestines

Recommended Formula: *Táo Huā Tāng* (桃花汤, Peach Blossom Decoction) from the *Treatise on Cold Damage* (*Shāng Hán Lùn*, 伤寒论) combined with *Zhēn Rén Yǎng Zàng Tāng* (真人养脏汤, Enlightened Master Viscera-Nourishing Decoction) from the *Beneficial Formulas from the Taiping Imperial Pharmacy* (*Tài Píng Huì Mín Hé Jì Jú Fāng*, 太平惠民和剂局方)

Substitute Formula: *Lǐ Zhōng Wán* (理中丸, Center-Regulating Pill)

Patent Formula: *Bǔ Pí Yì Cháng Wán* (补脾益肠丸, Spleen-Reinforcing Intestine-Benefiting Pill)

6. Recurrent Dysentery

Symptoms: Persistent and recurrent dysentery, decreased food intake quantity, lassitude, aversion to cold, abdominal pain, tenesmus with stools containing mucus or blood, a pale tongue with greasy coating and a soggy or deficient and weak pulse.

Treatment Principle:

- Warm the middle *jiao* and strengthen the spleen
- Clear the intestines and expel pathogen
- Circulate qi and stop pain

Main Acupuncture Points:

- ST 25 (*tiān shū*): Front-*mu* point of the large intestine to invigorate spleen and stomach, regulate qi and resolve dysentery

- ST 36 (*zú sān lǐ*): To invigorate spleen, tonify correct qi, alleviate diarrhea and promote circulation
- BL 20 (*pí shù*): Back-*shu* point of the spleen to regulate middle *jiao* qi, invigorate spleen, alleviate diarrhea and stop abdominal pain
- RN 12 (*zhōng wǎn*): Front-*mu* point of the stomach to harmonize spleen and stomach, warm middle *jiao* and regulate qi
- BL 25 (*dà cháng shù*): Back-*shu* point of the large intestine to regulate intestines and stomach, tonify qi and resolve dysentery and stop pain
- LV 13 (*zhāng mén*): Front-*mu* point of the spleen to invigorate spleen, regulate stomach and stop abdominal pain

Supporting Points:

- EX-CA 5 (*wèi shàng*): To tonify and raise the middle qi
- BL 30 (*bái huán shù*): To warm the uterus, regulate menstruation, leucorrhea and seminal emission

Recommended Formula: *Shēn Líng Bái Zhú Sǎn* (参苓白术散, Ginseng, Poria and Atractylodes Macrocephalae Powder) from the *Beneficial Formulas from the Taiping Imperial Pharmacy* (*Tài Píng Huì Mín Hé Jì Jú Fāng*, 太平惠民和剂局方)

Substitute Formula: *Lián Lǐ Tāng* (连理汤, Coptis Rectifying Decoction)

Patent Formula: *Shēn Líng Bái Zhú Wán* (参苓白术丸, Ginseng, Poria and Atractylodes Macrocephalae Pill)

Summary Chart for Dysentery

Patterns	Main Points	Supporting Points	Formulae
Damp-Heat Dysentery	ST 25, SP 10, ST 36, ST 44, LI 11, ST 37, ST 40	BL 27 for morbid leucorrhea GB 24 for gallbladder damp-heat	*Sháo Yào Tāng* or *Huáng Qín Tāng*
Toxic Heat Dysentery	ST 36, ST 44, LI 4, LI 11, LV 3, SP 10	HT 5 for mouth ulcers due to heart heat RN 10 for food stagnation	*Bái Tóu Wēng Tāng* or *Gé Gēn Huáng Qín Huáng Lián Tāng* plus *Huáng Lián Jiě Dú Tāng*
Damp-Cold Dysentery	ST 25, RN 12, RN 8, ST 36, RN 6, BL 20	BL 30 for uterine cold SP 14 for umbilical pain	*Wèi Líng Tāng* or *Bú Huàn Jīn Zhèng Qì Sǎn*
Yin Deficiency Dysentery	ST 25, ST 36, RN 12, KI 6, SP 6, KI 3	SP 14 for umbilical pain RN 4 for irregular menstruation	*Zhù Chē Wán* or *Huáng Lián Ē Jiāo Tāng*
Yang Deficiency Dysentery	ST 25, RN 8, ST 36, BL 20, BL 23, RN 12	RN 10 for food stagnation BL 27 for morbid leucorrhea and hemorrhoids	*Táo Huā Tāng* plus *Zhēn Rén Yǎng Zàng Tāng* or *Lǐ Zhōng Wán*
Recurrent Dysentery	ST 25, ST 36, BL 20, RN 12, BL 25, LV 13	EX-CA 5 for middle qi sinking BL 30 for uterine cold	*Shēn Líng Bái Zhú Sǎn* or *Lián Lǐ Tāng*

CASE STUDY 1: Acute Dysentery

Mr. Li, 18 years old.

Main Complaint: Stool containing pus and blood with abdominal pain for twelve hours.

Medical History: The patient swam in the river the day prior at noon and faced a thunder shower on the way home. He ate the remaining food from breakfast and suffered abdominal pain and urgency with rectal heaviness at night. The patient had been to the toilet three times since the night prior and the discharged stool contained pus and blood.

Presenting Symptoms: Abdominal pain, abdominal urgency with rectal heaviness, stool containing white pus and blood, thirst with preference to cold drinks, burning pain in the anus, scant dark urine, a red tongue with yellow greasy coating and a slippery and rapid pulse.

Physical Examination: Temperature: 37.2 ℃, pulse: 88 bpm, respiration: 20 bpm, blood pressure: 120/70 mmHg. The patient was lethargic and his facial complexion was red with dry lips. His neck was soft with no resistance. The chest was normal. His abdomen was slightly protruding and soft when pressed. There was tenderness in the middle and lower abdomen without rebound tenderness.

Pattern Differentiation

The patient contracted dampness during his walk in the rain after spending a day in the river. Since it was in the middle of summer, the weather was damp and hot. Since the patient also ate some unsanitary food, it injured the internal organs and lead to the internal accumulation of dampness and heat in the interior as well. Thus, both the external contraction and internal pathogens damaged the stomach and intestines which resulted in damp-heat type of dysentery. The scorching damp heat in the intestinal leads to the injury of the intestines causing qi stagnation and blood stasis manifested in the abdominal pain and urgency as well as in the blood and pus in the stools. Internal excess of heat injures the body fluids manifesting in the red facial complexion, dry lips, and thirst with a preference for cold drinks. Damp-heat pouring downward leads to the burning pain in anus and the scant dark urine. The red tongue with the yellow greasy coating and the slippery and rapid pulse are both manifestations of the accumulated and steaming of dampness and heat.

Diagnosis

TCM Diagnosis: Dysentery due to damp-heat accumulation

Western Medicine Diagnosis: Acute dysentery

Treatment

The main pathomechanism of this case is the accumulation and stagnation of dampness and heat in intestines.

Principles:

- Clear heat and remove stagnation
- Regulate qi and move blood
- Expel Dampness and stop pain

Formula: Modified *Sháo Yào Tāng* (Peony Decoction)

Ingredients:

白芍	*bái sháo*	15 g	Radix Paeoniae Alba
黄芩	*huáng qín*	12 g	Radix Scutellariae
黄连	*huáng lián*	12 g	Rhizoma Coptidis
大黄	*dà huáng*	10 g	Radix et Rhizoma Rhei
槟榔	*bīng láng*	12 g	Semen Arecae
当归	*dāng guī*	15 g	Radix Angelicae Sinensis
木香	*mù xiāng*	12 g	Radix Aucklandiae
金银花	*jīn yín huā*	15 g	Flos Lonicerae Japonicae
焦麦芽	*jiāo mài yá*	15 g	Fructus Hordei Germinatus (scorch-fried)
焦山楂	*jiāo shān zhā*	15 g	Fructus Crataegi (scorch-fried)
焦神曲	*jiāo shén qū*	15 g	Massa Medicata Fermentata (scorch-fried)
炙甘草	*zhì gān cǎo*	6 g	Radix et Rhizoma Glycyrrhizae Praeparata cum Melle

Formula Analysis:

In this formula, *bái sháo* and *dāng guī* are used to treat blood stasis by cooling and moving blood and harmonizing *ying*. *Mù xiāng, bīng láng* and *dà huáng* can relieve rectal heaviness by moving qi and removing stagnation. *Jīn yín huā, huáng qín* and *huáng lián* can clear heat, dry dampness and resolve toxins. *Jiāo shān zhā, jiāo shén qū* and *jiāo mài yá* can promote digestion and remove food stagnation. This formula can clear heat and dry dampness while regulating and harmonizing qi and blood. The patient was also administered a Chinese medicinal patent called *Xiāng Lián Wán* (Aucklandiae and Coptidis Pill), at the dosage of 6 g, three times a day and was told to eat only light food and avoid raw, cold, fatty, sweet, oily and greasy food.

Follow-up Consultations

After taking seven days of the formula, the abdominal pain and urgency with rectal heaviness were alleviated and the red and white purulent blood in the stools reduced. The fever remitted and gradually resumed health. The patient continued the formula for another week and recovered completely.

CASE STUDY 2: Dysentery
By Dr. Huang Zhi-qiang

Mr. Chen, 32 years old. 1st consultation on July 2nd, 2003.

Main Complaint: Diarrhea with white mucus for two months.

Medical History: The patient suffered from continual diarrhea 3 to 6 times a day with abdominal distension, fullness and dull pain, heavy and sagging feeling in the anus and poor appetite. This following a meal of sea food the patient made by himself over 2 months ago. His diarrhea was exacerbated by cold and the abdominal pain was severe. The stool contained white sticky mucus.

Presenting Symptoms: 3 to 6 episodes of diarrhea a day containing white mucus, abdominal urgency with rectal heaviness which worsens with cold, fatigue, poor appetite, a dull and moist tongue with thin, white and greasy coating and a wiry thin pulse. A stool test confirmed the presence of large amount of pus and a few RBC.

Diagnosis

TCM Diagnosis: Intermittent dysentery due to obstruction of dampness and cold

Western Medicine Diagnosis: Intermittent dysentery

Treatment

The main pathomechanism of this case of dysentery is the spleen and stomach yang qi deficiency with lingering intestinal food accumulation causing a qi stagnation and blood stasis with accumulation of damp-cold.

Principles:

- Warm the middle *jiao* and clear the intestine
- Drain and dry dampness
- Move qi and stop pain

Formula: Modified *Wēn Pí Tāng* (Spleen-Warming Decoction)

Ingredients:

生大黄	*shēng dà huáng*	6 g	Radix et Rhizoma Rhei (raw)
淡附子	*dàn fù zǐ*	4 g	Radix Aconiti Lateralis Praeparata
干姜	*gān jiāng*	5 g	Rhizoma Zingiberis
白芍	*bái sháo*	20 g	Radix Paeoniae Alba
当归	*dāng guī*	15 g	Radix Angelicae Sinensis
川连	*huáng lián*	5 g	Rhizoma Coptidis
广木香	*guǎng mù xiāng*	10 g	Radix Aucklandiae
厚朴	*hòu pò*	12 g	Cortex Magnoliae Officinalis
茯苓	*fú líng*	15 g	Poria
薏苡仁	*yì yǐ rén*	30 g	Semen Coicis
甘草	*gān cǎo*	5 g	Radix et Rhizoma Glycyrrhizae

Follow-up Consultations

After five doses of the formula, the frequency of the defecation reduced to one to two times a day, and the white sticky mucus appeared only occasionally and the rectal heaviness alleviated. After taking seven additional doses, all symptoms resolved.

Formula Analysis

The incomplete treatment of dysentery which lasted over 2 months might lead to chronic dysentery. In the treatment for chronic dysentery, we need to address the deficiency pattern. Ancient Chinese medicine experts noted that "stomach qi is the basis of health, and it is especially important when treating dysentery". This notion clearly states the importance of protecting the stomach qi. Additionally, the efficacy of the treatment can be more significant by also regulating qi and moving blood since there is always qi and blood stagnation in the intestine due to the inhibited intestinal function manifesting as abdominal urgency with rectal heaviness and stools containing sticky mucus and purulent blood. Dr. Liu He-jian noted that "Rectal heaviness can be eliminated naturally by regulating qi and the defecation of pus can be cured by moving blood".

In the formula, *dà huáng, fù zǐ, gān jiāng,* and *gān cǎo* are from *Wēn Pí Tāng* documented in the *Important Formulas Worth a Thousand Gold Pieces for Emergency* (*Bèi Jí Qiān Jīn Yào Fāng,* 备急千金要方) written by Sun Si-miao. *Fù zǐ, gān jiāng,* and *gān cǎo* are used to warm the center and to fortify the spleen. *Dà huáng* can clear heat, dissolve stasis and remove stagnation to clear the accumulation and remove stagnation in the intestines. *Huáng lián* is added to clear intestines and dry dampness. *Hòu pò, fú ling, yì yǐ rén* can dry dampness and fortify spleen. *Mù xiāng* can move qi and harmonize the stomach. *Dāng guī* and *bái sháo* serve to harmonize blood.

CASE STUDY 3: Pediatric Acute Dysentery
By Dr. Shi Xue-min

Mr. Xiao, 4 years old. 1st consultation on August 21th, 1981.

Main Complaint: Paroxysmal abdominal pain accompanied by emesis and diarrhea for four days.

Medical History: The patient suddenly suffered from a high fever of 40.5 ℃ in the afternoon of August 18th. There was absence of sweating and abdominal discomfort. He vomited fluids and food six times that day. He had diarrhea for three days and the stools were watery without pus and blood. He had taken antipyretics at home, but the fever did not resolve so he was taken to the Children's Hospital for emergency treatment. The patient was diagnosed with bacillary dysentery after examining his stool. He received intravenous injection of hydrocortisone and tetracycline and went home with some medicine after the fever remitted the next day. At noon of the following day (19th of August), his temperature rose to over 39 ℃ again. He had watery diarrhea containing mucus immediately following abdominal pain. He was taken to the hospital again for infusion, during which his abdominal pain aggravated intermittently. That afternoon the child had diarrhea over 20 times and maintained a temperature over 39 ℃. The symptoms were slightly relieved after he received another dose of hydrocortisone, atropine and tetracycline. He was admitted to the hospital for observation.

Physical Examination: Temperature: 38.2 ℃, pulse: 100 bpm, blood pressure: 90/60 mmHg. The child was alert but in low spirit. He was slightly undernourished. He had depressed eye sockets, wrinkled skin with poor elasticity, and no redness or swelling of the throat. The superficial lymph nodes were unpalpable. His neck was supple. No abnormal findings in the lungs. He had a regular heart beat, strong heart sounds, a little sunken and soft abdomen without obvious tenderness, unpalpable liver and spleen, active bowel sounds, redness of the anus, red tongue with a thin yellow coating and a thready and rapid pulse.

Blood Routine Test: WBC 13 400/mm^3, neutrophil 80%, lymphocyte 20%.

Stool Routine Test: RBC 10-15/HF, pyocytes all over the scope.

Diagnosis

TCM Diagnosis: Dysentery due to damp-heat retention

Western Medicine Diagnosis: Acute Dysentery

Treatment

Principles:

- Clear heat and resolve toxins
- Unblock the bowels and drain dampness

Acupuncture Point Combination: ST 37 (*shàng jù xū*), ST 25 (*tiān shū*), LI 11 (*qū chí*), PC 6 (*nèi guān*), ST 36 (*zú sān lǐ*), RN 4 (*guān yuán*).

Manipulations: Insert the needle one *cun* perpendicularly at ST 37 and stimulate to have a sensation radiating to the lower legs. Insert one *cun* perpendicularly at ST 25 and stimulate to have a sensation radiating to the lower abdomen. Insert one *cun* perpendicularly at LI 11 and PC 6 and stimulate to have a sensation radiating to the forearms. Apply the twirling, lifting and thrusting methods to purge all the points for one minute. Then apply the twirling method of even supplementation and drainage to ST 36 and RN 4 for one minute.

After one treatment, the abdominal pain and urgency with rectal heaviness resolved and after two treatments, the frequency of diarrhea decreased to two to three times a day. The patient was in better spirit and his appetite improved greatly. The body temperature reduced and all symptoms resolved. The patient received five more treatments to strengthen the body and consolidate the curative effect.

Notes

According to Western medicine, this case of acute dysentery is caused by the infection of dysentery bacillus and is easily contracted in the summer and autumn. According to Chinese medicine this case of dysentery is caused by the invasion of dampness and toxic heat. In serious cases, there might be signs of some critical symptoms such as fever, coma, convulsion and shock. In this case, the patient contracted an invasion of summer damp-heat which affected the spleen and stomach and damaged the body fluids. The pathogenic dampness and heat stagnate in the intestines causing qi stagnation manifested in the abdominal urgency and pain and the desire of defecation. The steaming of the dampness and heat results in fever.

In this acupuncture point selection, ST 37, ST 25 and LI 11 are the main points to treat intestinal diseases with heat clearing and dampness removing functions. RN 4 is the front-*mu* point of the small intestine channel and is used to regulate the spleen and stomach. After the middle *jiao* has been rectified, the acquired essence of food can be absorbed for nourishment and strength. When the source of qi and blood production is adequate, the healthy qi will return and be able to counteract with the pathogenic qi and the symptoms will resolve.

KEY CLINICAL POINTS

In the treatment of dysentery, we must treat the syndrome according to the pattern. First, unblock the intestines to remove and expel the pathogenic factors, warm in cold pattern and clear in heat patterns. Similarly, external treatment with herbal enemas can be used to quicken the effect. As for the bacillary dysentery and amebic dysentery, which are infectious, we should also prevent and control the spread of the disease. Furthermore, we should pay attention to the following clinical points:

1. For intermittent dysentery which breaks out recurrently and is chronic, if it is caused by amebic protozoa, *bái tóu wēng* and *shí liú pí* can be added to the treatment formula. In addition, 10 to 15 *yā dǎn zǐ* kernels can be made into capsules and taken after meals three times a day for 7 to 10 days as a course of treatment.

2. For acute dysentery which mainly appears in excess heat patterns, ancient Chinese medicine experts have said that we should not stop the bowels from moving and we should not apply the supplementing method. But in chronic dysentery or dysentery manifested mainly by chronic ulcerative colitis with cold-heat complex, the modified *Wū Méi Wán* (Mume Pill) formula can be used.

3. Using 30 g of the single medicinals *mǎ chǐ xiàn* and *xiǎo fēng wěi cǎo* have good effects on damp-heat dysentery when taken orally. One or both of these medicinals can also be added to the prescribed formulas. *Huáng lián* is bitter in flavor and cold in property and it has a good effect on treating dysentery where the dosage and application should be appropriate to the presenting case without harming the

stomach qi.

4. In chronic cases, with recurrent attacks, it is important to know that they are relatively difficult to treat. Hence, applying a Chinese medicinal enema with 100 ml decoction of *huáng lián, huáng bǎi, bái tóu wēng,* and *dà huáng,* is indicated for chronic ulcerative colitis, and chronic bacillary dysentery. Enema made of the decoction of *Xī Lèi Sǎn* (Tin-Like Powder) can also be applied to ulcerative colitis.

5. In epidemic toxic dysentery, if the case presents with syncope with continual diarrhea, no appetite, cold extremities and faint pulse, *Dú Shēn Tāng* (Single Ginseng Decoction) or *Shēn Fù Tāng* (Ginseng and Aconite Decoction) should be applied immediately to boost qi to consolidate yang.

6. In dysentery with inability to eat or dysentery with nausea mainly results from stomach disharmony and ascending-descending disorder of qi movement. They are critical and should be treated immediately. In excess patterns, modified *Kāi Jīn Sǎn* (Open Appetite Powder) or *Yù Shū Dān* (Jade Pivot Elixir) can be used. In deficiency patterns, *Liù Jūn Zǐ Tāng* (Six Gentlemen Decoction) plus *shí chāng pú* and *jiāng zhī* should be used to awaken the spleen and fortify the stomach.

COMPREHENSION QUESTIONS

1. What are the etiology and pathomechanism of dysentery?
2. What are the different causes and symptoms of dysentery and diarrhea?
3. What are the treatment principles for dysentery?
4. Multiple choice questions:

1) There are symptoms of abdominal pain and urgency with rectal heaviness, stool with red and white purulent blood sticky and smelly, burning sensation in the anus and scanty dark urine a yellow greasy coating and a slippery and rapid pulse. The differentiation pattern is:

A. Cold-damp dysentery
B. Epidemic toxin dysentery
C. Yin deficiency dysentery
D. Damp-heat dysentery
E. Intermittent dysentery

2) In the initial onset of damp-heat dysentery, when the exterior pathogen has not been released and there is excessive interior heat with symptoms of fever, sweating and a rapid pulse. What is the recommended formula:

A. *Sháo Yào Tāng* (Peony Decoction)
B. *Gé Gēn Qín Lián Tāng* (Pueraria, Scutellaria, and Coptis Decoction)
C. *Jīng Fáng Bài Dú Sǎn* (Schizonepeta and Saposhnikovia Toxin-Resolving Powder)
D. *Zhǐ Shí Dǎo Zhì Wán* (Immature Bitter Orange Stagnation-Moving Pill)

E. *Bái Tóu Wēng Tāng* (Pulsatilla Decoction)

Answers

1. The binding of damp-heat, epidemic toxin and cold-damp in the intestines cause qi and blood stagnation and damage the spleen and stomach as well as the intestinal vessels which causes the large intestine to fail to transport food residues manifesting as dysentery.

2. Both symptoms of dysentery and diarrhea occur more often in the summer and autumn and the location of the diseases is in the intestines and stomach. They are caused by external contraction of seasonal pathogens and internal injury due to improper diet. However, these two diseases manifest in different symptoms and pathomechanisms.

Dysentery is due to stagnation of damp-heat, epidemic toxin and food in intestines that bind with qi and blood which damage the spleen, stomach and intestinal vessels manifesting in frequent scanty defecation containing red and white purulent blood with severe abdominal urgency and rectal heaviness, incomplete or difficult defecation.

Diarrhea is due to interior retention of pathogenic dampness or spleen deficiency with dampness excess, leading to the failure of the spleen to transport and transform manifesting as loose or watery stool with possible undigested food, or fecal incontinence. In this case, the stool does not contain red and white purulent pus and there is no obvious sense of abdominal urgency with rectal heaviness.

3. The treatment principles of dysentery are directly related to their disease pattern. While it is proper to unblock the excess pathogens at the beginning stages we need to supplement deficiency in chronic cases. We need to clear for heat patterns, to warm for cold patterns, and to astringe in deficient patterns.

For dysentery with exterior pattern, it is better to add exterior-releasing formulas for dredging the exterior and unblocking the interior. If there is food stagnation, medicinals to promote digestion and guide out stagnation can be added. If there is rectal heaviness, it can be treated by regulating qi while the defecation of pus can be treated by moving blood. These two treatment principles are the main ones to treat dysentery. During the treatment of dysentery, it is important to always protect the stomach qi.

4. 1) D, 2) B.

4.7 Bloody Stool

Bloody stool is a kind of disease caused by the injury of stomach and intestines with clinical manifestations of stool containing blood or black stools. Bloody stool is a commonly seen symptom in internal medicine which is due to diseases such as gastrointestinal inflammation, ulcers, tumors, diverticulitis, and polyps.

In Chinese medicine, there are various patterns associated with the symptoms of bloody stools. There are the invasion of exogenous pathogens, disturbances due to internal emotional disorders, intake of improper diet, overstrain and overwork, prolonged illness or febrile diseases. These patterns lead to the injury of stomach and intestines and cause the irregular flow of blood out of the vessels. The two main pathomechanisms are: the irregular flow of blood outside of the vessel due to internal fire and heat and blood spilling out of vessels due to qi deficiency failing to contain reflecting the excessive and deficient patterns respectively. Qi deficiency is further divided into righteous qi deficiency and yang deficiency. Although the causes of the excessive and deficient patterns hold very different roots, the change of the excessive pattern to a deficient pattern is commonly seen in clinic. For example, if excessive pathogenic damp-heat retention in the intestines drives blood out of vessels during a long period of time, it will render to the depletion of yin and blood as well as the internal generation of deficient fire consuming qi of the middle *jiao* leading the qi failing to control the blood. Below is a list of the commonly seen patterns and their respective treatment principles, acupuncture points and formulas.

CLINICAL PATTERNS DIFFERENTIATION AND TREATMENTS

1. Damp-Heat Retention in the Intestines

Symptoms: Foul-smelling bright red bloody stools, stools which are either difficult to pass or loose, tenesmus, burning sensation around the anus, abdominal pain, bitter taste, dry mouth, a red tongue with yellow and greasy coating and a soft and rapid or slippery and rapid pulse.

Treatment Principle:

- Clear heat and drain dampness
- Cool blood and stop bleeding

Main Acupuncture Points:

- ST 37 (*shàng jù xū*) and LI 11 (*qū chí*): Upper and lower *he*-sea points of the large intestine to resolve stagnation, expel damp-heat, cool blood, regulate qi and stop pain

- PC 4 (*xì mén*): *Xi*-cleft point of the pericardium to promote blood circulation, cool blood and stop bleeding
- ST 40 (*fēng lóng*): To expel phlegm and dampness
- ST 44 (*nèi tíng*): To clear toxic heat, drain dampness and regulate *yang ming* channels
- LI 4 (*hé gǔ*): To clear *yang ming* heat, activate the channel and stop pain
- SP 10 (*xuè hǎi*): To promote blood flow and dispel stasis, invigorate the spleen and cool blood

Supporting Points:

- BL 27 (*xiǎo cháng shù*): To expel damp-heat, morbid leucorrhea, alleviate diarrhea, stop abdominal pain and regulate intestines
- GB 24 (*rì yuè*): Front-*mu* point of the gallbladder to resolve hypochondriac pain, expel damp-heat and benefit the gallbladder

Recommended Formula: *Dì Yú Sǎn* (地榆散, Sanguisorba Powder) from the *[Yang] Ren-zhai's Direct Guidance on Formulas* (*Rén Zhāi Zhí Zhǐ Fāng*, 仁斋直指方)

Substitute Formula: *Huái Jiǎo Wán* (槐角丸, Sophora Pill)

Patent Formula: *Huái Jiǎo Wán* (槐角丸, Sophora Pill)

2. Qi Failing to Control the Blood

Symptoms: Recurring bloody stools with red or dark purple blood, either mild or profuse in volume, pale complexion, shortness of breath, lassitude, dull epigastric pain which likes pressure, emaciation, palpitations, insomnia, disinclination to speak, a pale tongue and a thready and weak pulse.

Treatment Principle:

- Invigorate spleen and warm the middle *jiao*
- Tonify qi and control blood

Main Acupuncture Points:

- BL 17 (*gé shù*): Influential point of the blood to nourish and harmonize blood, promote circulation and treat bloody stools
- SP 6 (*sān yīn jiāo*): To harmonize spleen and nourish yin, invigorate blood and improve digestion
- SP 8 (*dì jī*): *Xi*-cleft point of the spleen to invigorate blood, regulate spleen, improve digestion and benefit appetite
- ST 36 (*zú sān lǐ*): To invigorate spleen, tonify correct qi and promote blood circulation
- BL 20 (*pí shù*): Back-*shu* point of the spleen to invigorate spleen, control bleeding and stop abdominal pain
- RN 6 (*qì hǎi*): To invigorate spleen, tonify original qi, harmonize blood and promote circulation

Supporting Points:

- BL 35 (*huì yáng*): To treat bloody stools and hemorrhoids
- BL 54 (*zhì biān*): To treat hematuria and bloody stools

Recommended Formula: *Guī Pí Tāng* (归脾汤, Spleen-Restoring Decoction) from the *Formulas to Aid the Living* (*Jì Shēng Fāng*, 济生方)

Substitute Formula: *Bŭ Zhōng Yì Qì Tāng* (补中益气汤, Center-Supplementing and Qi-Boosting Decoction)

Patent Formula: *Guī Pí Wán* (归脾丸, Spleen-Restoring Pill)

3. Deficient Cold of the Spleen and Stomach

Symptoms: Dark purple or black bloody loose stools, cold limbs, aversion to cold, dull abdominal pain which likes warmth and pressure, preference for hot drinks, emaciation, poor appetite, pale complexion, lassitude, a pale tongue and a thready and weak pulse.

Treatment Principle:

- Strengthen the spleen and warm the middle *jiao*
- Nourish blood and stop bleeding

Main Acupuncture Points:

- RN 8 (*shén què*): Apply moxibustion to warm the yang and regulate fluid passages
- ST 25 (*tiān shū*): Front-*mu* point of the large intestine to invigorate spleen and stomach, regulate qi and stop pain
- ST 36 (*zú sān lĭ*): To invigorate spleen, tonify qi and blood, promote circulation and stop pain
- RN 12 (*zhōng wăn*): Front-*mu* point of the stomach to harmonize spleen and stomach, warm middle *jiao* and regulate qi
- BL 20 (*pí shù*): Back-*shu* point of the spleen to invigorate spleen, control bleeding and stop abdominal pain
- BL 17 (*gé shù*): Influential point of the blood to nourish and harmonize blood, promote circulation and treat bloody stools

Supporting Points:

- RN 10 (*xià wăn*): To regulate qi, dispel food stagnation and stop abdominal pain
- BL 27 (*xiăo cháng shù*): To treat morbid leucorrhea, cure hemorrhoids, stop abdominal pain and regulate intestines

Recommended Formula: *Huáng Tŭ Tāng* (黄土汤, Yellow Earth Decoction) from the *Essentials from the Golden Cabinet* (*Jīn Guì Yào Lüè*, 金匮要略)

Substitute Formula: *Lĭ Zhōng Wán* (理中丸, Center-Regulating Pill) combined with *Chì Xiăo Dòu Dāng Guī Săn* (赤小豆当归散, Semen Phaseoil and Chinese Angelica Powder)

Patent Formula: *Lĭ Zhōng Wán* (理中丸, Center-Regulating Pill)

4. Wind Damaging Intestinal Collaterals

Symptoms: Bloody stools with fresh blood or dry stools or diarrhea, anal pruritus, hemorrhoids, a red tongue with a yellow coating and a wiry pulse.

Treatment Principles:

- Clear intestines and stop bleeding
- Dispel wind and harmonize collaterals

Main Acupuncture Points:

- RN 12 (*zhōng wǎn*): Front-*mu* point of the stomach to harmonize spleen and stomach, regulate middle *jiao* and tonify qi
- ST 36 (*zú sān lǐ*): To invigorate spleen, tonify qi and blood, promote circulation and stop pain
- BL 20 (*pí shù*): Back-*shu* point of the spleen to invigorate spleen, control bleeding and stop abdominal pain
- LI 4 (*hé gǔ*): To expel wind, harmonize collaterals, activate the channel and stop pain
- GB 31 (*fēng shì*): To expel wind, activate channel
- ST 25 (*tiān shū*): Front-*mu* point of the large intestine to invigorate spleen and stomach, regulate qi and stop pain

Supporting Points:

- SI 3 (*hòu xī*): To treat fever due to wind attacking upwards, benefit the head and neck
- BL 8 (*luò què*): To clear vision and dizziness due to heat attacking upwards

Recommended Formula: *Huái Huā Sǎn* (槐花散, Flos Sophorae Powder) from the *Experiential Formulas for Universal Relief* (*Pǔ Jì Běn Shì Fāng*, 普济本事方)

Substitute Formula:

- *Huái Jiǎo Wán* (槐角丸, Sophora Pill)
- *Liáng Xuè Dì Huáng Tāng* (凉血地黄汤, Rehmannia Blood-Cooling Decoction)

Patent Formula:

- *Huái Jiǎo Wán* (槐角丸, Sophora Pill)
- *Dì Yú Huái Jiǎo Wán* (地榆槐角丸, Sanguisorba and Sophora Fruit Pill)

5. Heat Retention in the Stomach and Intestines

Symptoms: Bloody stools with viscous and fresh or dark purple blood, distending and burning epigastric and abdominal pain, halitosis, fever, thirst with desire to drink cold drinks, bitter taste, vexation, emaciation, a red tongue with a yellow greasy coating and a slippery and rapid or rapid and surging pulse.

Treatment Principles:

- Clear heat and drain fire
- Invigorate blood and stop bleeding

Main Acupuncture Points:

- ST 36 (*zú sān lǐ*): To invigorate spleen, tonify qi and blood, promote circulation and stop pain

- ST 37 (*shàng jù xū*) and LI 11 (*qū chí*): Upper and lower *he*-sea points of the large intestine to resolve stasis, clear heat, cool blood, regulate qi and stop pain
- BL 21 (*wèi shù*): Back-*shu* point of the stomach to invigorate spleen and harmonize stomach, alleviate diarrhea, promote digestion and stop hypochondriac pain
- ST 41 (*jiě xī*): To clear stomach heat, stop abdominal pain and calm the spirit
- ST 44 (*nèi tíng*): To clear toxic heat and dampness, regulate *yangming* channels
- BL 17 (*gé shù*): Influential point of the blood to nourish and harmonize blood, promote circulation and treat bloody stools

Supporting Points:

- LV 3 (*tài chōng*): *Yuan*-source point of the liver to clear liver and gallbladder heat, nourish blood and yin
- RN 10 (*xià wǎn*): To regulate qi, dispel food stagnation and stop abdominal pain

Recommended Formula: *Shí Huī Sǎn* (十灰散, Ten Charred Substances Powder) from the *Divine Book of Ten Medicinal Formulas* (*Shí Yào Shén Shū*, 十药神书)

Substitute Formula: *Xiè Xīn Tāng* (泻心汤, Heart-Draining Decoction)

Patent Formula: *Sān Huáng Piàn* (三黄片, Three Yellows Tablet)

Summary Chart for Bloody Stool

Patterns	Main Points	Supporting Points	Formulae
Damp-Heat Retention in the Intestines	ST 37, LI 11, PC 4, ST 40, ST 44, LI 4, SP 10	BL 27 for morbid leucorrhea GB 24 for damp-heat in the gallbladder	*Dì Yú Sǎn* or *Huái Jiǎo Wán*
Qi Failing to Control the Blood	BL 17, SP 6, SP 8, ST 36, BL 20, RN 6	BL 35 for hemorrhoids BL 54 for hematuria	*Guī Pí Tāng* or *Bǔ Zhōng Yì Qì Tāng*
Deficient Cold of the Spleen and Stomach	RN 8, ST 25, ST 36, RN 12, BL 20, BL 17	RN 10 for food stagnation and indigestion BL 27 for hemorrhoids and morbid leucorrhea	*Huáng Tǔ Tāng* or *Lǐ Zhōng Wán* plus *Chì Xiǎo Dòu Dāng Guī Sǎn*
Wind Damaging Intestinal Collaterals	RN 12, ST 36, BL 20, LI 4, GB 31, ST 25	SI 3 for fever due to wind BL 8 for blurry vision and dizziness due to wind	*Huái Huā Sǎn*, *Huái Jiǎo Wán* or *Liáng Xuè Dì Huáng Tāng*
Heat Retention in the Stomach and Intestines	ST 36, ST 37, LI 11, BL 21, ST 41, ST 44, BL 17	LV 3 for liver and gallbladder heat RN 10 for food stagnation and indigestion	*Shí Huī Sǎn* or *Xiè Xīn Tāng*

CASE STUDY 1: Acute Bloody Stools

Mr. Wang, 74 years old.

Main Complaint: Dark stools for one week.

Medical History: The patient suffered from chronic gastritis for 20 years. In the past 6 months, he suffered an important weight loss, lack of strength, palpitations, poor appetite, and dull pain in the stomach area for half a year. Recently, the patient experienced black stools everyday for a week with increased pain in the abdomen which refused pressure.

Presenting Symptoms: Black stools, shortness of breath, reluctance to speak, discomfort in the stomach, a pale purple tongue and a deep, thin and weak pulse.

Physical Examination: Temperature: 36.5 ℃, pulse: 87 bpm, respiration: 20 bpm, blood pressure: 130/80 mmHg. The patient was conscious and very thin with sallow yellow facial complexion. His abdomen was flat and there is obvious tenderness in epigastric region. Stool examination confirmed high level of blood cells in the stool.

Pattern Differentiation

Symptoms such as emaciation, lack of strength, and poor appetite are caused by qi deficiency of the spleen and stomach. Spleen and stomach are the foundation of acquired constitution and the source of qi and blood production. Qi deficiency of the spleen and stomach leads to insufficiency of qi and blood manifesting as shortness of breath, sallow yellow complexion and a thin and weak pulse. Furthermore, the spleen manages the blood; hence, qi deficiency of the spleen causes the blood to flow outside of the vessels and move out of the body with the stool. The black colour of the stool is actually static blood combined with the stool spilling out of vessels. This is a deficient case due to a long standing excessive pattern.

Diagnosis

TCM Diagnosis: Bloody stool due to spleen failing to control the blood

Western Medicine Diagnosis: Bloody stools

Treatment

The chief pathomechanism of this case is the spleen and stomach qi deficiency unable to control blood flow causing bleeding.

Principles:

- Fortify the spleen to contain the blood
- Tonify qi and regulate stool

Formula: Modified *Guī Pí Tāng* (Spleen-Restoring Decoction)

Ingredients:

人参	*rén shēn*	15 g	Radix et Rhizoma Ginseng
黄芪	*huáng qí*	20 g	Radix Astragali
白术	*bái zhú*	15 g	Rhizoma Atractylodis Macrocephalae
当归	*dāng guī*	15 g	Radix Angelicae Sinensis

阿胶	*ē jiāo*	15 g	Colla Corii Asini
白芍	*bái sháo*	15 g	Radix Paeoniae Alba
五灵脂	*wǔ líng zhī*	10 g	Faeces Trogopterori
蒲黄	*pú huáng*	10 g	Pollen Typhae
龙眼肉	*lóng yǎn ròu*	15 g	Arillus Longan
甘草	*gān cǎo*	5 g	Radix et Rhizoma Glycyrrhizae

Formula Analysis

In the formula, *rén shēn, huáng qí* and *bái zhú* fortify the spleen, tonify qi and contain blood to treat the root. *Dāng guī* and *bái sháo,* serve to nourish blood. *Pú huáng, ē jiāo* and *wǔ líng zhī* are combined to stop bleeding. As this type of bleeding of the deficient type is accompanied with blood stasis, it is proper to add *ē jiāo* which can supplement deficiency and astringe bleeding, as well as *wǔ líng zhī* and *pú huáng* which can stop bleeding and invigorate blood.

Chinese Patent Medicine: *Guī Pí Wán* (Spleen-Restoring Pill).

This patent formula can be made into three different kinds of preparations with different doses. Water-honey pills can be taken 6 g three times a day, small honey pills can be taken 9 g three times a day; big honey pills can be taken at 1 pill three times a day to be taken with warm water or fresh ginger soup.

Follow-up Consultations

After seven doses of the formula, the abdominal pain was alleviated, the appetite improved and there was no black stools. The patient was advised to eat more rich food in nutrition and avoid cold and difficult to digest food during the treatment.

CASE STUDY 2: Bloody Stool
By Dr. Zhang Bo-yu

Mr. Mao, 18 years old.

Main Complaint: Epigastric pain for 7 years and bloody stools for a week.

Medical History: The patient suffered from epigastric pain for 7 years which occurred every winter and spring.

Presenting Symptoms: During the last week, the abdominal pain aggravated especially at night with acid regurgitation, nausea, black stools, a pale tongue with a white coating and a thin pulse.

Diagnosis

TCM Diagnosis: Bloody stool due to spleen yang deficiency

Western Medicine Diagnosis: Bloody stools

Treatment

The pathogenesis of this case is mainly due to spleen deficiency generating deficient cold failing to contain blood with liver deficiency generating heat failing to store blood leading to bloody stools.

Principles:

- Warm yang and fortify the spleen
- Regulate the intestines and stop bleeding

Formula: Modified *Huáng Tǔ Tāng* (Yellow Earth Decoction)

Ingredients:

党参	*dǎng shēn*	12 g	Radix Codonopsis
炒白术	*bái zhú*	9 g	Rhizoma Atractylodis Macrocephalae
熟附片	*shú fù piàn*	9 g	Radix Aconiti Lateralis Praeparata (added first)
熟地黄	*shú dì huáng*	12 g	Radix Rehmanniae Praeparata
炒黄芩	dry-fried *huáng qín*	9 g	Radix Scutellariae
阿胶	*ē jiāo*	9 g	Colla Corii Asinie (melted in decoction)
仙鹤草	*xiān hè cǎo*	30 g	Herba Agrimoniae
灶心土	*zào xīn tǔ*	30 g	Terra Flava Usta (wrapped)

Follow-up Consultations

After taking four doses of the formula, the stool test confirmed no occult blood was present.

Notes

Bloody stools can be divided into upper and lower intestinal bleeding. Generally, bright red colour indicates lower intestinal bleeding and the dark purple stools indicates upper area bleeding of the stomach. In this case, the blood is darkish, which falls into the upper area of the stomach. Since the patient suffered from epigastric pain for 7 years, it is a chronic case of stomach deficiency which has weakened his healthy qi. Therefore, there are manifestations of spleen failing to transport nutrients and spleen and stomach deficient cold manifested as epigastric pain severe at night, a pale tongue with white coating and a thin pulse. The symptoms of nausea and acid regurgitation are signs of liver hyperactivity caused by spleen deficiency and liver fire damaging the spleen. These clinical manifestations clearly demonstrate a deficient cold of the spleen with excessive heat of the liver. The treatment should be in accordance with the intention of *Huáng Tǔ Tāng* recorded in *Essentials from the Golden Cabinet* (*Jīn Guì Yào Lüè*, 金匮要略), warming the middle *jiao*, stopping bleeding and clearing pathogenic heat.

In the formula, *zào xīn tǔ* is used to stop bleeding. *Dǎng shēn*, *bái zhú* and *shú fù piàn* can warm spleen yang and supplement the center qi. *Shú dì huáng* and *ē jiāo* enrich yin and astringe the blood. They are combined with *xiān hè cǎo* to supplement deficiency, and *huáng qín* to clear heat of liver.

These ingredients can warm yang without impairing yin and nourish yin without hindering the spleen yang.

CASE STUDY 3: Chronic Ulcerative Pancolitis
By Dr. Li Bo-ning

Ms. Wang, 40 years old. Technician. 1st consultation on June 11th, 1989.

Main Complaint: Diarrhea and bloody stool for six months.

Medical History: Six months ago, the patient suddenly began to have abdominal pain, diarrhea, and 10 days later bloody stool occurred. The symptoms gradually aggravated and she had to be hospitalized one month later due to massive bloody stools. At the time, it was diagnosed as ulcerative pancolitis. She was given hormones, antibiotics, hemostatic, blood transfusion and a variety of symptomatic treatments. The symptoms gradually improved, but her stool was still loose containing lots of blood for 1 to 2 times a day. Four months after the treatment, a colonoscopy showed no improvement of the colon lesions so the doctor suggested surgery. The patient refused and turned to acupuncture and moxibustion.

Presenting Symptoms: Chronic moon face with a dull yellow complexion, listlessness, low voice with a thin white tongue coating and a weak pulse.

Diagnosis

TCM Diagnosis: Bloody stool due to qi failing to control blood

Western Medicine Diagnosis: Ulcerative Pancolitis

Principles:

- Warm yang and consolidate the root
- Tonify qi and contain the blood to stop bleeding

Acupuncture Point Combination:

Body Points: RN 12 (*zhōng wǎn*), ST 25 (*tiān shū*), ST 36 (*zú sān lǐ*), RN 4 (*guān yuán*).

Ear Points: liver (*gān*), spleen (*pí*), stomach (*wèi*), sanjiao (*sān jiāo*).

Manipulations: Apply 5 moxa cones to each body point to supplement, 3 times a day. Gua sha technique was given on the bladder channel and *du mai*. The patient was also given the Chinese medicinal decoction *Lǐ Zhōng Tāng* (Center-Regulating Pill) as a supportive treatment. The point selection varied slightly according to presenting symptoms.

Point Analysis

In this case, the treatment is to strengthen the spleen and qi, clear heat and drain dampness as well as warm the middle *jiao* to dissipate cold.

RN 12 is the front-mu point of the stomach channel, BL 25 is the back-*shu* point of the large intestine channel, and ST 36 is the lower *he*-sea point of the stomach channel. These three points are selected to benefit the spleen and rectify the intestines. SP 6, the intersection point of three yin channels of foot, is selected to regulate qi of three yin channels of foot, strengthen spleen and stomach, and supplement qi and blood. SP 10 is an important point of the spleen channel to regulate intestines and stop diarrhea. BL 17 is the point of blood convergence which can regulate the bleeding.

Follow-up Consultations

After receiving 12 treatments, the symptoms resolved and there was no more blood in the stools, the patient had more energy and had a normal appetite. Her complexion was rosy, and there was a pink tongue with a thin and white coating and a thin and forceful pulse. Afterwards, the patient was discharged from the hospital and continued to receive moxibustion treatment twice a week for about 2 months to consolidate the treatment. In 4 month follow-up visits, the patient was healthy and had no recurrence of the symptoms.

Notes

This case of bloody stools is due to yang qi deficiency with deficient internal cold causing the spleen weakness and failing to control the blood flow. The blood spills out of vessels and seeps into the intestines. The pale complexion and thin pulse manifest this qi and blood deficiency. Moxibustion therapy is effective to tonify the yang and warm the channels. Chronic diarrhea will definitely injure the kidney yang, so tonifying the kidney is always applied in the course of treatment for chronic diarrhea. Application of the *Gua Sha* technique to the cutaneous areas of related channels on the back can strengthen yang, consolidate the root and rectify the balance of *zang-fu* organs. Though the *Lǐ Zhōng Tāng* decoction is taken intermittently, it can assist the treatment in this chronic and severe case. The patient was able to avoid surgery and recuperate fully within 20 days.

KEY CLINICAL POINTS

Generally speaking, the pattern of bloody stool should be determined according to different disease causes, pathomechanisms, excess or deficiency by observing the signs and symptoms.

In cases of intestinal damp-heat, we must clear heat and drain dampness, cool the blood and stop bleeding. In cases of qi deficiency failing to contain the blood, we need to tonify qi to contain blood. In cases of deficient cold of the spleen and stomach, we need to fortify the spleen and warm the center, nourish blood and stop bleeding. In chronic cases, we notice there is often the declination of *zang* qi, or failure of the liver to store the blood, failure of the spleen to contain the blood due to yang deficiency, and kidney failing to secure the lower part of the body due to yang deficiency. In these cases, the treatment should reinforce the healthy qi while dispelling the pathogenic factors. Additionally, these clinical points are noteworthy:

1. Pay attention to differential diagnosis of bloody stool

First, we must differentiate it from dysentery with additional signs of fever and aversion to cold at its initial stage with pus and blood in the stools. Dysentery will also have symptoms of abdominal pain and urgency with rectal heaviness and heat burning sensation around the anus. In contrast, bloody stool does not have pus in the stools nor experiences abdominal urgency with tenesmus. Secondly, we must differentiate it from hemorrhoids. Hemorrhoids belongs to an external disease that is also characterized by bleeding during or after defecation. However, it is usually associated with foreign body sensation or pain of the anus where the blood will have a bright red color. A physical examination of the anus can detect internal or external hemorrhoids.

2. In the modern Chinese medicinals formulas for acute upper gastrointestinal bleeding, the medicinals *dà huáng, bái jí, sān qī* and *dì yú* are often applied since they are safe, effective and non-toxic. Modern pharmacology study suggests that *dà huáng* has many hemostatic effects and is regarded as an important ingredient to treat acute upper gastrointestinal bleeding. It can be grounded into powder and taken with warm water, 3 to 5 g, 4 times a day.

3. Once the bleeding has stopped, Chinese medicine is also a good treatment approach in the convalescence period to stabilize the condition, prevent recurrence of the bleeding and restore strength. As bleeding consumes qi, this disease often presents with qi deficiency and blood depletion. Powerful qi and blood supplementing medicinals such as *rén shēn, huáng qí, dāng guī* and *gǒu qǐ zǐ* can be used when necessary.

4. Prognosis of bloody stool is mainly related to three factors. The first factor is the cause of bleeding. Generally, the externally contracted illness is easier to be cured, while the bleeding due to internal damage is more difficult. Secondly, it is closely related to the amount of bleeding. A small amount indicates a mild case, while a massive loss of blood denotes a severe case which can cause a critical life threatening situation. Thirdly, the severity of the accompanied symptoms will also demonstrate the condition of the healthy qi. In a mild case, the patient will be able to talk and has a good spirit. However in severe cases, the patient will be extremely weak and in some cases will not be able to walk or talk. Furthermore, the frequency and colour of defecation will all be considered in the prognosis evaluation.

COMPREHENSION QUESTIONS

1. What are the characters of the spleen and stomach deficient cold pattern and the treatment principles and recommended formula?

2. How can you differentiate upper and lower bleeding in the symptom of bloody stool?

3. Multiple choice questions:

1) Mr. Xia, 53 years old. His symptoms are red bloody stools, ungratifying defecation or loose stools, occasional abdominal pain, bitter taste in the mouth, red tongue with yellow greasy coating and a soggy and rapid pulse. The recommended formula is:

A. Modified *Huáng Tŭ Tāng* (Yellow Earth Decoction)
B. Modified *Huái Jiăo Wán* (Pagoda Tree Pod Pill) or *Dì Yú Săn* (Sanguisorbae Powder)
C. Modified *Bái Tóu Wēng Tāng* (Pulsatillae Decoction)
D. Modified *Sháo Yào Tāng* (Peony Decoction)
E. Modified *Gé Gēn Huáng Qín Huáng Lián Tāng* (Pueraria, Scutellaria, and Coptis Decoction)

2) Mr. Guo, 44 years old. His symptoms are red bloody stools or dark purple stools, poor appetite, fatigue, sallow yellow complexion, palpitations, sleeplessness, a pale tongue and a thin pulse. The disease pattern is:

A. Qi deficiency failing to contain blood
B. Intestinal damp-heat retention
C. Spleen-stomach deficient cold
D. Qi stagnation and blood stasis
E. Yin deficiency and yang hyperactivity

Answers

1. The clinical manifestations of the spleen and stomach deficient cold pattern are dark purple or black bloody stools, abdominal dull pain, a preference for hot drinks, lusterless complexion, mental fatigue, reluctance to speak, loose stools, a pale tongue and a thin pulse. The treatment principles are to fortify the spleen, warm the center, nourish blood and stop bleeding. The recommended formula is *Huáng Tŭ Tāng* (Yellow Earth Decoction). In this formula, *zào xīn tŭ* warms the center and stops bleeding. *Bái zhú, fù zĭ* and *gān căo* warm the center and fortify the spleen. *Dì huáng* and *ē jiāo* nourish blood and stop bleeding. *Huáng qín* is bitter and cold and clears deficient fire. For serious yang deficiency with aversion to cold with cold extremities, we can add *lù jiăo shuāng, páo jiāng, ài yè* and so on to warm yang and stop bleeding.

2. The theory of upper and lower gastrointestinal bleeding derives from the classical medical text *Essentials from the Golden Cabinet* (*Jīn Guì Yào Lüè*, 金匮要略) written by Zhang Zhong-jing. It is classified accordingly due to the location of the bleeding. Lower gastrointestinal bleeding is close to the anus and is identified by bright blood in the stool, while upper gastrointestinal bleeding is far away from the anus and is characterized by dark or purplish blood in the stools and often has

a recurrent history of stomach diseases, jaundice, tympanites and so on, while the lower gastrointestinal bleeding mostly have a history of hemorrhoids. The upper gastrointestinal bleeding is commonly due to deficient cold of the spleen and stomach, while the lower gastrointestinal bleeding is often caused by intestinal dampness and heat retention.

3. 1) B, 2) A.

4.8 *Wěi* Syndrome

Wěi Syndrome is characterized by flaccidity and weakness of the limbs being unable to move voluntarily sometimes accompanied by muscle atrophy. Clinically, it often affects the lower limbs causing the inability to walk.

This syndrome is initially recorded in the *Inner Classic* (*Nèi Jīng*, 内经); the chapter *Discussion on Wěi* mentions that its main pathomechanism is lung heat and dryness. As dryness of the lung causes the lung to fail to distribute the essence to the five *zang* organs, the body becomes malnourished and the limbs become flaccid. The *wěi* syndrome can be further classified into five types, namely *wěi* of the skin, vessels, sinews, bones and flesh, which denotes its severity and relation to the five *zang* organs. Its etiology mainly includes external contraction of heat and warm toxins, chronic retention of dampness, internal damage due to excessive emotions, damage due to excessive or improper food intake and over exhaustion, congenital deficiency all of which contribute to the depletion of the five *zang* organs, depletion of essence and body fluids, consumption of qi and blood, or qi and blood stagnation, causing the lack of nourishment of the muscles, sinews and vessels resulting in the *wěi* syndrome. In Western medicine the symptom of flaccid and weak limbs is often associated to diseases such as polyneuritis, motor neurone disease, spinal lesions, myasthenia gravis, multiple sclerosis and periodic paralysis.

CLINICAL PATTERNS DIFFERENTIATION AND TREATMENTS

1. Dampness Attacking the Spleen and Stomach

Symptoms: Ptosis or swelling of eyelids, limb heaviness, lethargy, glomus and stuffy sensation in the chest and diaphragm, abdominal distension and fullness, poor appetite, loose stools, pale complexion, a pale and enlarged tongue with teeth marks and a white greasy coating with a soggy or slippery pulse.

Treatment Principle:

- Invigorate spleen and harmonize stomach
- Resolve dampness and regulate qi circulation

Main Acupuncture Points:

- BL 20 (*pí shù*): Back-*shu* point of the spleen to regulate middle *jiao* qi, invigorate spleen, alleviate diarrhea and stop abdominal pain
- BL 21 (*wèi shù*): Back-*shu* point of the stomach to invigorate spleen and

harmonize stomach, alleviate diarrhea, promote digestion and stop hypochondriac pain

- ST 40 (*fēng lóng*): To expel phlegm and dampness
- ST 36 (*zú sān lǐ*): To expel dampness, strengthen qi, invigorate spleen, alleviate diarrhea and promote circulation
- SP 9 (*yīn líng quán*): To harmonize middle *jiao*, expel dampness and resolve edema
- ST 25 (*tiān shū*): Front-*mu* point of the large intestine to invigorate spleen and stomach, expel dampness, regulate qi and resolve diarrhea

Supporting Points:

- EX-CA 5 (*wèi shàng*): To tonify and raise the middle qi
- RN 10 (*xià wǎn*): To regulate qi, dispel food stagnation and stop abdominal pain

Recommended Formula: *Bú Huàn Jīn Zhèng Qì Săn* (不换金正气散, Priceless Qi-Righting Powder) from the *Beneficial Formulas from the Taiping Imperial Pharmacy* (*Tài Píng Huì Mín Hé Jì Jú Fāng*, 太平惠民和剂局方)

Substitute Formula: *Huò Pò Xià Líng Tāng* (藿朴夏苓汤, Agastache, Pinellia and Poria Decoction)

Patent Formula: *Huò Xiāng Zhèng Qì Ruăn Jiāo Náng* (藿香正气软胶囊, Agastache Qi-Correcting Soft Capsule)

2. Damp-Heat Obstructing the Collaterals

Symptoms: Four-limb flaccidity and weakness, drooping of the eyelids, generalized heaviness, limb numbness or mild swelling, fever, chest or abdominal discomfort, dark-yellow complexion, lethargy, scanty and dark-yellow urine burning, hesitant and painful urination, a yellow and greasy tongue coating and a slippery and rapid pulse.

Treatment Principle:

- Clear heat and drain dampness
- Clear channels and activate qi

Main Acupuncture Points:

- LI 11 (*qū chí*): *He*-sea point of the large intestine to clear damp-heat, treat upper limb paralysis, reduce fever and stop abdominal pain
- ST 31 (*bì guān*): To resolve dampness, benefit lumbus and knees, benefit lower extremities and activate the channel
- GB 31 (*fēng shì*): To resolve dampness and treat lower limb paralysis
- ST 36 (*zú sān lǐ*): To support correct qi, resolve dampness and improve circulation, treat abdominal distention and benefit lower limbs
- GB 34 (*yáng líng quán*): *He*-sea point of the gallbladder to clear damp-heat, unbind the chest, treat lower limb weakness and numbness, relax sinews, benefit joints and stop pain
- SP 9 (*yīn líng quán*): *He*-sea point of the spleen to resolve damp-heat, harmonize

spleen and stomach, tonify kidney, regulate fluid passages

• DU 14 (*dà zhuī*): To clear heat, tonify deficiencies, activate yang qi, treat pain and stiffness of the neck, shoulders and back

Supporting Points:

• BL 27 (*xiǎo cháng shù*): To expel damp-heat, resolve morbid leucorrhea, alleviate diarrhea, stop abdominal pain and regulate intestines

• GB 24 (*rì yuè*): Front-*mu* point of the gallbladder to resolve hypochondriac pain, expel damp-heat and benefit the gallbladder

Recommended Formula: *Èr Miào Sǎn* (二妙散, Two Mysterious Powder) from the *Teachings of [Zhu] Dan-xi* (*Dān Xī Xīn Fǎ*, 丹溪心法)

Substitute Formula: *Xuān Bì Tāng* (宣痹汤, Painful Obstruction Resolving Decoction)

Patent Formula: *Èr Miào Wán* (二妙丸, Two Mysterious Pill)

3. Spleen and Stomach Deficiency

Symptoms: Gradual flaccidity and weakness of the limbs, drooping of the eyelids, poor appetite, loose stools, abdominal distension, pale complexion, facial edema, shortness of breath, lethargy, disinclination to speak, a thin white tongue coating and a thready pulse.

Treatment Principle:

• Supplement qi and warm the channels

• Strengthen the spleen and nourish muscles

Main Acupuncture Points:

• LI 4 (*hé gǔ*): *Yuan*-source point of the large intestine to treat upper limb disorders and stop pain

• ST 36 (*zú sān lǐ*): To tonify spleen and nourish the healthy qi

• GB 34 (*yáng líng quán*): To treat lower limb weakness and numbness, relax sinews, benefit joints and stop pain

• BL 20 (*pí shù*): Back-*shu* point of the spleen to invigorate spleen and benefit qi, harmonize middle *jiao* and improve digestion

• RN 12 (*zhōng wǎn*): Front-*mu* point of the stomach to invigorate spleen and harmonize stomach, regulate qi and stop pain

• SP 6 (*sān yīn jiāo*): To invigorate spleen and stomach, improve appetite and regulate digestion

Supporting Points:

• EX-CA5 (*wèi shàng*): To treat middle qi sinking and abdominal disharmony

• ST 40 (*fēng lóng*): To expel phlegm and dampness

Recommended Formula: *Shēn Líng Bái Zhú Sǎn* (参苓白术散,Ginseng, Poria and Atractylodes Macrocephalae Powder) from the *Beneficial Formulas from the Taiping Imperial Pharmacy* (*Tài Píng Huì Mín Hé Jì Jú Fāng*, 太平惠民和剂局方)

Substitute Formula: *Bǔ Zhōng Yì Qì Tāng* (补中益气汤, Center-Supplementing and

Qi-Boosting Decoction)

Patent Formula:

- *Shēn Líng Bái Zhú Wán* (参苓白术丸, Ginseng, Poria and Atractylodes Macrocephalae Pill)
- *Xiāng Shā Liù Jūn Wán* (香砂六君丸, Costusroot and Amomum Six Gentlemen Pill)

4. Spleen and Kidney Yang Deficiency

Symptoms: Pale complexion, poor appetite, cold limbs and aversion to cold, weakness of the limb, fatigue, shortness of breath, loose stools with undigested food, early morning diarrhea, borborygmus, abdominal pain, soreness and pain of the lumbus, seminal emission, impotence, profuse urination or urinary incontinence or scanty clear urine with edema, a pale and swollen tongue with teeth marks and a white and moist coating, a deep, slow and weak pulse.

Treatment Principle:

- Warm the middle *jiao* and strengthen spleen
- Warm kidney yang and nourish essence and blood

Main Acupuncture Points:

- BL 20 (*pí shù*): Back-*shu* point of the spleen to invigorate spleen and benefit qi, harmonize middle *jiao* and improve digestion
- BL 23(*shèn shù*): Back-*shu* point of the kidney to benefit the original qi and kidney yang
- KI 3 (*tài xī*): *Yuan* point of the kidney to nourish kidney yin and yang and strengthen the lumbus
- DU 20 (*bǎi huì*): To raise qi and yang
- RN 6 (*qì hǎi*): To tonify kidney and spleen, fortify yang, invigorate qi and harmonize blood
- ST 36 (*zú sān lǐ*): To tonify spleen, benefit the healthy qi, nourish blood and strengthen lumbus and knees

Supporting Points:

- RN 8 (*shén què*): Apply moxibustion to warm the yang and resolve edema
- ST 27 (*dà jù*): To nourish essence

Recommended Formula: *Yòu Guī Wán* (右归丸, Right-Restoring Pill) from *The Complete Works of [Zhang] Jing-yue* (*Jǐng Yuè Quán Shū*, 景岳全书)

Substitute Formula: *Jīn Guì Shèn Qì Wán* (金匮肾气丸, Golden Cabinet's Kidney Qi Pill)

Patent Formula: *Yòu Guī Wán* (右归丸, Right-Restoring Pill)

5. Liver and Kidney Yin Deficiency

Symptoms: A slow and gradual onset of lower limb flaccidity and weakness, drooping of the eyelids, lower back soreness, inability to stand for long duration of time, lethargy, alopecia, blurry vision, dry eyes, dry throat, tinnitus, vertigo, nocturnal emissions, enuresis, irregular menstruation, insomnia or profuse dreaming, vexing heat in the five centers, muscular atrophy, a red tongue with a scanty coating and a thready and rapid pulse.

Treatment Principle:

- Tonify the liver and kidney
- Nourish yin and supplement the blood
- Clear empty heat and cool blood

Main Acupuncture Points:

- BL 43 (*gāo huāng*): To tonify kidney and liver, nourish yin and clear heat
- GB 34 (*yáng líng quán*): To treat lower limb weakness and numbness, relax sinews, benefit joints and stop pain
- BL 23 (*shèn shù*): Back-*shu* point of the kidney to tonify kidney yin and original qi, strengthen lumbar region, regulate lower fluid passages, benefit vision and hearing
- SP 6 (*sān yīn jiāo*): To invigorate liver and kidney, improve circulation, astringe lower fluid passages, treat lower limb pain, spasms and paralysis
- KI 3 (*tài xī*): *Yuan*-source point of kidney to tonify kidney yin, clear deficient heat and treat heel and foot disorders
- LV 3 (*tài chōng*): *Yuan*-source point of the liver to clear heat, nourish liver yin, benefit vision and strengthen lower limb weakness

Supporting Points:

- RN 4 (*guān yuán*): To harmonize menstruation, tonify kidney-essence, supplement deficiencies and weakness
- EX-LE 6 (*dăn náng xué*): To treat muscular atrophy and lower limb numbness

Recommended Formula: *Hŭ Qián Wán* (虎潜丸, Hidden Tiger Pill) from the *Teachings of [Zhu] Dan-xi* (*Dān Xī Xīn Fă*, 丹溪心法)

Substitute Formula:

- *Zuŏ Guī Wán* (左归丸, Left-Restoring Pill)
- *Liù Wèi Dì Huáng Wán* (六味地黄丸, Six Ingredients Rehmannia Pill)

Patent Formula: *Liù Wèi Dì Huáng Wán* (六味地黄丸, Six Ingredients Rehmannia Pill)

6. Qi and Blood Deficiency

Symptoms: Limb heaviness, shortness of breath, dizziness or vertigo which are induced by fatigue and aggravated with exertion, pale complexion, lusterless lips, fingernails and hair, palpitations, insomnia, lethargy, poor memory, disinclination to speak, poor appetite, a pale tongue with a thready and weak or knotted and intermittent pulse.

Treatment Principle:

- Tonify qi and nourish blood
- Calm the spirit and activate blood

Main Acupuncture Points:

- RN 12 (*zhōng wǎn*): To regulate qi and invigorate spleen
- ST 25 (*tiān shū*): Front-*mu* point of the large intestine to harmonize intestines, regulate qi and invigorate the spleen
- ST 36 (*zú sān lǐ*): To tonify spleen and benefit the healthy qi, nourish blood and resolve insomnia
- ST 40 (*fēng lóng*): To nourish the spleen, clear phlegm, calm the spirit, treat dizziness and alleviate pain
- ST 45 (*lì duì*): To calm the spirit, dredge the channel and resolve insomnia

Supporting Points:

- SP 4 (*gōng sūn*): To harmonize the middle *jiao*, regulate the *chong* and *ren* vessels, regulate qi and invigorate spleen
- HT 2 (*qīng líng*): To regulate qi and blood, activate the channel and stop pain

Recommended Formula: *Bā Zhēn Tāng* (八珍汤, Eight Gem Decoction) from the *Categorized Synopsis of the Whole* (*Zhèng Tǐ Lèi Yào*, 正体类要)

Substitute Formula: *Rén Shēn Yǎng Róng Tāng* (人参养荣汤, Ginseng Supporting and Nourishing Decoction)

Patent Formula: *Guī Pí Wán* (归脾丸, Spleen-Restoring Decoction)

Summary Chart for *Wĕi* Syndrome

Patterns	Main Points	Supporting Points	Formulae
Dampness Attacking the Spleen and Stomach	BL 20, BL 21, ST40, ST 36, SP 9, ST 25	EX-CA 5 for middle qi sinking RN 10 for food stagnation	*Bú Huàn Jīn Zhèng Qì Sǎn* or *Huò Pò Xià Líng Tāng*
Damp-Heat Obstructing the Collaterals	LI 11, ST 31, GB 31, ST 36, GB 34, SP 9, DU 14	BL 27 for morbid leucorrhea and diarrhea GB 24 for gallbladder damp-heat	*Èr Miào Sǎn* or *Xuān Bì Tāng*
Spleen and Stomach Deficiency	LI 4, ST 36, GB 34, BL 20, RN 12, SP 6	EX-CA 5 for middle qi sinking ST 40 for dampness and phlegm due to spleen deficiency	*Shēn Líng Bái Zhú Sǎn* or *Bǔ Zhōng Yì Qì Tāng*
Spleen and Kidney Yang Deficiency	BL 20, BL 23, KI 3, DU 20, RN 6, ST 36	RN 8 for middle and cold due to yang deficiency ST 27 for essence deficiency and impotence	*Yòu Guī Wán* or *Jīn Guì Shèn Qì Wán*
Liver and Kidney Yin Deficiency	BL 43, GB 34, BL 23, SP 6, KI 3, LV 3	RN 4 for irregular menstruation EX-LE 6 for muscular atrophy and lower limb disorders	*Hǔ Qián Wán* or *Zuǒ Guī Wán* or *Liù Wèi Dì Huáng Wán*
Qi and Blood Deficiency	RN 12, ST 25, ST 36, ST 40, ST 45	SP 4 for *chong* and *ren* vessels insufficiency HT 2 for heart qi and blood deficiency	*Bā Zhēn Tāng* or *Rén Shēn Yǎng Róng Tāng*

CASE STUDY 1: Chronic Ocular Myasthenia

Ms. Zhang, 16 years old.

Main Complaint: Bilateral drooping of the eye lids for 3 years.

Medical History: Three yeas ago, the patient's parents noticed the patient was always squinted her eyes and was unable to fully open her eyes. She received treatment from an ophthalmologist but there was no effect. In April 2009, neostigmine test was positive and the patient was diagnosed with ocular myasthenia. After being treated in many hospitals, the drooping slightly alleviated but soon relapsed after treatment. She also experienced poor appetite, scanty stools and normal urine since the beginning of this disease.

Presenting Symptoms: Drooping of both eyelids with swelling on the right side, poor vision, diplopia, aggravation in the afternoon, slightly yellow complexion, lack of strength, moderate constitution, a light colored tongue with a thin white coating and a thin and weak pulse.

Physical Examination: Temperature: 36.1 ℃, pulse: 88 bpm, respiration: 19 bpm, blood pressure: 120/75 mmHg. The patient was young, alert, low spirited, cooperative, with a fluent speech and normal responses. An examination of the nervous system showed cranial nerves (−), normal strength of both hands and of the upper and lower limbs. Neostigmine Test: (+)

Pattern Differentiation

In this case, the spleen and stomach weakness leads to the failure to transport nutrients to the muscles, tendons and vessels causing the *wěi* syndrome. The light coloured tongue with thin white coating and thin and weak pulse are signs of spleen and stomach weakness and qi and blood deficiency. The disease location is in the muscles and the related organs are the spleen, stomach, liver and kidney. This pattern demonstrates deficiency at the root with an excess in the branch.

Diagnosis

TCM Diagnosis: *Wěi* syndrome due to spleen and stomach deficiency

Western Medicine Diagnosis: Ocular myasthenia

Treatment

Principles:

- Supplement the middle *jiao* and tonify qi
- Fortify the spleen and raise the clear yang

Formula: Modified *Shēn Líng Bái Zhú Săn* (Ginseng, Poria and Atractylodes Macrocephalae Powder) combined with *Bŭ Zhōng Yì Qì Tāng* (Center-Supplementing and Qi-Boosting Decoction).

Ingredients:

党参	*dǎng shēn*	15 g	Radix Codonopsis
白术	*bái zhú*	15 g	Rhizoma Atractylodis Macrocephalae
茯苓	*fú líng*	10 g	Poria
山药	*shān yào*	10 g	Rhizoma Dioscoreae
扁豆	*biǎn dòu*	15 g	Semen Lablab Album
莲子	*lián zǐ*	15 g	Semen Nelumbinis
黄芪	*huáng qí*	15 g	Radix Astragali
当归	*dāng guī*	15 g	Radix Angelicae Sinensis
薏苡仁	*yì yǐ rén*	10 g	Semen Coicis
砂仁	*shā rén*	10 g	Fructus Amomi
陈皮	*chén pí*	15 g	Pericarpium Citri Reticulatae
升麻	*shēng má*	15 g	Rhizoma Cimicifugae
柴胡	*chái hú*	15 g	Radix Bupleuri
神曲	*shén qū*	5 g	Massa Medicata Fermentata
炙甘草	*zhì gān cǎo*	5 g	Radix et Rhizoma Glycyrrhizae Praeparata cum Melle
大枣	*dà zǎo*	20 g	Fructus Jujubae

Formula Analysis

This syndrome is due to spleen and stomach weakness with qi and blood deficiency failing to nourish the limbs sinews and tendons. The formula suggested is a modification of *Shēn Líng Bái Zhú Sǎn* (Ginseng, Poria and Atractylodes Macrocephalae Powder) and *Bǔ Zhōng Yì Qì Tāng* (Center-Supplementing and Qi-Boosting Decoction). *Shēn Líng Bái Zhú Sǎn* has the effect of fortifying the spleen, boosting qi and draining dampness and is indicated for spleen and stomach deficiency with internal accumulation of dampness. *Bǔ Zhōng Yì Qì Tāng* can fortify the spleen, tonify qi and nourish blood, and it is indicated for spleen and stomach deficiency, depletion of middle *jiao*, and qi and blood deficiency. The commonly used medicinals include *rén shēn, bái zhú, shān yào, biǎn dòu, lián zǐ, gān cǎo* and *dà zǎo* to fortify the spleen and boost qi; *huáng qí* and *dāng guī* are added to boost qi and nourish blood; *yì yǐ rén, shā rén, fú líng* and *chén pí* are used to fortify the spleen, rectify qi and remove dampness; *shēng má* and *chái hú* are added to lift clear yang; and *shén qū* can promote digestion and guide out food stagnation.

Follow-up Consultations

After 15 doses, the drooping of the eye lip was better and the patient was less fatigued and weak. After taking another 20 doses, all symptoms resolved completely. In a follow-up consultation 3 months later, the eye lids were normal and she was asked to take *Bǔ Zhōng Yì Qì Wán* (Center-Supplementing and Qi-Boosting Pill) in patent form to consolidate the treatment.

CASE STUDY 2: Weakness and Numbness of the Hands and Feet

Ms. Luo, 54 years old. 1st consultation on February 17th, 2011.

Main Complaint: Weakness and numbness of hands and feet for 2 weeks.

Medical History and Symptoms: The patient suffered from nasal congestion without fever and sore throat after catching a cold 2 weeks prior. The symptoms relieved by self medicating common cold patents. However, the following day, she was afflicted by numbness and weakness of both hands and feet which aggravated progressively and started to spread proximally. At the same time, the weakness of the limbs worsened and her wrists and ankles started to become flaccid. The patient had no history of deviated mouth, drooling, sluggish speech or choking. Her urine was normal, stools were dry, appetite was normal and sleep was poor.

Physical Examination: Her heart rate was regular at 68 bpm. The heart sound was low and dull, A2=P2, and no murmurs were found. Her tongue was in the middle when stretched out, the nasolabial groove symmetric and pharyngeal reflex normal. Her muscle strength of upper and lower limbs was grade 5, of the fingers and toes grade 3. The muscle tone was normal, and the tendon reflex was slightly weak. Babinski sign (−). No other pathological reflexes were found. The blood test showed TG 1.98 mmol/L.

Diagnosis

TCM Diagnosis: *Wěi* syndrome due to turbid phlegm obstructing the collaterals

Western Medicine Diagnosis: Weakness and numbness of the hands and feet

Principles:

- Activate blood and remove blood stasis
- Drain dampness and clear heat
- Nourish the liver and kidney yin
- Tonify qi and fortify the spleen

Acupuncture Point Combination:

For upper limbs: LI 15 (*jiān yú*), LI 11 (*qū chí*), LI 10 (*shǒu sān lǐ*), LI 4 (*hé gǔ*), SJ 5 (*wài guān*), chest *jiā jǐ* (EX-B2);

For lower limbs: ST 31 (*bì guān*), ST 32 (*fú tù*), ST 36 (*zú sān lǐ*), ST 40 (*fēng lóng*), GB 31 (*fēng shì*), GB 34 (*yáng líng quán*), SP 6 (*sān yīn jiāo*) and lumbar *jiā jǐ* (EX-B2).

Manipulations: Insert the needle into the selected points and apply supplementing method by twisting and rotating the needles. Electro-stimulation is given to the upper and lower limbs. The acupuncture treatment is given once a day lasting 30 min. Ten days make one treatment course, and altogether 3 treatment courses were given. During the acupuncture treatment course, we can supplement with Chinese herbal decoction such as modified *Èr Chén Tāng* (Two Matured Substances

Decoction) to fortify the spleen and dissolve phlegm, activate blood and unblock the collaterals.

Notes

The *wěi* syndrome is characterized by flaccid and weak limbs and muscle atrophy as limbs are unable to move voluntarily for an extended amount of time. It is related to the invasion of exogenous pathogens combined with irregular or inappropriate diet. The pathomechanism is turbid phlegm obstructing the collaterals. The *yang ming* channels normally have a large amount of qi and blood, so points from the *yang ming* channels of the upper and lower limbs are selected to dredge the channels and rectify qi and blood. The *jiā jĭ* points located on both sides of the *du mai* connect with the back-*shu* points of the *zang-fu* organs and are able to rectify yin and yang of *zang-fu* organs, and unblock and move qi and blood. Both SJ 5 and GB 31 pertain to the *shao yang* channel of the hand and foot and can assist the *yang ming* channels to unblock and move qi and blood. GB 34 is the influential point of tendons and can rectify tendons. SP 6 is used to fortify the spleen, supplement the liver and boost the kidney to strengthen the tendons and relieve the *wěi* syndrome.

KEY CLINICAL POINTS

1. Avoid impairing the healthy qi when expelling pathogens and avoid increasing pathogenic factors when supplementing.

Since this disease is due to a complex pattern of both deficiency and excess, the treatment principles need to address both patterns simultaneously to be effective. When expelling the pathogenic factors of dampness, heat, phlegm and cold, we should prevent from draining the healthy qi of the spleen and stomach. Additionally, when nourishing the yang and yin of the organ, we need to avoid increasing the pathogenic dampness, heat, cold and phlegm.

2. Treating the *wěi* syndrome by selecting the *yang ming* channels

Selecting acupuncture points of the *yang ming* channels mainly refers to fortifying the spleen and stomach to treat the *wěi* syndrome. The lung fluid is derived from the spleen and stomach, and the essence and blood of the liver and kidney are also dependent on the generation and transformation of the spleen and stomach. Therefore, in any patterns with fluid deficiency, it is important to nourish yang and fortify the spleen and stomach. If the function of the spleen and stomach is vigorous, the appetite will be normal and the qi, blood and fluids will be sufficient, thus nourishing the sinews and vessels and the patient will recover from the *wěi* syndrome. By selecting the points on the *yang ming* channels we also clear heat from its channels.

3. Be cautious when applying wind-expelling medicinals to treat the *wěi* syndrome.

The *wěi* syndrome usually results from deficiency and its excess pattern is often

affected by heat pathogen. Wind-expelling medicinals can disperse the wind and open interstitial space causing the dryness of the blood to aggravate the syndrome.

BRIEF SUMMARY

The disease location of the *wěi* syndrome is in the tendons, vessels and muscles. The channels and collaterals are passageways of the flow of qi and blood. If the *wěi* syndrome lasts for a long time, the normal flow of qi and blood will be affected, contributing to obstruction in the channels thus causing the lack of nourishment of the tendons and vessels while the movements of the joint will become difficult and the muscles will atrophy. The pattern of this disease is deficiency in the root with an excess in the branch. The treatment principles are mainly to boost qi and blood, nourish channels, clear heat and eliminate phlegm and dampness, unblock qi and move blood.

COMPREHENSION QUESTIONS

1. What is the pathomechanism of the *wěi* syndrome?
2. How can we treat the *wěi* syndrome by selecting the *yang ming* channels?
3. Multiple choice questions.

1) For the liver and kidney depletion pattern of the *wěi* syndrome, the recommended formula is:

A. *Èr Miào Săn* (Two Mysterious Powder)

B. *Qīng Zào Jiù Fèi Tāng* (Dryness Clearing and Lung Rescuing Decoction)

C. *Shēn Líng Bái Zhú Săn* (Ginseng, Poria and Atractylodes Macrocephalae Powder) with *Bŭ Zhōng Yì Qì Tāng* (Center-Supplementing and Qi-Boosting Decoction)

D. *Hŭ Qián Wán* (Hidden Tiger Pill)

E. *Shèng Yù Tāng* (Sage Recovery Decoction) combined with *Bŭ Yáng Huán Wŭ Tāng* (Yang-Supplementing and Five-Returning Decoction)

2) For the chronic *wěi* syndrome with weakness of the extremities, emaciation, and scaly nails, the recommended formula is:

A. *Shèng Yù Tāng* (Sage Recovery Decoction) combined with *Xuè Fŭ Zhú Yū Tāng* (Blood Mansion Stasis-Expelling Decoction)

B. *Shèng Yù Tāng* (Sage Recovery Decoction) combined with *Dà Huáng Zhè Chóng Wán* (Rhubarb and Eupolyphaga Pill)

C. *Shèng Yù Tāng* (Sage Recovery Decoction) combined with *Bŭ Yáng Huán Wŭ Tāng* (Yang-Supplementing and Five-Returning Decoction)

D. *Shèng Yù Tāng* (Sage Recovery Decoction) combined with *Liù Wèi Dì Huáng Wán* (Six-Ingredient Rehmannia Pill)

E. *Shèng Yù Tāng* (Sage Recovery Decoction) combined with *Shēn Tòng Zhú Yū Tāng* (Generalized Pain Stasis-Expelling Decoction)

Answers

1. The disease location of *wěi* syndrome lies in the sinews, vessels and muscles, but the disease has a deficient root of the five *zang* organs. Various factors can consume essential qi of five *zang* organs, leading to declination of the essence, blood and fluids. As the five *zang* organs have been impaired, their functions will be weak and the generation of qi and essence, blood and body fluids deficient. Therefore, sinews, vessels and muscles will lack of nourishment and become weak resulting in muscle weakness and flaccidity.

Generally, patterns of deficiency with excess heat are more common. When the *wěi* syndrome is due to external contraction of warm pathogen and damp-heat at the initial stage it causes a slight depletion of fluids and a strong pathogenic heat, so it is an excess pattern. If this situation lasts for a longer time, the fluids of the lung and stomach will be impaired and blood and essence of the kidney and liver will be consumed becoming a deficiency or a deficiency-excess complex pattern. When the *wěi* syndrome is due to internal damage of the spleen and stomach, liver and kidney depletion, deficiency of qi, blood and body fluids, it falls under a deficiency pattern, but it can also be complicated with the later formation of dampness, heat, phlegm and stasis, manifesting as a root deficiency and branch excess pattern.

2. Selecting the *yang ming* channels refers to choosing acupuncture points along both the hand and foot *yang ming* channels to fortify the spleen and stomach to treat the *wěi* syndrome. The lung fluids and the essence and blood of the liver and kidney derive from and depend on the transformation of food from the spleen and stomach. Therefore, for any kind of body fluid deficiency, it is important to fortify the spleen and stomach as well as nourish yin. When the function of the spleen and stomach is vigorous, the appetite will be normal and the formation of qi, blood and body fluids will be sufficient, thus the sinews and vessels will recover from the *wěi* syndrome. In addition, selecting acupuncture points from *yang ming* channels also involves the ability of dispelling pathogens. The Spiritual Pivot (*Líng Shū*, 灵枢) records: "For the *wěi* syndrome, select points from the *yang ming* channels because it is the channel where righteous qi and pathogenic qi constantly stay regardless excess and deficiency". Moreover, as the classical text the *Symptoms, Causes, Pulses, and Treatment* (*Zhèng Yīn Mài Zhì*, 症因脉治) mentions, "For only selecting the *yang ming*, it means to treat the *wěi* syndrome and diseases caused by excess *yang ming* heat. As the heat accumulation is cleared, the urination and defecation will become normal, the spleen and stomach will resume their functions in transforming food, producing essence and nourishing blood, thus moistening all the sinews and benefiting joints." Therefore, clearing heat from the *yang ming* also pertains to

clearing as well as tonifying. In conclusion, it is vitally important to strengthen the spleen and stomach with medicinal or acupuncture points to effectively treat the *wěi* syndrome.

3. 1) D, 2) C.

4.9 Deficiency & Consumption Syndrome

The term "deficiency and consumption" is a direct translation form the Chinese term "*xū láo* (虚痨)". This term describes the general depletion of multiple *zang-fu* organs accompanied by insufficient qi, blood, yin and yang. The syndrome of deficiency and consumption is often due to constitutional deficiency, mental and physical exhaustion over a long period of time, chronic insomnia, pregnancy, prolonged severe loss of blood combined with poor rest and improper diet. In Chinese medicine, it is categorized as three main types: mental consumption, blood consumption and marrow consumption. In western medicine, it can be associated to many various western diseases which involve the endocrine, immunity, and circulatory systems. Iron deficiency anemia in the western medicine falls into the category of blood consumption.

The common clinical manifestations of deficiency and consumption syndrome are pale or sallow yellow complexion, mental fatigue, lack of strength, vertigo, palpitations, a pale tongue, and thin and weak pulse. The disease location lies in the heart, liver and kidney. They are often seen in complex patterns of a combination of deficiency and excess patterns. Here is a list of the commonly seen patterns in clinic with their respective treatment principles, acupuncture points and formulas.

CLINICAL PATTERNS DIFFERENTIATION AND TREATMENTS

1. Qi and Yin Deficiency

Symptoms: Pale complexion, shortness of breath, lethargy, malar flush, vexing heat in the five centers, disinclination to speak, spontaneous sweating or night sweating, or hemoptysis with light red blood, a pink tongue with teeth marks with a scanty coating and a thin and weak or thin and rapid pulse.

Treatment Principle:

- Invigorate qi and nourish yin
- Tonify yang and support the righteous qi

Main Acupuncture Points:

- ST 36 (*zú sān lǐ*): To tonify spleen, support the correct qi and tonify deficiency
- RN 6 (*qì hǎi*): To support the original qi, tonify kidney and treat general weakness
- BL 20 (*pí shù*): Back-*shu* point of the spleen to regulate middle *jiao* qi, invigorate spleen, resolve hemoptysis

- SP 6 (*sān yīn jiāo*): To invigorate spleen, liver and kidney, tonify yin and harmonize lower *jiao*
- KI 3 (*tài xī*): *Yuan*-source point of kidney to tonify spleen and kidney yin, clear deficient heat and resolve hemoptysis
- RN 4 (*guān yuán*): To tonify the original qi, nourish kidney, supplement deficiencies and treat general weakness

Supporting Points:

- LV 3 (*tài chōng*): *Yuan*-source point of the liver to spread liver qi, clear heat, nourish liver yin, treat lower limb weakness
- BL 43 (*gāo huāng*): To tonify kidney and liver, nourish yin and clear heat

Recommended Formula: *Shēng Mài Săn* (生脉散, Pulse-Engendering Powder) from the *Clarifying Doubts about Damage from Internal and External Causes* (*Nèi Wài Shāng Biàn Huò Lùn*, 内外伤辨惑论)

Substitute Formula: *Wŭ Wèi Zĭ Tāng* (五味子汤, Fructus Schisandrae Sphenantherae Decoction)

Patent Formula: *Shēng Mài Yĭn* (生脉饮, Pulse-Engendering Beverage)

2. Lung and Kidney Qi Deficiency

Symptoms: Shortness of breath aggravated by exertion, shallow breathing with more exhalation than inhalation, deep breathing requires raising of shoulders, lower back and knee soreness and pain, inhibited urination or incontinence, pale complexion, mental fatigue, low voices, aversion to wind, spontaneous sweating, susceptibility to catch common colds, orthopnea, incessant cold sweats, cold limbs, purple lips, a pale and enlarged tongue with a white coating and a deep and weak or floating, big and rootless pulse.

Treatment Principle:

- Tonify lung qi and kidney yang
- Nourish essence and astringe qi leakage

Main Acupuncture Points:

- ST 36 (*zú sān lĭ*): To tonify spleen, support the correct qi and tonify deficiency
- RN 6 (*qì hăi*): To support the original qi, tonify kidney and treat general weakness
- BL 13 (*fèi shù*): Back-*shu* point of the lung to nourish lung, descend qi, release exterior, regulate sweating and harmonize breathing
- KI 3 (*tài xī*): *Yuan*-source point of kidney to tonify kidney, benefit lung, regulate lower fluid passage and anchor inhalation
- RN 17 (*dàn zhōng*): Front-*mu* point of the pericardium and sea of qi to invigorate pectoral qi
- DU 20 (*băi huì*): To nourish the sea of marrow, pacify wind, raise yang and treat collapse

Supporting Points:

- LU 7 (*liè quē*): Confluent point of the *ren mai* to harmonize the *ren mai* and unbind the chest, regulate upper fluid passage, promote lung descending function, release exterior and expel wind
- KI 27 (*shù fǔ*): To alleviate cough and wheezing, descend rebellious qi and harmonize breathing

Recommended Formula: *Bǔ Fèi Tāng* (补肺汤, Tonifying Lung Decoction) from the *Formulae by Li Zhong-nan* (*Yǒng Lèi Qián Fāng*, 永类钤方) combined with *Rén Shēn Gé Jiè Sǎn* (人参蛤蚧散, Ginseng and Gecko Powder) from the *Precious Mirror of Health* (*Wèi Shēng Bǎo Jiàn*, 卫生宝鉴)

Substitute Formula: *Bǔ Fèi Sǎn* (补肺散, Tonifying Lung Powder) combined with *Jīn Guì Shèn Qì Wán* (金匮肾气丸, Golden Cabinet's Kidney Qi Pill)

Patent Formula: *Yù Píng Fēng Sǎn* (玉屏风散, Jade Wind-Barrier Powder) combined with *Jīn Guì Shèn Qì Wán* (金匮肾气丸, Golden Cabinet's Kidney Qi Pill)

3. Heart Blood and Spleen Qi Deficiency

Symptoms: Poor appetite, epigastric discomfort after eating, lassitude, loose stools, sallow complexion, palpitations, poor memory, insomnia, profuse dreaming, a pale tongue with thin white coating and a weak, thready or knotted-intermitted pulse.

Treatment Principle:

- Strengthen the spleen and supplement qi
- Nourish blood and calm the heart

Main Acupuncture Points:

- ST 36 (*zú sān lǐ*): To invigorate spleen, tonify qi and nourish blood, resolve palpitation and calm the spirit
- RN 6 (*qì hǎi*): To support the original qi and treat general weakness
- BL 20 (*pí shù*): Back-*shu* point of the spleen to regulate middle *jiao* qi, invigorate spleen to nourish qi and blood
- BL 15 (*xīn shù*): Back-*shu* point of the heart to calm the spirit, clear heat and unbind the chest
- HT 7 (*shén mén*): *Yuan*-source point of the heart to tonify the original qi of the heart, stop palpitations and calm the spirit
- BL 17 (*gé shù*): Influential point of the blood to nourish and harmonize blood and promote circulation

Supporting Points:

- EX-HN 24 (*ān mián*): To calm the spirit and resolve insomnia
- RN 4 (*guān yuán*): To harmonize menstruation, supplement deficiencies and resolve general weakness

Recommended Formula: *Guī Pí Tāng* (归脾汤, Spleen-Restoring Decoction) from the *Formulas to Aid the Living* (*Jì Shēng Fāng*, 济生方)

Substitute Formula:

- *Bā Zhēn Tāng* (八珍汤, Eight Gem Decoction)
- *Rén Shēn Yǎng Róng Tāng* (人参养荣汤, Ginseng Supporting and Nourishing Decoction)

Patent Formula: *Rén Shēn Guī Pí Wán* (人参归脾丸, Ginseng Spleen-Restoring Pill)

4. Liver Blood and Kidney Yin Deficiency

Symptoms: Headache, vertigo, dizziness, deafness, tinnitus, dry eyes with photophobia, blurry vision, dry mouth, sore throat, irritability, limb numbness, weakness and flaccidity, muscle spasms, malar flush, lower back soreness, nocturnal emissions, a dry and red tongue with a scant or no coating and a wiry, thready and rapid or deep and thready pulse.

Treatment Principle:

- Nourish liver and kidney yin
- Cool blood and clear deficient heat

Main Acupuncture Points:

- SP 6 (*sān yīn jiāo*): To invigorate liver and kidney, improve circulation, astringe lower fluid passages, treat lower limb pain, spasms and paralysis
- BL 18 (*gān shù*): Back-*shu* point of the liver to nourish liver, clear heat, benefit sight and hearing, calm the spirit
- BL 23 (*shèn shù*): Back-*shu* point of the kidney to tonify kidney yin and original qi, strengthen lumbar region, regulate lower fluid passages and benefit vision and hearing
- LV 3 (*tài chōng*): *Yuan*-source point of the liver to clear heat, nourish liver yin, benefit vision and strengthen lower limb weakness
- KI 3 (*tài xī*): *Yuan*-source point of kidney to tonify kidney yin, clear deficient heat and treat heel and foot disorder
- GB 34 (*yáng líng quán*): To treat lower limb weakness and numbness, relax sinews, benefit joints and stop pain

Supporting Points:

- EX-LE 6 (*dǎn náng xué*): To treat muscular atrophy and lower limb numbness
- DU 21 (*qián dǐng*): To subdue liver yang, clear eyes and calm spirit

Recommended Formula: *Liù Wèi Dì Huáng Wán* (六味地黄丸, Six Ingredients Rehmannia Pill) from the *Key to Diagnosis and Treatment of Children's Diseases* (*Xiǎo Ér Yào Zhèng Zhí Jué*, 小儿药证直诀) combined with *Bǔ Gān Tāng* (Liver-Supplementing Decoction) from the *Golden Mirror of the Medical Tradition* (*Yī Zōng Jīn Jiàn*, 医宗金鉴)

Substitute Formula: *Qǐ Jú Dì Huáng Wán* (杞菊地黄丸, Lycium Berry, Chrysanthemum and Rehmannia Pill)

Patent Formula: *Qǐ Jú Dì Huáng Wán* (杞菊地黄丸, Lycium Berry, Chrysanthemum and Rehmannia Pill)

5. Spleen and Kidney Yang Deficiency

Symptoms: Pale complexion, poor appetite, cold limbs, aversion to cold, lassitude, shortness of breath, loose stools containing undigested food or early morning diarrhea, borborygmus, abdominal pain, lower back soreness and pain, seminal emission, impotence, profuse urination or incontinence or scanty clear urine with edema, all symptoms being aggravated by cold or improper diet, a pale swollen tongue with teeth marks and a white coating and a weak, deep and slow pulse.

Treatment Principle:

- Warm the middle *jiao* and strengthen the spleen
- Warm and reinforce kidney yang and nourish essence and blood

Main Acupuncture Points:

- SP 6 (*sān yīn jiāo*): To invigorate spleen and kidney, improve circulation, astringe lower fluid passages, benefit lower limbs and stop diarrhea
- KI 3 (*tài xī*): *Yuan*-source point of kidney to tonify kidney yang, benefit spleen and alleviate breathing, regulate menstruation and treat lower limb disorders
- RN 8 (*shén què*): Apply moxibustion to warm the yang and resolve edema
- RN 12 (*zhōng wǎn*): Front-*mu* point of the stomach to harmonize spleen and stomach, warm middle *jiao* and regulate qi
- DU 4 (*mìng mén*): To tonify kidney, regulate *du mai*, strengthen lumbar region, treat sexual dysfunction, secure essence and benefit lower limbs
- RN 4 (*guān yuán*): Front-*mu* point of the small intestine to benefit the uterus, tonify original qi, supplement deficiencies, treat diarrhea and regulate menstruation

Supporting Points:

- EX-CA 5 (*wèi shàng*): To tonify and raise the middle qi
- ST 27 (*dà jù*): To nourish essence

Recommended Formula: *Fù Zǐ Lǐ Zhōng Wán* (附子理中丸, Aconite Center-Regulating Pill) from the *Beneficial Formulas from the Taiping Imperial Pharmacy* (*Tài Píng Huì Mín Hé Jì Jú Fāng*, 太平惠民和剂局方) combined with *Jīn Guì Shèn Qì Wán* (金匮肾气丸, Golden Cabinet's Kidney Qi Pill) from the *Essentials from the Golden Cabinet* (*Jīn Guì Yào Lüè*, 金匮要略)

Substitute Formula: *Yòu Guī Wán* (右归丸, Right-Restoring Pill)

Patent Formula:

- *Jīn Guì Shèn Qì Wán* (金匮肾气丸, Golden Cabinet's Kidney Qi Pill)
- *Yòu Guī Wán* (右归丸, Right-Restoring Pill)

6. Heart and Kidney Yang Deficiency

Symptoms: Palpitations, spontaneous sweating, lassitude, chest tightness or pain, cold limbs, aversion to cold, pale complexion, lower back soreness, seminal emission, impotence, profuse urination or incontinence or scanty clear urine with edema, stools containing undigested food or early morning diarrhea, a pale and swollen tongue body with teeth marks with a white moist coating or a dark-purple tongue and a thready and weak or deep slow and weak pulse.

Treatment Principle:

- Supplement and warm heart yang
- Warm and reinforce kidney yang
- Nourish original qi and supplement essence and blood

Main Acupuncture Points:

- BL 15 (*xīn shù*): Back-*shu* point of the heart to tonify and nourish the heart, calm the spirit, unbind the chest and treat palpitations
- BL 23 (*shèn shù*): Back-*shu* point of the kidney to tonify kidney yang and original qi, strengthen lumbar region, regulate lower fluid passages and treat sexual dysfunction
- RN 14 (*jù quē*): Front-*mu* point of the heart to calm the spirit, unbind the chest, treat palpitations and nourish the heart
- DU 4 (*mìng mén*): To tonify kidney, regulate *du mai*, strengthen lumbar region, treat sexual dysfunction and secure essence
- RN 8 (*shén què*): Apply moxibustion to warm the yang and resolve edema
- HT 7 (*shén mén*): *Yuan*-source point of the heart to regulate and tonify heart, unbind the chest and treat palpitations

Supporting Points:

- DU 20 (*bǎi huì*): To raise the yang, benefit the mind, calm spirit, nourish the sea of marrow and rescue from prolapse
- RN 4 (*guān yuán*): Front-*mu* point of the small intestine to benefit the uterus, tonify original qi, supplement deficiencies, treat diarrhea and regulate menstruation

Recommended Formula: *Zhěng Yáng Lǐ Láo Tāng* (拯阳理劳汤, Yang-Saving and Deficiency Taxation-Regulating Decoction) from the *Required Readings from the Medical Ancestors* (*Yī Zōng Bì Dú*, 医宗必读) combined with *Yòu Guī Yǐn* (右归饮, Right-Restoring Beverage) from *The Complete Works of [Zhang] Jing-yue* (*Jǐng Yuè Quán Shū*, 景岳全书)

Substitute Formula: *Jīn Guì Shèn Qì Wán* (金匮肾气丸, Golden Cabinet's Kidney Qi Pill)

Patent Formula: *Jīn Guì Shèn Qì Wán* (金匮肾气丸, Golden Cabinet's Kidney Qi Pill)

7. Kidney Yin and Yang Deficiency

Symptoms: Lower back soreness and cold pain, tinnitus, dry hair, malar flush, night sweating, cold limbs, dizziness and blurry vision, afternoon fever, frequent and turbid urination, nocturnal seminal emission, spermatorrhea, impotence, amenorrhea, a red tongue with scanty coating or a pale and plump tongue body with teeth marks and a weak and thin pulse.

Treatment Principle:

- Warm and reinforce kidney yang
- Nourish kidney yin and supplement essence and blood

Main Acupuncture Points:

- BL 23 (*shèn shù*): Back-*shu* point of the kidney to tonify kidney yin and yang, support original qi, strengthen lumbar region, regulate lower fluid passages and treat sexual dysfunction
- DU 4 (*mìng mén*): To tonify kidney, regulate *du mai*, strengthen lumbar region, treat sexual dysfunction and secure essence
- BL 28 (*páng guāng shù*): Back-*shu* point of the bladder to tonify original qi, benefit essence, strengthen lumbus and lower limbs, regulate urination and lower *jiao*
- RN 8 (*shén què*): Apply moxibustion to warm the yang and resolve edema
- KI 3 (*tài xī*): *Yuan*-source point of kidney to tonify kidney yin and yang and regulate menstruation
- KI 10 (*yīn gǔ*): To tonify kidney and benefit yang, harmonize lower *jiao* and treat sexual dysfunction

Supporting Points:

- RN 4 (*guān yuán*): Front-*mu* point of the small intestine to benefit the uterus, tonify original qi, supplement deficiencies and regulate menstruation
- ST 27 (*dà jù*): To nourish essence and treat impotence

Recommended Formula: To treat severe yin deficiency take *Yòu Guī Wán* (右归丸, Right-Restoring Pill) from *The Complete Works of [Zhang] Jing-yue* (*Jǐng Yuè Quán Shū*, 景岳全书); to treat severe yang deficiency take *Zuǒ Guī Wán* (左归丸, Left-Restoring Pill) from *The Complete Works of [Zhang] Jing-yue* (*Jǐng Yuè Quán Shū*, 景岳全书)

Substitute Formula: *Gù Zhēn Yǐn Zi* (固真饮子, Vitality Reinforcing Liquid)

Patent Formula:

- *Yòu Guī Wán* (右归丸, Right-Restoring Pill)
- *Zuǒ Guī Wán* (左归丸, Left-Restoring Pill)

8. Kidney Essence Deficiency

Symptoms: Lethargy, dull consciousness, shaking of the limbs, loosing teeth, male and female infertility, amenorrhea, dizziness, blurry vision, forgetfulness, absent mindedness, deafness, tinnitus, foot flaccidity with lack of strength, pale complexion, a flaccid tongue without any coating and a deep and weak pulse.

Treatment Principle:

- Tonify kidney and secure essence
- Nourish yin and supplement essence and blood

Main Acupuncture Points:

- KI 3 (*tài xī*): *Yuan*-source point of the kidney to nourish yin and resolve insomnia
- ST 36 (*zú sān lǐ*): To invigorate spleen, tonify qi and nourish blood, resolve palpitation and calm the spirit

- DU 20 (*bǎi huì*): To raise yang and nourish the sea of marrow
- RN 4 (*guān yuán*): To tonify original qi and benefit essence
- RN 6 (*qì hǎi*): To tonify original qi and blood, benefit essence and fortify yang
- DU 4 (*mìng mén*): To regulate *du mai* and benefit *ming men*

Supporting Points:

- KI 10 (*yīn gǔ*): To tonify kidney yang and treat impotence
- BL 52 (*zhì shì*): To tonify kidney essence
- ST 27 (*dà jù*): To nourish essence and resolve sexual dysfunctions

Recommended Formula: *Hé Chē Dà Zào Wán* (河车大造丸, Placenta Great Creation Pill) from the *Essential Formula to Support Longevity* (*Fú Shòu Jīng Fāng*, 扶寿精方)

Substitute Formula: *Bǔ Tiān Dà Zào Wán* (补天大造丸, Heaven-Supplementing Great Creation Pill)

Patent Formula: *Hé Chē Dà Zào Wán* (河车大造丸, Placenta Great Creation Pill)

9. Essence Deficiency and Blood Stasis

Symptoms: Yellow or dark complexion, muscular, skin and nail deterioration, emaciation and muscle atrophy, abdominal distention and fullness or lumps, reduced food intake, in severe cases refusal of eating, epistaxis, bleeding gums, dark-pale lips and fingernails, a dark purple tongue and a thin and rapid or thin and choppy pulse.

Treatment Principle:

- Tonify qi and nourish blood
- Supplement essence and resolve bleeding
- Move blood to resolve stasis

Main Acupuncture Points:

- BL 17 (*gé shù*): Influential point of the blood to activate the blood circulation, dispel stasis, unbind the chest, treat heart pain and palpitations
- ST 36 (*zú sān lǐ*): To tonify qi and nourish blood
- RN 17 (*dàn zhōng*): Front-*mu* point of the pericardium and sea of qi to invigorate chest qi
- SP 10 (*xuè hǎi*): To promote blood flow, dispel blood stasis, harmonize menstruation and calm the spirit
- LV 3 (*tài chōng*): *Yuan*-source point of the liver to promote qi circulation, nourish liver blood and strengthen lower limb weakness
- ST 25 (*tiān shū*): Front-*mu* point of the large intestine to invigorate spleen and stomach, regulate qi, stop abdominal pain and distension

Supporting Points:

- PC 4 (*xì mén*): *Xi*-cleft point of the pericardium to activate blood circulation, dispel stasis, stop bleeding, calm the spirit, treat palpitations and heart pain
- EX-LE 6 (*dǎn náng xué*): To treat muscular atrophy and lower limb numbness

Recommended Formula: *Dà Huáng Zhè Chóng Wán* (大黄䗪虫丸, Rhubarb and Eupolyphaga Pill) from the *Essentials from the Golden Cabinet* (*Jīn Guì Yào Lüè*, 金匮要略)

Substitute Formula: *Xuè Fǔ Zhú Yū Tāng* (血府逐瘀汤, Blood Stasis Expelling Decoction)

Patent Formula: *Dà Huáng Zhè Chóng Wán* (大黄䗪虫丸, Rhubarb and Eupolyphaga Pill)

Summary Chart for Deficiency-Consumption

Patterns	Main Points	Supporting Points	Formulae
Qi and Yin Deficiency	ST 36, RN 6, BL 20, SP 6, KI 3, RN 4	LV 3 for lower limb weakness BL 43 for deficient heat due to kidney and liver yin deficiency	*Shēng Mài Sǎn* or *Wǔ Wèi Zǐ Tāng*
Lung and Kidney Qi Deficiency	ST 36, RN 6, BL 13, KI 3, RN 17, DU 20	LU 7 for exterior wind attacking lung KI 27 for cough and wheezing	*Bǔ Fèi Tāng* plus *Rén Shēn Gé Jiè Sǎn* or *Bǔ Fèi Sǎn*
Heart Blood and Spleen Qi Deficiency	ST 36, RN 6, BL 20, BL 15, HT 7, BL 17	EX-HN 24 for insomnia RN 4 for irregular menstruation	*Guī Pí Tāng* or *Bā Zhēn Tāng* or *Rén Shēn Yǎng Róng Tāng*
Liver Blood and Kidney Yin Deficiency	SP 6, BL 18, BL 23, LV 3, KI 3, GB 34	EX-LE 6 for muscular atrophy DU 21 for liver yang rising due to yin deficiency	*Liù Wèi Dì Huáng Wán* plus *Bǔ Gān Tāng* or *Qǐ Jú Dì Huáng Wán*
Spleen and Kidney Yang Deficiency	SP 6, KI 3, RN 8, RN 12, DU 4, RN 4	EX-CA 5 for middle qi sinking ST 27 for kidney-essence deficiency	*Fù Zǐ Lǐ Zhōng Wán* plus *Jīn Guì Shèn Qì Wán* or *Yòu Guī Wán*
Heart and Kidney Yang Deficiency	BL 15, BL 23, RN 14, DU 4, RN 8, HT 7	DU 20 for prolapse due to yang collapse RN 4 for uterine cold and irregular menstruation	*Zhěng Yáng Lǐ Láo Tāng* plus *Yòu Guī Yǐn* or *Jīn Guì Shèn Qì Wán*
Kidney Yin and Yang Deficiency	BL 23, DU 4, BL 28, RN 8, KI 3, KI 10	RN 4 for irregular menstruation ST 27 for impotence due to essence deficiency	Yin deficiency: *Yòu Guī Wán*; Yang deficiency: *Zuǒ Guī Wán* or *Gù Zhēn Yǐn Zǐ*
Kidney Essence Deficiency	KI 3, ST 36, DU 20, RN 4, RN 6, DU 4	KI 10 for impotence BL 52 for essence deficiency ST 27 for sexual dysfunction	*Hé Chē Dà Zào Wán* or *Bǔ Tiān Dà Zào Wán*
Essence Deficiency and Blood Stasis	BL 17, ST 36, RN 17, SP 10, LV 3, ST 25	PC 4 for blood stasis and bleeding EX-LE 6 for muscular atrophy	*Dà Huáng Zhè Chóng Wán* or *Xuè Fǔ Zhú Yū Tāng*

CASE STUDY 1: Iron Deficiency Anemia

Mr. Zhang, 12 years old.

Main Complaint: Headache, tinnitus, weakness and palpitations relapse for nearly a month.

Medical History: The patient gradually suffered from increasing symptoms of headache, blurry vision, occasional tinnitus, fatigue, weakness, palpitations and flustered complexion after exertion, lack of concentration and memory loss which obviously affected his grades. Blood test showed Hb level at 74 g/L and the patient was diagnosed with iron deficiency anemia. He was immediately administered blood nourishing Chinese medications and vitamin C. Blood tests done every two weeks confirmed the gradual increase of the Hb volume. He maintained this therapy for half a year and his Hb peaked at 118 g/L while symptoms relieved significantly. At that time, the patient stopped his medication. Last month, the patient had a relapse of his previous symptoms and went for a consultation. Blood test indicated Hb level of 75 g/L. He was asked to take iron supplements in oral liquid form for a month. However, the blood test remained at Hb 78 g/L at the next follow-up visit. Therefore, he decided to take Chinese medicine. The patient had no history of contagious diseases such as hepatitis or tuberculosis and no history of blood diseases.

Presenting Symptoms: Headache, blurry vision, tinnitus, weakness, palpitations, vexation, poor sleep, poor appetite, abdominal distension and loose stool. The patient was thin and tall with no vitality in the eyes, a pale and lustreless complexion and lips, pale eyelids and nails, edema of the eyelid with a dark bluish colour, a thin, pale and small tongue with a white and greasy coating and thin pulse.

Other Medical Test Results:

Blood routine test: WBC 8.6×10^9/L, RBC 5.1×10^{12}/L, Hb 75 g/L, PLT 84×10^9/L, HCT 30.3%, MCV 57.6fl, MCHC 242.2 g/L, MCH 14.3pg. A marrow aspiration test confirmed the proliferative anemia with possible iron deficiency anemia. There were no abnormal findings in the stool and urine tests.

Pattern Differentiation

This patient demonstrated a low appetite for a long time which led to malnutrition and poor absorption of nutrients. This condition impaired the normal function of the spleen and stomach to transport and transform food. This lack of absorption caused qi and blood deficiency failing to nourish the heart and developed into blood consumption manifesting as headache, dizziness, palpitations, vexation, insomnia and lack of strength. The weakness of the spleen and stomach failed to transform food and transport liquids which caused a stagnation of qi and dampness manifesting as fatigue, poor appetite, abdominal distension, loose stool and edema of the eyelid. In this case, the condition lasted for a long time which affected the kidney essence inhibiting the marrow from producing blood increasing the deficiency of qi and blood. The qi and blood deficiency combined with the dampness stagnation prevented the healthy yang to ascend to the head and face causing a lack of nourishment manifesting in the symptoms of lustreless complexion, headache, tinnitus and the lack of vitality in the eyes. The signs of thin, pale and small tongue body and the thin pulse are signs of qi and blood deficiency. This case belongs to the deficiency and consumption syndrome due to spleen qi and heart blood deficiency with kidney essence depletion.

Diagnosis

TCM Diagnosis: Deficiency and consumption syndrome due to spleen qi and heart blood deficiency with kidney essence depletion

Western Medicine Diagnosis: Iron deficiency anemia

Treatment

Principles:

- Tonify the spleen qi and supplement the heart blood
- Strengthen the kidney and nourish the essence

Formula: Modified *Guī Pí Tāng* (Spleen-Restoring Decoction) from the *Formulas to Aid the Living* (*Jì Shēng Fāng*, 济生方)

Ingredients:

黄芪	*huáng qí*	30 g	Radix Astragali
当归	*dāng guī*	10 g	Radix Angelicae Sinensis
党参	*dǎng shēn*	15 g	Radix Codonopsis
白术	*bái zhú*	10 g	dry-fried Rhizoma Atractylodis Macrocephalae
茯苓	*fú líng*	10 g	Poria
龙眼肉	*lóng yǎn ròu*	10 g	Arillus Longan
肉苁蓉	*ròu cōng róng*	15 g	Herba Cistanches
桑椹	*sāng shèn*	15 g	Fructus Mori
补骨脂	*bǔ gǔ zhī*	15 g	Fructus Psoraleae
木香	*mù xiāng*	10 g	Radix Aucklandiae
白蔻仁	*bái kòu rén*	6 g	Fructus Amomi Rotundus
谷芽	*gǔ yá*	30 g	dry-fried Fructus Setariae Germinatus
麦芽	*mài yá*	30 g	dry-fried Fructus Hordei Germinatus
丹参	*dān shēn*	30 g	Radix et Rhizoma Salviae Miltiorrhizae
川芎	*chuān xiōng*	9 g	Rhizoma Chuanxiong
红花	*hóng huā*	6 g	Flos Carthami
肉桂	*ròu guì*	6 g	Cortex Cinnamomi
大枣	*dà zǎo*	15 g	Fructus Jujubae
生姜	*shēng jiāng*	10 g	Rhizoma Zingiberis Recens
甘草	*gān cǎo*	9 g	Radix et Rhizoma Glycyrrhizae

Formula Analysis

The main cause of this case of deficiency and consumption syndrome is the spleen qi deficiency and heart blood depletion. As it is said in the Spiritual Pivot (*Líng Shū*, 灵枢): "The middle *jiao* takes in qi and liquids which are then transformed into red blood." In this formula, the medicinals *huáng qí, dǎng shēn, bái zhú* and *gān cǎo* are warm and sweet, which can boost the spleen qi to promote the production of blood. *Dāng guī* and *lóng yǎn ròu* are warm and sweet and they directly supplement the blood and nourish the heart. *Fú líng* calms the mind and, combined with *bái zhú,* can drain the accumulated dampness. *Ròu cōng róng, sāng shèn* and *bǔ gǔ zhī* are added to strengthen the kidney and supplement essence to produce marrow and blood. *Dān shēn, chuān xiōng, hóng huā* and *ròu guì* are added to activate blood, remove stagnation, and dispel stasis to warm the channels. *Mù xiāng* and *bái kòu rén* are acrid and aromatic which can regulate qi and stimulate the spleen. *Gǔ yá* and *mài yá* promote digestion and expel food stagnation. They can also assist in tonifying the spleen qi to restore the food transportation and transformation functions as they also protect the stomach qi and prevent the other medicinals from hindering the stomach. *Shēng jiāng* and *dà zǎo* harmonize and protect the spleen and stomach to promote the source of qi and blood production. The combination of these ingredients can tonify the spleen qi, remove stagnated qi and dampness and nourish heart blood.

Chinese Patent Medicine: The patient also took a daily dose of 60 g (30 g/twice a day) of *Lǘ Jiāo Bǔ Xuè Chōng Jì* (Donkey Hide Blood Supplementing Infusion Granules) to greatly nourish the blood deficiency. This patent is often given to patients suffering from iron deficiency anemia.

Follow-up Consultations

Second Consultation: After taking 20 doses of the medication, most of the symptoms were alleviated and his mental state improved. His complexion was rosy, appetite and sleep were normal, but he still felt a slight abdominal distention and had loose stool. Blood test showed Hb 98 g/L. The same prescription was given for 20 more days.

Third Consultation: After another 20 doses, all symptoms were resolved. Blood test showed Hb 125 g/L.

CASE STUDY 2: Aplastic Anemia
By Dr. Fu Ru-lin①

Female, 31 years old. 1st consultation on November 21st, 2003.

Main Complaint: Weakness of the lower extremities, general lack of strength and

① Wu Xiao-yong. Fu Ru-lin's Experience on Treating Chronic Aplastic Anemia (傅汝林治疗慢性再生障碍性贫血经验介绍), Beijing Journal of Traditional Chinese Medicine, 2008; 27 (6).

pale complexion for 3 years with aggravation for 3 months.

Medical History: Three years ago, the patient experienced weakness of the lower extremities with a general lack of strength, fatigue, headache and dizziness without any obvious cause of onset. The patient also had a pale complexion with subcutaneous dark macules. At consultation, blood test results showed WBC 2.3×10^9/L, Hb 45 g/L, and PLT 30×10^9/L. Bone marrow aspiration indicated aplastic anemia. The patient was hospitalized and given Stanozolol and testosterone medication. The symptoms improved but the patient had to stop the treatment due to lack of finances. During the last 3 months, the patient's condition worsened and she had to receive an emergency blood transfusion. She then consulted Chinese medicine for treatments.

Presenting Symptoms: Headache, weakness of the lower extremities, general lack of strength, bleeding from the gums and nose, subcutaneous macules all over the body, pale and lustreless complexion, poor appetite, enlarged purplish tongue with a scanty coating and weak and a large and rapid pulse.

Physical Examination: Normal heart and lung, soft abdomen, no palpable liver and spleen and no abnormal findings in the nervous system.

Other Medical Test Results: Blood test showed Hb 38 g/L, WBC 2.1×10^9/L, PLT 15×10^9/L.

Diagnosis

TCM Diagnosis: Deficiency and consumption syndrome due to spleen qi and kidney essence deficiency with blood depletion and blood stasis

Western Medicine Diagnosis: Aplastic anemia

Treatment

The pathomechanism of this case is mainly due to the deficiency of the spleen qi and heart blood. The weak spleen qi is unable to produce the necessary amount of blood and is unable to keep the blood within the vessels causing the bleeding of the gums and nose. The continual bleeding and lack of production of the blood increases the blood deficiency. The internal bleeding under the skin causes blood stasis manifesting as the maculae and creates stagnation within the channels. The kidney qi and essence deficiency is manifested in the general lack of strength and the weakness in the extremities as well as the headache.

Principles:

- Tonify the spleen qi and kidney essence
- Nourish the blood and supplement essence
- Invigorate blood and stop bleeding

Ingredients:

淫羊藿	*yín yáng huò*	30 g	Herba Epimedii
旱莲草	*hàn lián cǎo*	30 g	Herba Ecliptae
鸡血藤	*jī xuè téng*	30 g	Caulis Spatholobi
黄芪	*huáng qí*	20 g	Radix Astragali
枸杞子	*gǒu qǐ zǐ*	15 g	Fructus Lycii
菟丝子	*tù sī zǐ*	15 g	Semen Cuscutae
紫河车	*zǐ hé chē*	15 g	Placenta (powder, infused separately)
女贞子	*nǚ zhēn zǐ*	15 g	Fructus Ligustri Lucidi
熟地黄	*shú dì huáng*	12 g	Radix Rehmanniae Praeparata
当归	*dāng guī*	12 g	Radix Angelicae Sinensis
巴戟天	*bā jǐ tiān*	10 g	Radix Morindae Officinalis
阿胶	*ē jiāo*	10 g	Colla Corii Asini (melted in decoction)
龟板胶	*guī bǎn jiāo*	8 g	Colla Testudinis Plastri (melted in decoction)
鹿角胶	*lù jiǎo jiāo*	8 g	Colla Cornus Cervi (melted in decoction)
甘草	*gān cǎo*	6 g	Radix et Rhizoma Glycyrrhizae

In addition to this formula, the patient was asked to decoct 60 g of fresh *bái máo gēn* with water for drinking as tea.

Follow-up Consultations

After taking 4 doses, the bleeding of the gum and nose stopped and the skin macules faded away while the appetite improved. After another 14 doses, the blood test showed Hb 67 g/L, WBC 3.3×10 g/L, and PLT 56×10 g/L. The mental state of the patient was normal and she was able to move around freely. The patient continued taking the formula for half a year and the blood test showed Hb 81 g/L, and WBC 3.8×10 g/L, and PLT 85×10 g/L.

In the follow-up visits 2 years later, the patient's condition was stable and the blood analysis showed no abnormal findings.

CASE STUDY 3: Chronic Anemia
By Dr. Li Shou-shan

Ms. Li, 43 years old. 1st consultation on May 27th, 2006.

Main Complaint: Fatigue, weakness, headache, shortness of breath for nearly 10 years with aggravation for 2 months.

Medical History: The patient was weak since she gave birth to her first child 10 years ago. Since then, the patient also suffered from general fatigue, lack of strength, headache, shortness of breath and flustered complexion after exertion. Bone marrow testing diagnosed iron deficiency anemia. She was given various blood generating medications without any improvements. In recent 2 months, all the symptoms aggravated due to overstrain. The patient suffered from hyperthyroidism in 1988 which was successfully treated and had not relapsed.

Presenting Symptoms: General fatigue, lack of strength, headache, shortness of breath, flustered complexion after exertion, lower back pain, lumbar and knee weakness, poor appetite, insomnia, scanty pale menstruation which lasted over a week. The patient was emaciated with lustreless complexion, pale lips and nails, a pale tongue with white coating and a deficient and thin pulse.

Diagnosis

TCM Diagnosis: Deficiency and consumption syndrome due to spleen and kidney depletion

Western Medicine Diagnosis: Iron deficiency anemia

Treatment

Principles:

- Tonify spleen qi and kidney essence
- Strengthen qi and nourish blood

Formula: *Dāng Guī Bǔ Xuè Tāng* (Chinese Angelica Blood-Supplementing Decoction)

Ingredients:

黄芪	*huáng qí*	30 g	Radix Astragali
当归	*dāng guī*	10 g	Radix Angelicae Sinensis
鸡血藤	*jī xuè téng*	30 g	Caulis Spatholobi
熟地黄	*shú dì huáng*	30 g	Radix Rehmanniae Praeparata
山药	*shān yào*	15 g	Rhizoma Dioscoreae
山茱萸	*shān zhū yú*	10 g	Fructus Corni
丹参	*dān shēn*	10 g	Radix et Rhizoma Salviae Miltiorrhizae
龟板胶	*guī bǎn jiāo*	5 g	Colla Testudinis Plastri (melted in decoction)
鹿角胶	*lù jiǎo jiāo*	5 g	Colla Cornus Cervi (melted in decoction)

Formula Analysis

In this case, the patient had prenatal deficiency and postnatal malnourishment which resulted in the deficiency of both the spleen and kidney leading to the lack of production of blood and essence. In this case the formula, *Dāng Guī Bǔ Xuè Tāng* (Chinese Angelica Blood-Supplementing Decoction) is able to supplement the spleen qi to produce the blood and strengthen the kidney qi to support the spleen. This formula can also directly nourish the blood and support the essence to support the postnatal root.

Follow-up Consultations

After 20 doses of the formula and taking porridge with *dà zăo, lóng yăn ròu, gŏu qĭ zĭ, bái mù ĕr* and sugar in her daily diet, the patient showed significantly more strength. The symptoms of back pain and shortness of breath resolved and the menses were more abundant. However, she was still very weak with diarrhea and slight abdominal distension after meal. Her tongue was pale with white coating and a thin pulse. The medicinals *shā rén* 7.5 g, *bái zhú* 15 g and *gé gēn* 15 g were added to the original formula to strengthen the spleen and drain dampness. After 20 more doses, the patient showed a great relief of all the symptoms.

CASE STUDY 4: Monocytic Anemia

Ms. Chen, 47 years old.

Main Complaint: Repeated fever, anemia, purpura and soreness of the bones for over a year.

Medical History: On May 10th, 2006, the patient suffered from fever, sore throat, pale complexion, macules over the skin, and bone soreness. She was treated in a local hospital with antibiotics which improved her symptoms, but the disease relapsed on June 4th. Therefore, she was hospitalized for further testing. A bone marrow aspiration showed 60% monocytes and the patient was diagnosed with acute monocytic leukemia. She received 3 sessions of chemotherapy of IA and Arc-C without complete remission. On the fourth session, the patient went into complete remission. However later on, the disease reoccured and she was treated with chemotherapy 10 more times. Recently, marrow test showed 78% blast cells and the symptoms worsened so she decided to try Chinese medicine.

Presenting Symptoms: Headache, lack of strength, sallow yellow complexion, low fever, night sweat, general bone ache, sore and itching throat, occasional cough, skin macules, masses below the rib-side, poor appetite, poor sleep, loose stools twice a day, normal urination, a pale red tongue with a thin coating and a thin and rapid pulse.

The patient had no past history of hepatitis or tuberculosis, no contact with toxic matters and no family history of cancer. Blood test showed: WBC 2.51 $\times 10^9$/L, N 0.6 $\times 10^9$/L, blast cells 21%, RBC 2.65$\times 10^{12}$/L, Hb 65 g/L, PLT 52$\times 10^9$/L.

Diagnosis

TCM Diagnosis: Deficiency and consumption syndrome due to qi and yin depletion with toxic heat

Western Medicine Diagnosis: Monocytic anemia

Treatment

Principles:

- Tonify qi and nourish yin
- Clear heat and resolve toxins

Formula: Modified *Sān Cái Fēng Suĭ Dān* (Heaven, Human, and Earth Marrow-Retaining Elixir) combined with *Sì Jūn Zĭ Tāng* (Four Gentlemen Decoction)

Ingredients:

太子参	*tài zĭ shēn*	20 g	Radix Pseudostellariae
天冬	*tiān dōng*	10 g	Radix Asparagi
生地	*shēng dì*	15 g	Radix Rehmanniae
白术	*bái zhú*	12 g	Rhizoma Atractylodis Macrocephalae
茯苓	*fú líng*	15 g	Poria
白芍	*bái sháo*	12 g	Radix Paeoniae Alba
北沙参	*běi shā shēn*	12 g	Radix Glehniae
菟丝子	*tù sī zĭ*	15 g	Semen Cuscutae
牡丹皮	*mŭ dān pí*	12 g	Cortex Moutan (dry-fried)
黄柏	*huáng băi*	6 g	Cortex Phellodendri Chinensis (dry-fried)
黄连	*huáng lián*	3 g	Rhizoma Coptidis
景天三七	*jĭng tiān sān qī*	15 g	Herba Sedi Aizoon
半枝莲	*bàn zhī lián*	15 g	Herba Scutellariae Barbatae
白花蛇舌草	*bái huā shé shé căo*	15 g	Herba Hedyotis Diffusae
防风	*fáng fēng*	15 g	Radix Saposhnikoviae (dry-fried)
桔梗	*jié gĕng*	10 g	Radix Platycodonis
砂仁	*shā rén*	6 g	Fructus Amomi (added later)
陈皮	*chén pí*	6 g	Pericarpium Citri Reticulatae
白蔻仁	*bái kòu rén*	6 g	Fructus Amomi Rotundus
谷芽	*gŭ yá*	6 g	Fructus Setariae Germinatus
麦芽	*mài yá*	6 g	Fructus Hordei Germinatus
甘草	*gān căo*	6 g	Radix et Rhizoma Glycyrrhizae

Formula Analysis

This is a case of healthy qi deficiency and lingering pathogenic factors of toxic heat. The treatment is to mainly supplement deficiency and secondarily dispel pathogenic toxic heat. Thus, the formulas of *Sān Cái Fēng Suĭ Dān* (Heaven, Human, and Earth Marrow-Retaining Elixir) and *Sì Jūn Zĭ Tāng* (Four Gentlemen Decoction) are used to tonify qi and nourish yin while eliminating residual toxins. In the formula, *tài zĭ shēn, bái zhú, fú líng,* and *gān căo* are used to fortify the spleen and boost qi. *Tiān dōng, shēng dì, shā shēn,* and *bái sháo* are to nourish yin and supplement the blood. *Tù sī zǐ* boosts the kidney and replenishes essence. The application of these medicinals aims at reinforcing healthy qi. *Mǔ dān pí, huáng bǎi, huáng lián, bàn zhī lián* and *bái huā shé shé cǎo* can clear heat and resolve toxins as well as eliminate residual pathogens. *Jǐng tiān sān qī* resolves stasis and stops bleeding. *Fáng fēng* and *jié gěng* diffuse the lung and relieve cough. *Shā rén, chén pí, bái kòu rén, gǔ yá,* and *mài yá* can remove dampness and awaken the spleen, promote digestion and guide out food stagnation to protect stomach qi, assist qi boosting and yin nourishing herbs without creating stagnation or damaging the stomach.

Chinese Patent Medicine:

The Chinese medicinal patent of *Liù Shén Wán* (Six Spirits Pill) was also taken orally with the dosage of 20 pills, 3 times a day. This patent is often indicated to treat leukemia due to exuberant toxic heat pattern. The patent *Dāng Guī Lóng Huì Wán* (Chinese Angelica, Gentian and Aloe Pill) was taken with red date soup, at the dosage of 2 pills, 3 times a day. This patent is indicated for leukemia due to exuberant toxic heat and liver and gallbladder excessive fire pattern.

The patent *Zhēn Qí Fú Zhèng Jiāo Náng* (Ligustrum and Astragalus Health Reinforcing Capsule) was also taken at the dosage of 3 capsules, 3 times a day. The patent is indicated for leukemia due to deficiency of both qi and yin.

Follow-up Consultations

After 7 days of the treatment, the sore and itching throat, appetite, and defecation all improved, but there were still night sweats, lack of strength, hot sensation in the palm, pale red tongue with thin with yellow and slightly greasy coating and a thin and rapid pulse.

At that time the blood test showed: WBC 3.6×10^9/L, N 1.7×10^9/L, blast cells 13%, RBC 3.15×10^{12}/L, Hb 88 g/L, PLT 84×10^9/L.

As the patient had a weak constitution and her healthy qi had been impaired with deficiency of yin essence and internal toxic heat, the treatment was to eliminate toxic pathogens. Based on the previous formula, we removed *fáng fēng* and *jié gěng*, and added *wǔ wèi zǐ* 10 g and *guī bǎn jiāo* 10 g. Low dosages of the chemotherapy of MAG was applied according to the patient's constitution.

After 2 months of treatment, all the symptoms were cured and her mental state improved. The blood test showed: WBC 4.6×10^9/L, N 2.5×10^9/L, Hb 120 g/L, PLT 86×10^9/L and the marrow test was CR.

The patient continued to take Chinese herbs with 3 more sessions of chemotherapy to consolidate the treatment. The marrow test showed CR and the patient lived 4 more years with a high quality of life.

Clinical Analysis

The patient had a weak constitution and after contracting toxic heat, the pathogenic factors prevailed and entered the bone marrow causing pathogenic heat stagnation in the marrow. As the toxic pathogens lingered for a long time, the kidney essence was consumed and kidney qi was damaged. When the kidney failed to govern the bone and produce marrow, the marrow became more deficient and production of essence and blood was short of source, resulting in deficiency-consumption. Toxic pathogens invading the exterior causes struggle between healthy qi and pathogenic qi resulting in fever. As the toxic pathogens accumulate in the throat, there is a sore and itching throat. When the pathogenic heat enters the *ying*-blood level, it consumes and stirs the blood frenetically and together with the failure of qi to control blood due to qi deficiency, the blood spills out of vessels, manifesting as skin purpura and macules. Accumulation of pathogenic toxins and static blood in the bone marrow and channels leads to general bone ache and scrofula. Insufficiency of kidney essence and marrow results in failure of qi and blood production which is manifested in anemia. The patient has experienced many sessions of chemotherapy which also has impaired the qi and blood. Therefore, the lack of nourishment to the *zang-fu* organs and the spleen and stomach failing to transport further weakens the qi and blood manifesting as the symptoms of headache, lack of strength, sallow yellow complexion, poor appetite, and loose stool. Insufficient body fluid and internal generation of deficient fire bring forth the symptoms of low fever, insomnia and night sweats. The pale red tongue with a thin coating and the thin and rapid pulse are signs of both qi and yin depletion. This case of deficiency and consumption syndrome is a combination of depletion of healthy qi as the main pattern with a secondary pattern of pathogenic excess.

Notes

Leukemia is also known as cancer of the blood and it is a complex and life threatening disease. It is usually caused by prenatal constitution deficiency, mental or physical overstrain, prolonged illness, or febrile disease which lead to the depletion of the healthy qi combined with pathogenic toxins which enter the marrow and stagnate; or it is caused by toxic substance injuring the *ying*-blood level and kidney essence which in turn affect the bone marrow and bring about the disorder of qi and blood production. Leukemia has a root deficiency and branch excess. Its disease location lies in the bone marrow and it relates to the kidney, liver and spleen.

Clinically, it is featured as fever, bleeding, anemia, bone ache and scrofula. When leukemia is at the stage of the deficiency and consumption syndrome, it usually belongs to the middle and late stages or it is after a few sessions of chemotherapy. At this time, the healthy qi is deficient and the pathogenic toxin lingers, manifesting as deficiency signs like pale complexion, fatigue, lack of strength, shortness of breath, reluctant to speak, low fever, night sweat, or cold limbs, poor appetite, and abdominal distention.

CASE STUDY 5: Leukemia

Mr. Wang, 39 years old. 1st consultation on May 23rd, 1960.

Main Complaint: Abdominal masses accompanied with fatigue and lack of strength for a year.

Medical History: One year ago, the patient felt abdominal fullness and distension, and masses could be palpated. He gradually lost weight and felt flustered accompanied with night sweats for more than half a year. He was hospitalized due to fever and blood routine test showed WBC 140×10^{9}/L. His spleen was enlarged with the transverse diameter 1 cm over the navel. He was diagnosed with leukemia and the patient was hospitalized.

A peripheral hemogram showed: WBC 24.6×10^{9}/L, RBC 1.78×10^{12}/L, Hb 44 g/L, neutrophil 57%, polymorphonuclears 20%, lymphocyte 6%, neutrophilic promyelocyte 7%, myelocyte 3%, and promyelocyte 7%.

Six sessions of deep X-ray radiation were applied twice a week and the WBC decreased to a normal level while the spleen slightly reduced in size so he was discharged from the hospital. Afterwards, the hemogram was stable for a month, but it gradually rose. At that time the chemotherapy and blood transfusion were not effective so he was hospitalized again.

Presenting Symptoms: Sallow yellow and lusterless complexion, lethargic appearance, fatigue, lack of strength, abdominal fullness and distension, weak limbs, poor appetite, a thin and white tongue coating with thin and rapid pulse with softness in the *cùn* position.

Diagnosis

TCM Diagnosis: Deficiency and consumption syndrome due to qi and blood deficiency and stasis

Western Medicine Diagnosis: Leukemia

Treatment

In this case, the symptoms indicate qi and blood deficiency as well as accumulation of blood and toxic stasis.

Principles:

- Tonify qi and dissolve stasis
- Reinforce healthy qi and soften hardness

Ingredients:

熟地黄	*shú dì huáng*	12 g	Radix Rehmanniae Praeparata
党参	*dǎng shēn*	12 g	Radix Codonopsis
黄芪	*huáng qí*	15 g	Radix Astragali
白芍	*bái sháo*	6 g	Radix Paeoniae Alba
鳖甲	*biē jiǎ*	24 g	Carapax Trionycis
莪术	*é zhú*	9 g	Rhizoma Curcumae
牡蛎	*mǔ lì*	24 g	Concha Ostreae

丹参	*dān shēn*	9 g	Radix et Rhizoma Salviae Miltiorrhizae
砂仁	*shā rén*	2.4 g	Fructus Amomi
牛膝	*niú xī*	9 g	Radix Achyranthis Bidentatae
白术	*bái zhú*	9 g	Rhizoma Atractylodis Macrocephalae
茯苓	*fú líng*	12 g	Poria
当归	*dāng guī*	6 g	Radix Angelicae Sinensis
生地	*shēng dì*	12 g	Radix Rehmanniae

In addition, the patient also took the patent formula *Rén Shēn Biē Jiă Jiān Wán* (Ginseng Turtle Shell Decocted Pill) at 4.5 g twice a day. The patient was also told to apply locally over the spleen area the plaster of *Gŏu Pí Xiāo Pĭ Gāo* (Mass Dissipating Dogskin Plaster) combined with *ā wèi* 1.5 g and change the plaster once a week.

Follow-up Consultations

After one month of this treatment, the appetite and complexion improved and the spleen shrunk in size. His pulse was moderate and tongue coating thin. Blood routine test showed that the total count of WBC had lowered. It requires patience to treat such a severe case of internal damage and the previous formula was given again.

After one more month of the same formula, the WBC count was at 30×10^9/L, RBC improved, the spleen shrunk some more and other symptoms alleviated, so he was discharged from the hospital.

KEY CLINICAL POINTS

1. In the treatment of anemia we need to address the cause of the disease. We will need to supplement the diet in malnutrition and expel parasites if the anemia is due to intestinal parasites. In some cases, anemia is due to either internal or external bleeding. In these cases, the bleeding must be stopped and treated. Sometimes, the bleeding is due to chronic gastrointestinal diseases or profuse menstruation and spotting (*bēng lòu*, 崩漏). In these cases, they need to be treated according to their corresponding pattern differentiation. In addition, we need to support the spleen function by producing blood as well as nourishing the blood.

2. It is important to notice that the western diagnosis of "anemia" does not equal to the blood deficiency in the Chinese medicine since anemia is often more complex than a singular blood deficiency syndrome. It often involves the deficiency of the spleen qi failing to transform and transport the nutrient to produce blood manifesting as fatigue, lack of strength, shortness of breath, reluctance to speak, poor appetite and loose stool. It sometimes involves the deficiency of spleen qi in holding the blood inside the vessels causing bleeding. Essentially, strengthening the spleen function with formulas such as *Bā Zhēn Tāng* (Eight-Gem Decoction), *Shēn Líng Bái Zhú Săn* (Ginseng, Poria and Atractylodes Macrocephalae Powder), *Bŭ Zhōng Yì Qì Tāng* (Center-

Supplementing and Qi-Boosting Decoction), and *Guī Pí Tāng* (Spleen-Restoring Decoction) are appropriate. Other medicinals can be added to promote transformation and transportation of the food as well as remove stagnation such as *mù xiāng, shā rén, bái kòu rén*, fried *gŭ yá*, fried *mài yá, jī nèi jīn* and *shén qū*.

3. It is important to notice that in chronic cases of anemia, the liver blood and kidney essence will also be depleted manifesting as headache, blurry vision, vexation, lumbago, lumbar and knee weakness with a thin tongue body and thin and deep pulse. The kidney governs the bone and generates marrow as well as essence and blood. The liver stores the blood and shares the same source of yin with the kidney. Thus, in order to produce essence and blood, the body needs to have the support of both the liver and kidney. When considering the formula combination we can add medicinals to supplement the kidney essence to stimulate marrow to produce blood, such as *gŏu qĭ zĭ, ròu cōng róng, sāng shèn, bŭ gŭ zhī, tù sī zĭ, guī băn jiāo* and *lù jiăo jiāo*.

4. Prolonged illness inevitably leads to static blood. In the treatment of deficiency-consumption syndrome with blood depletion we not only need to nourish the blood but also we must activate the blood circulation to remove blood stasis with formulas such as *Dà Huáng Zhè Chóng Wán* (Rhubarb and Eupolyphaga Pill) or medicinals such as *dān shēn, chuān xiōng*, and *hóng huā*. These medicinals will help to dispel blood stasis to nourish blood.

5. Chemotherapy is the fundamental treatment in western medicine for leukemia. In elderly patient, weak or patients with liver and kidney disorders, the dosage of chemotherapy can not be overused. During the period of chemotherapy, the practitioner needs to pay close attention to blood and marrow tests. Supportive treatment with Chinese medicine and acupuncture can be provided according to the pattern but should always focus on reinforcing healthy qi and consolidating the root by especially boosting the spleen and kidney since the kidney is the prenatal root, and the spleen is the postnatal root which assures the production of qi and blood.

COMPREHENSION QUESTIONS

1. List the symptoms associated with acute and chronic anemia.

2. List the common pattern differentiations and treatment of deficiency and consumption syndrome.

3. What is the etiology and pathomechanism of leukemia in Chinese medicine?

4. Multiple choice questions:

1) The Chinese medical canon which names the five kinds of deficiency and consumptive syndromes, seven damages and six excesses is:

A. *The Yellow Emperor's Inner Classic* (*Huáng Dì Nèi Jīng*, 黄帝内经)

B. *Essentials from the Golden Cabinet* (*Jīn Guì Yào Lüè*, 金匮要略)

C. *Treatise on the Origins and Manifestations of Various Diseases* (*Zhū Bìng Yuán Hòu Lùn*, 诸病源候论)

D. *The Classic of Difficult Issues* (*Nàn Jīng*, 难经)
E. *Non-Resident Collection* (*Bù Jū Jí*, 不居集)

2) The main etiopathology of blood deficiency is due to the defiency of spleen and stomach not producing the blood. Which other *zang* organs are also closely related to this disease?
A. Lung, spleen and kidney
B. Heart, liver and kidney
C. Heart, lung and kidney
D. Liver, spleen and kidney
E. Lung, liver and kidney

3) The most important physical condition to identify an accurate prognosis of the deficiency and consumption syndrome lies in:
A. The state of qi and blood deficiency
B. The abundance of body fluids
C. The strength of spleen and stomach
D. The consolidation of qi
E. The disassociation of yin and yang

4) For chronic deficiency and consumption syndrome due to internal static blood, it is necessary to combine the treatment according to the pattern while adding a formula to dispel blood stasis and nourish blood such as:
A. *Xuè Fŭ Zhú Yū Tāng* (Blood Mansion Stasis-Expelling Decoction)
B. *Biē Jiă Jiān Wán* (Turtle Shell Decocted Pill)
C. *Dà Huáng Zhè Chóng Wán* (Rhubarb and Eupolyphaga Pill)
D. *Shŭ Yù Wán* (Dioscoreae Pill)
E. *Dĭ Dāng Tāng* (Resistance Decoction)

5) In Chinese medicine, the main disease causing leukemia include healthy qi deficiency and
A. Phlegm turbidity
B. Heat toxin retention
C. Static blood
D. Qi stagnation
E. Food stagnation

Answers

1. The symptoms associated with acute anemia are general weakness, lack of strength, dizziness, pale and lustreless complexion, lack of concentration, memory loss, insomnia, palpitations, pale tongue with a thin and deep pulse. In chronic

anemia, these symptoms also appear with the addition of gum or nose bleeding, skin maculae, purplish or purple spot on the tongue and a choppy pulse manifesting a blood stasis pattern.

2. The common patterns of deficiency and consumption syndrome and their corresponding treatments are:

- For spleen and stomach deficiency syndrome, use *Xiāng Shā Liù Jūn Zǐ Tāng* (Costusroot and Amomum Six Gentlemen Decoction) and *Dāng Guī Bǔ Xuè Tāng* (Chinese Angelica Blood-Supplementing Decoction) to fortify the spleen and harmonize the stomach, tonify qi and nourish blood.
- For heart and spleen deficiency, use *Guī Pí Tāng* (Spleen-Restoring Decoction) or *Bā Zhēn Tāng* (Eight-Gem Decoction) to tonify qi and blood, nourish the heart and calm the mind.
- For spleen and kidney yang deficiency, use *Bā Zhēn Tāng* (Eight-Gem Decoction) with *Wú Bǐ Shān Yào Wán* (Incomparable Yam Pill) to warm and supplement the spleen and stomach.
- For liver and kidney yin deficiency, use *Zhī Bǎi Dì Huáng Wán* (Anemarrhena, Phellodendron and Rehmannia Pill) to nourish liver and kidney yin and essence as well as subdue deficiency heat.
- For worm accumulation, combine *Huà Chóng Wán* (Worm-Expelling Pill) with *Bā Zhēn Tāng* (Eight-Gem Decoction) to kill worms, remove accumulation and nourish qi and blood.

3. Leukemia is usually caused by a constitutional insufficiency, physical or mental overstrain, prolonged illness, or febrile disease which lead to a severe depletion of healthy qi combined with the retention of toxins which enters the marrow and causes stagnation of qi and blood; or causes the retention of toxins which injure the *yin*-blood level and kidney essence affecting the bone marrow. At the initial stage of acute leukemia or at the last critical moment of late stage leukemia, the excess patterns play a leading role. During the progression of the disease, the combination of the deficiency and excess complex pattern often occurs. Patients treated with chemotherapy or at the late stage of leukemia usually demonstrate a deficiency and consumption syndrome with the consumption of qi, blood, yin and yang with the binding retention of toxin and blood stasis.

4. 1) C, 2) B, 3) C, 4) C, 5) B.

4.10 *Bì* Syndrome

Bì syndrome is a series of diseases mainly characterized by joint and muscle aching pain, numbness, heaviness, and inhibited movement, or even swelling and burning sensation of the joints. It is resulted from blocked channels and inhibited flow of qi and blood due to the external invasion of pathogenic wind, cold, dampness, and heat. In mild cases, it occurs in joints of the limbs, while in severe cases, the internal organs are inflicted. In the Western medicine, rheumatoid arthritis is similar to the *bì* syndrome and pain of multiple joints, called *lì jié* in Chinese and also a symptom of this syndrome.

This disease is both related to external contraction of pathogenic wind, cold, damp and heat, combined with the weakness of the healthy or the righteous qi. As it is said in the *Basic Questions — About Bì* (*Sù Wèn — Bì Lùn*, 素问・痹论): "The pathogenic wind, cold and dampness are mixed together which results in the *bì* syndrome". In the *Formulas to Aid the Living — Bì* (*Jì Shēng Fāng — Bì*, 济生方・痹), it also states, "The cause of *bì* is related to a weak body with an insecure interstitial space contracting pathogenic wind, cold and dampness". *The Personal Standards for the 'Essentials from the Golden Cabinet* (*Jīn Guì Yào Lüè Xīn Diǎn*, 金匮要略心典) states: "The pain of multiple joints (*lì jié*) may not come to be if there is only deficiency of the liver and kidney without the invasion of water-dampness".

Being exposed to exterior conditions of pathogenic wind, cold, heat and dampness while sweating, over exhausted, or over working might cause the pathogenic factors to enter the body and channels and stagnate in the joints and block channels causing a stagnation of qi and blood flow leading to painful joints, swelling, redness and limited movement. The invasion of pathogenic wind, cold and dampness is the external cause of this disease, while weak *zang-fu* functions, a weak constitution or weak healthy qi is the internal cause. Below is a list of the common patterns of *bì* syndrome and their corresponding acupuncture and formula treatments.

CLINICAL PATTERNS DIFFERENTIATION AND TREATMENTS

1. Wind Cold Damp Obstruction

Symptoms: Swelling and pain with a possible feeling of heaviness, difficulty in bending and stretching of the joints, morning stiffness, exacerbated by exposure to cold, fever, slight aversion to wind and cold, a bland taste in the mouth and an absence of thirst, a sunken tight or floating tight pulse.

Treatment Principle:

- Dispel wind and dissipate cold
- Eliminate dampness and unblock collateral vessels

Main Acupuncture Points:

- DU 14 (*dà zhuī*): Sea of qi point to clear heat, tonify deficiency, activate yang qi, treat pain and stiffness of the neck, shoulders and back
- LI 11 (*qū chí*): *He*-sea point of the large intestine to resolve stagnation, expel dampness, alleviate diarrhea and stop pain
- SJ 5 (*wài guān*): To release the exterior and clear heat
- ST 36 (*zú sān lĭ*): To tonify spleen, support the correct qi and tonify deficiency
- BL 23 (*shèn shù*): Back-*shu* point of the kidney to benefit the original qi and kidney yin
- KI 3 (*tài xī*): *Yuan*-source point of kidney to tonify spleen and kidney yin, clear deficient heat and resolve hemoptysis
- RN 4 (*guān yuán*): To tonify the original qi, nourish kidney, supplement deficiency and treat general weakness
- GB 34 (*yáng líng quán*): To treat lower limb weakness and numbness, relax sinews, benefit joints and stop pain
- GB 30 (*huán tiào*): To activate the channel, alleviate pain, benefit the lumbar region and lower limbs, dispel wind and drain dampness
- SP 5 (*shāng qiū*): To invigorate spleen and resolve dampness, harmonize the intestines and stomach, benefit the sinews and bones
- SJ 14 (*jiān liáo*): To dispel wind and damp, activate the channel and alleviate pain, regulate blood and qi, benefit the shoulder joint

Supporting Points:

- BL 20 (*pí shù*): Back-*shu* point of the spleen to regulate middle *jiao* qi, invigorate spleen, resolve hemoptysis
- ST 40 (*fēng lóng*): To expel phlegm and dampness

Recommended Formula: *Juān Bì Tāng* (蠲痹汤, Rheumatism-Relieving Decoction) from the *Medical Revelations* (*Yī Xué Xīn Wù*, 医学心悟)

Substitute Formula:

- *Wū Tóu Tāng* (乌头汤, Aconite Decoction) combined with *Zhú Fù Tāng* (术附汤, White Atractylodes and Aconite Decoction)
- *Fáng Jĭ Huáng Qí Tāng* (防己黄芪汤, Stephania Root and Astragalus Decoction) combined with *Fáng Fēng Tāng* (防风汤, Saposhnikovia Decoction)

Patent Formula:

- *Fēng Shī Gŭ Tòng Jiāo Náng* (风湿骨痛胶囊, Capsules for Rheumatic Bone Pain)
- *Hán Shī Bì Chōng Jì* (寒湿痹冲剂, Granules for Cold-Damp Impediment)

2. Wind Damp Heat Binding

Symptoms: Swelling, pain or heaviness limbs and joints, difficulty bending and stretching, morning stiffness which is exacerbated by heat, aversion to wind, fever, thirst, a red tongue with a yellow and greasy or dry coating.

Treatment Principle:

- Disperse wind and clear heat
- Eliminate dampness and unblock collaterals

Main Acupuncture Points:

- DU 14 (*dà zhuī*): To clear heat, activate yang qi, treat pain and stiffness of the neck, shoulders and back
- SJ 14 (*jiān liáo*): To dispel wind, drain damp, activate the channel, alleviate pain, regulate blood and qi and benefit the shoulder joint
- LI 11 (*qū chí*): *He*-sea point of the large intestine to resolve stagnation, expel dampness, alleviate diarrhea and stop pain
- SJ 5 (*wài guān*): To release the exterior and clear heat
- KI 3 (*tài xī*): *Yuan*-source point of kidney to tonify spleen and kidney yin, clear deficient heat and resolve hemoptysis
- GB 34 (*yáng líng quán*): To treat lower limb weakness and numbness, relax sinews, benefit joints and stop pain
- GB 30 (*huán tiào*): To activate channels, alleviate pain, benefit the lumbar region and lower limbs, dispel wind and drain damp
- LI 4 (*hé gǔ*): *Yuan*-source point of the large intestine to treat upper limb disorders and stop pain

Supporting Points:

- BL 20 (*pí shù*): Back-*shu* point of the spleen to regulate middle *jiao* qi, invigorate spleen, resolve hemoptysis
- SP 9 (*yīn líng quán*): To harmonize middle *jiao*, expel dampness and resolve edema

Recommended Formula: *Dà Qín Jiāo Tāng* (大秦艽汤, Large Gentian Decoction) from the *Medical Illumination* (*Yī Xué Fā Míng*, 医学发明)

Substitute Formula:

- *Sì Miào Sǎn* (四妙散, Wonderfully Effective Four Powder)
- *Xuān Bì Tāng* (宣痹汤, Painful Obstruction Resolving Decoction)

Patent Formula: *Shī Rè Bì Chōng Jì* (湿热痹冲剂, Granules for Damp-Heat Impediment)

3. Binding of Pathogenic Cold and Heat

Symptoms: Swelling and pain of the joints in the extremities with difficulty bending and stretching, local area feels hot to the touch but the patient has a subjective aversion to cold; or there is no local heat but the patient has a subjective feeling of having a fever, vexation and reddish urine, thirst with a desire to drink (heat syndrome is more severe) or no desire to drink (cold syndrome is more severe), a string-like and rapid pulse or a string-like and tight pulse.

Treatment Principle:

- Disperse wind and warm cold
- Clear heat and drain dampness
- Unblock channels and stop pain

Main Acupuncture Points:

- DU 14 (*dà zhuī*): To clear heat, activate yang qi, treat pain and stiffness of the neck, shoulders and back
- SJ 14 (*jiān liáo*): To dispel wind, drain damp, activate the channel and alleviate pain, regulate blood and qi and benefit the shoulder joint
- LI 11 (*qū chí*): *He*-sea point of the large intestine to resolve stagnation, expel dampness, alleviate diarrhea and stop pain
- SJ 5 (*wài guān*): To release the exterior and clear heat
- GB 30 (*huán tiào*): To activate the channel and alleviate pain, benefit the lumbar region and lower limbs, dispel wind and drain dampness
- KI 3 (*tài xī*): *Yuan*-source point of kidney to tonify spleen and kidney yin, clear deficient heat and resolve hemoptysis
- GB 34 (*yáng líng quán*): To treat lower limb weakness and numbness, relax sinews, benefit joints and stop pain
- SP 6 (*sān yīn jiāo*): To invigorate spleen, liver and kidney, tonify yin and harmonize lower *jiao*

Supporting Points:

- ST 36 (*zú sān lǐ*): To tonify spleen, support the correct qi and tonify deficiency
- EX-LE 5 (*xī yǎn*): To dispel wind damp, reduce swelling and alleviate pain, benefit the knee joint

Recommended Formula: *Guì Zhī Sháo Yào Zhī Mǔ Tāng* (桂枝芍药知母汤, Cinnamon Twig, Peony and Anemarrhena Decoction) from the *Essentials from the Golden Cabinet* (*Jīn Guì Yào Lüè*, 金匮要略)

Substitute Formula: *Juān Bì Tāng* (蠲痹汤, Rheumatism-Relieving Decoction)

4. Turbid Phlegm Obstructing Collaterals

Symptoms: Prolonged swelling of the joints with a fixed stabbing pain, morning stiffness, joint deformity, a dark purple tongue, or tongue is with petechiae and a wiry, thready and choppy pulse.

Treatment Principle:

- Move blood circulation and resolve stasis
- Dispel phlegm and dredge collaterals

Main Acupuncture Points:

- DU 14 (*dà zhuī*): To clear heat, activate yang qi, treat pain and stiffness of the neck, shoulders and back
- SJ 14 (*jiān liáo*): To dispel wind, drain damp, activate the channel and alleviate pain, regulate blood and qi, benefit the shoulder joint

• LI 11 (*qū chí*): *He*-sea point of the large intestine to resolve stagnation, expel dampness, alleviate diarrhea and stop pain

• SJ 5 (*wài guān*): To release the exterior and clear heat

• GB 30 (*huán tiào*): To activate the channel and alleviate pain, benefit the lumbar region and lower limbs, dispel wind and drain damp

• KI 3 (*tài xī*): *Yuan*-source point of kidney to tonify spleen and kidney yin, clear deficient heat and resolve hemoptysis

• GB 34 (*yáng líng quán*): To treat lower limb weakness and numbness, relax sinews, benefit joints and stop pain

• SP 10 (*xuè hăi*): To promote blood flow and dispel stasis, invigorate the spleen and cool blood

• ST 40 (*fēng lóng*): To expel phlegm and dampness

Supporting Points:

• SP 9 (*yīn líng quán*): To harmonize middle *jiao*, expel dampness and resolve edema

• BL 20 (*pí shù*): Back-*shu* point of the spleen to regulate middle *jiao* qi, invigorate spleen, resolve hemoptysis

Recommended Formula: *Shēn Tòng Zhú Yū Tāng* (身痛逐瘀汤, Generalized Pain Stasis-Expelling Decoction) from the *Correction of Errors in Medical Works* (*Yī Lín Găi Cuò*, 医林改错) combined with *Zhĭ Mí Fú Líng Wán* (指迷茯苓丸, Pathfinder Poria Pill) from the *Formulas for Maintaining Healthy and Puzzling Diseases* (*Quán Shēng Zhĭ Mí Fāng*, 全生指迷方)

Substitute Formula: *Dí Tán Tāng* (涤痰汤, Phlegm-Flushing Decoction) combined with *Juān Bì Tāng* (蠲痹汤, Rheumatism-Relieving Decoction)

Patent Formula: *Pán Lóng Qī Piàn* (盘龙七片, Crag Bergenia Tablet)

5. Liver Blood and Kidney Yin Deficiency

Symptoms: Chronic swelling, pain and deformity of joints with a heat sensation, difficulty in bending and stretching, aching pain and weakness in the lumbus and knees, emaciation, dizziness, tinnitus, a red tongue with a scanty coating and a thin rapid pulse.

Treatment Principle:

• Nourish blood and tonify the liver

• Strengthen kidney and nourish the essence

• Strengthen the sinews and bones

Main Acupuncture Points:

• DU 14 (*dà zhuī*): To clear heat, activate yang qi, treat pain and stiffness of the neck, shoulders and back

• SJ 14 (*jiān liáo*): To dispel wind and damp, activate the channel and alleviate pain, regulate blood and qi, benefit the shoulder joint

• LI 11 (*qū chí*): *He*-sea point of the large intestine to resolve stagnation, expel dampness, alleviate diarrhea and stop pain

- SJ 5 (*wài guān*): To release the exterior and clear heat
- GB 30 (*huán tiào*): To activate the channel and alleviate pain, benefit the lumbar region and lower limbs, dispel wind and drain damp
- GB 34 (*yáng líng quán*): To treat lower limb weakness and numbness, relax sinews, benefit joints and stop pain
- KI 3 (*tài xī*): *Yuan*-source point of kidney to tonify spleen and kidney yin, clear deficient heat and resolve hemoptysis
- BL 23 (*shèn shù*): Back-*shu* point of the kidney to benefit the original qi and kidney yin
- BL 18 (*gān shù*): Back-*shu* point of the liver to spread liver qi, clear liver and gallbladder heat, unbind the chest and promote circulation

Supporting Points:

- LV 3 (*tài chōng*): *Yuan* point of the liver to relieve chest congestion and irritability
- SP 6 (*sān yīn jiāo*): To invigorate spleen, liver and kidney, tonify yin and harmonize lower *jiao*

Recommended Formula: *Zuǒ Guī Wán* (左归丸, Left-Restoring Pill) from *The Complete Works of [Zhang] Jing-yue* (*Jǐng Yuè Quán Shū*, 景岳全书)

Substitute Formula:

- *Dà Bǔ Yīn Wán* (大补阴丸, Major Yin-Supplementing Pill) combined with *Hǔ Qián Wán* (虎潜丸, Hidden Tiger Pill)
- *Liù Wèi Dì Huáng Wán* (六味地黄丸, Six Ingredients Rehmannia Pill)

Patent Formula:

- *Qiáng Jīn Jiàn Gǔ Wán* (强筋健骨丸, Sinew-and-Bone Strengthening Pill)
- *Liù Wèi Dì Huáng Wán* (六味地黄丸, Six Ingredients Rehmannia Pill)

6. Kidney Yang Deficiency with Congealing Cold

Symptoms: Cold pain and swelling of the joints with difficulty in bending and stretching, joint deformity, morning stiffness, aversion to cold, pale complexion, a pale enlarged tongue and a deep and thin pulse.

Treatment Principle:

- Warm the kidney yang and dissipate cold
- Eliminate dampness and dredge collaterals

Main Acupuncture Points:

- BL 23 (*shèn shù*): Back-*shu* point of the kidney to benefit the original qi and kidney yin
- DU 14 (*dà zhuī*): To clear heat, activate yang qi, treat pain and stiffness of the neck, shoulders and back
- SJ 14 (*jiān liáo*): To dispel wind, drain damp, activate the channel and alleviate pain, regulate blood and qi, benefit the shoulder joint
- LI 11 (*qū chí*): *He*-sea point of the large intestine to resolve stagnation, expel

dampness, alleviate diarrhea and stop pain

- SJ 5 (*wài guān*): To release the exterior and clear heat
- GB 30 (*huán tiào*): To activate the channel and alleviate pain, benefit the lumbar region and lower limbs, dispel wind and damp
- GB 34 (*yáng líng quán*): To treat lower limb weakness and numbness, relax sinews, benefit joints and stop pain
- KI 3 (*tài xī*): *Yuan*-source point of kidney to tonify spleen and kidney yin, clear deficient heat and resolve hemoptysis
- RN 4 (*guān yuán*): To tonify the original qi, nourish kidney, supplement deficiency and treat general weakness

Supporting Points:

- SP 4 (*gōng sūn*): To invigorate spleen, harmonize middle *jiao* and regulate qi
- DU 4 (*mìng mén*): To tonify kidney, regulate *du mai*, strengthen lumbar region, treat sexual dysfunction, secure essence and benefit lower limbs

Recommended Formula: *Dú Huó Jì Shēng Tāng* (独活寄生汤, Pubescent Angelica and Mistletoe Decoction) from the *Important Formulas Worth a Thousand Gold Pieces for Emergency* (*Bèi Jí Qiān Jīn Yào Fāng*, 备急千金要方)

Substitute Formula: *Guì Zhī Fù Zǐ Tāng* (桂枝附子汤, Cinnamon Twig and Aconite Decoction)

Patent Formula: *Yì Shèn Juān Bì Wán* (益肾蠲痹丸, Kidney-Replenishing and Rheumatism-Relieving Pill)

Summary Chart for *Bì* Syndrome

Patterns	Main Points	Supporting Points	Formulae
Wind Cold Damp Obstruction	DU 14, LI 11, SJ 5, ST 36, BL 23, KI 3, RN 4, GB 34, GB 30, SP 5, SJ 14	BL 20 for strengthening the spleen, invigorating qi ST 40 for expelling phlegm and dampness	*Juān Bì Tāng* or *Wū Tóu Tāng* plus *Zhú Fù Tāng* or *Fáng Jǐ Huáng Qí Tāng* plus *Fáng Fēng Tāng*
Wind Damp Heat Binding	DU 14, SJ 14, LI 11, SJ 5, KI 3, GB 34, GB 30, LI 4	BL 20 for strengthening the spleen and invigorating qi SP 9 for clearing heat and draining dampness	*Dà Qín Jiāo Tāng* or *Sì Miào Sǎn* or *Xuān Bì Tāng*
Binding of Pathogenic Cold and Heat	DU 14, SJ 14, LI 11, SJ 5, GB 30, KI 3, GB 34, SP 6	ST 36 for fortifying qi and tonifying healthy qi EX-LE5 for treating knee pain	*Guì Zhī Sháo Yào Zhī Mǔ Tāng* or *Juān Bì Tāng*
Turbid Phlegm Obstructing Collaterals	DU 14, SJ 14, LI 11, SJ 5, GB 30, KI 3, GB 34, SP 10, ST 40	SP 9 for clearing heat and draining dampness BL 20 for strengthening the spleen and invigorating qi	*Shēn Tòng Zhú Yū Tāng* plus *Zhǐ Mí Fú Líng Wán* or *Dí Tán Tāng*

Continued

Patterns	Main Points	Supporting Points	Formulae
Liver Blood and Kidney Yin Deficiency	DU 14, SJ 14, LI 11, SJ 5, GB 30, GB 34, KI 3, BL23, BL 18	LV 3 for nourishing liver blood and clearing liver heat SP 6 for nourishing yin and clearing empty heat	*Zuǒ Guī Wán* or *Dà Bǔ Yīn Wán* or *Liù Wèi Dì Huáng Wán*
Kidney Yang Deficiency with Congealing Cold	BL 23, DU 14, SJ 14, LI 11, SJ 5, GB 30, GB 34, KI 3, RN 4	SP 4 for strengthening spleen DU 4 to tonify kidney and secure yang	*Dú Huó Jì Shēng Tāng* or *Guì Zhī Fù Zǐ Tāng*

CASE STUDY 1: Chronic *Bì* Syndrome

Ms. Wang, 58 years old. 1st consultation on February 18th, 2006.

Main Complaints: Painful and enlarged finger joints of both hands for 5 years with stiffness and deformation for over a year.

Medical History: The patient lives in the countryside and has a rigorous life style. 5 years ago, she suffered from fever, joint pain and swelling of the four extremities after working on the farm in the rain. Her symptoms were relieved with Chinese and Western medical treatment in a local hospital. However, these symptoms occurred repeatedly due to weather changes to cold and damp weather. The year prior, her finger joints gradually became stiff and deformed. She sought help from many hospitals without any curative effects.

Presenting Symptoms: Swelling and stiffness of the finger joints with stabbing pain, inhibited movement and numbness aggravated by cold weather and slightly relieved by heat, occasionally accompanied by palpitations, shortness of breath, normal appetite, sleep, urine and stool, a darkish red tongue with a white and greasy coating and a deep and thin pulse. The patient had a history of hypertension for 3 years which was under control by taking Dogbane Tablet twice a day.

Physical Examinations: Temperature: 36.5 ℃, pulse: 88 bpm, respiration: 20 bpm, blood pressure: 135/80 mmHg. There were no other abnormal findings of the general condition besides the swelling and deformation of the finger joints of both hands with pain that aggravated with pressing and limited movement. Blood test showed: RF (+), ESR 40mm/h, ASO 252 Iu/ml.

Pattern Differentiation

The patient was in her fifties and had a difficult life of working in the fields under harsh weather conditions. She showed clear signs of liver and kidney deficiency with qi and blood deficiency seen in the shortness of breath and palpitation. After being exposed to exterior cold and dampness, the patient suffered from *bì* syndrome since the healthy qi was not strong enough to expel the pathogens, which penetrated in the interior and stagnated in the channels and bones. This stagnation of pathogenic cold and dampness in the channels and vessels produced static blood binding with the phlegm leading to joint stiffness, swelling, stabbing pain, deformation, and difficulty in treatment. Since the pathogenic cold and dampness belongs to a yin pathogen, the disease worsened in cold weather and is slightly relieved in warm conditions. The darkish red tongue with white and greasy coating and deep and thin pulse are signs of liver and kidney deficiency with internal cold-dampness obstruction.

Diagnosis

TCM Diagnosis: *Bì* syndrome due to liver and kidney deficiency with cold and dampness obstruction in the joints

Western Medicine Diagnosis: Rheumatoid arthritis

Treatment

In this case, the deficiency of the liver, spleen and kidney is the root of the disease, while the pathogenic wind, cold, dampness and static blood are the branch. The pathomechanism is inhibited channels and obstruction of qi and blood flow due to retention of cold and dampness. This is a complex pattern of both deficiency and excess.

Principles:

- Supplement the liver blood and kidney yin
- Dispel wind and unblock collaterals
- Disperse cold and relieve pain

Formula: Modified *Dú Huó Jì Shēng Tāng* (Pubescent Angelica and Mistletoe Decoction).

Ingredients:

独活	*dú huó*	10 g	Radix Angelicae Pubescentis
桑寄生	*sāng jì shēng*	10 g	Herba Taxilli
秦艽	*qín jiāo*	10 g	Radix Gentianae Macrophyllae
防风	fáng fēng	10 g	Radix Saposhnikoviae
当归	*dāng guī*	10 g	Radix Angelicae Sinensis
川芎	*chuān xiōng*	6 g	Rhizoma Chuanxiong
白芍	*bái sháo*	10 g	Radix Paeoniae Alba
熟地黄	*shú dì huáng*	10 g	Radix Rehmanniae Praeparata
牛膝	*niú xī*	10 g	Radix Achyranthis Bidentatae
茯苓	*fú líng*	10 g	Poria
党参	*dǎng shēn*	15 g	Radix Codonopsis
桂枝	*guì zhī*	6 g	Ramulus Cinnamomi
杜仲	*dù zhòng*	10 g	Cortex Eucommiae
甘草	*gān cǎo*	6 g	Radix et Rhizoma Glycyrrhizae

Formula Analysis

In the formula, *dú huó, sāng jì shēng, shú dì huáng, niú xī* and *dù zhòng* are used to to supplement the liver and kidney, and strengthen sinews and bones. *Fú líng* and *gān cǎo* are used to promote the transformation and formation of body fluids. *Dāng guī, bái sháo* and *chuān xiōng* harmonize *yin* and nourish blood. *Dǎng shēn* and *fú líng* are to boost qi and fortify the spleen. *Qín jiāo* and *fáng fēng* can dispel wind and drain dampness. *Guì zhī* disperses cold and relieves pain. *Gān cǎo* harmonizes the actions of other medicinals. All the medicinals are combined to boost the kidney, unblock collaterals, reinforce healthy qi and dispel pathogens.

Chinese Patent Medicine:

The patient was also given the patent medicine of *Fēng Shī Gǔ Tòng Jiāo Náng* (Wind-Dampness Bone Ache Capsule) at the dosage of 2 to 4 capsules, twice a day to warm channels, disperse cold, unblock collaterals and relieve pain.

This patent contains *chuān wū* (Radix Aconiti) and *cǎo wū* (Radix Aconiti Kusnezoffii), which are poisonous. Avoid taking this formula patent over the recommended dosages and it is contraindicated for pregnant women.

Follow-up Consultations

After she taking 3 doses of the medication, the joint pain was slightly relieved. She continued to take 7 more doses and the joint pain continued to improve. However, there was still morning stiffness and the pain aggravated in cloudy days. On the basis of the former formula, *hǎi tóng pí* 10 g, *hǎi fēng téng* 10 g, *fáng jǐ* 10 g and *yín yáng huò* 15 g were added. She took this formula for over a month and the joint pain and swelling significantly remitted, the morning stiffness was not obvious, and there was only mild pain during climate changes. Then, *hǎi tóng pí* and *fáng jǐ* were removed from the formula, while *guì zhī* 9 g was added to strengthen the effect of warming yang and dispersing cold. After she took 15 more doses, all the symptoms resolved and ESR was 20mm/h. She continued to take this formula for another month which resolved the disease and blood test showed RF (−).

CASE STUDY 2: Rheumatoid Arthritis
By Dr. Zhang Ji

Ms. Pei, 24 years old. 1st consultation on December 12th, 2004.

Main Complaints: Bilateral limbs joint pain, stiffness and inhibited movement for over 2 years.

Medical History: The patient suffered from bilateral limbs joint pain, stiffness and inhibited movement 2 years ago. The pain of wrists was the most significant. In the summer of 2003, the blood test showed ESR 80mm/h and RF (+) and the treatments given were not very effective.

Presenting Symptoms: Difficulty in walking and needing help to move around, bilateral wrists, interphalangeal joints and ankles were swollen, painful and were unable to move which worsened with pressure and on cloudy and cold days. There was a thin and small tongue with a red tip and a yellow and greasy coating with a thin wiry pulse.

Physical Examination: Temperature 37.5 ℃. The patient was conscious, but was very lethargy and depressed. There was no abnormal finding in the heart and lung examination.

Diagnosis

TCM Diagnosis: *Bì* syndrome due to qi and blood deficiency with the retention of pathogenic cold and dampness stagnation in the joints

Western Medicine Diagnosis: Rheumatoid arthritis

Treatment

The patomechanism of *bì* syndrome is deficiency of qi, blood, liver and kidney at the root and obstruction of pathogenic wind, cold, dampness, static blood and phlegm-turbidity at the branch. A combination of Chinese medicinals and acupuncture was given for the treatment.

Principles:

- Tonify qi and warm the kidney
- Expel cold and drain dampness
- Dispel wind and remove phlegm
- Move qi and stop pain

Ingredients:

独活	*dú huó*	12 g	Radix Angelicae Pubescentis
桑寄生	*sāng jì shēng*	12 g	Herba Taxilli
青风藤	*qīng fēng téng*	12 g	Caulis Sinomenii
海风藤	*hǎi fēng téng*	12 g	Caulis Piperis Kadsurae
制川乌	*zhì chuān wū*	5 g	Radix Aconiti Praeparata (decocted first)
炙黄芪	*zhì huáng qí*	12 g	Radix Astragali Praeparata cum Melle
丹参	*dān shēn*	12 g	Radix et Rhizoma Salviae Miltiorrhizae
炙甘草	*zhì gān cǎo*	6 g	Radix et Rhizoma Glycyrrhizae Praeparata cum Melle
连翘	*lián qiào*	12 g	Fructus Forsythiae
杜仲	*dù zhòng*	12 g	(dry fried) Cortex Eucommiae
威灵仙	*wēi líng xiān*	10 g	Radix et Rhizoma Clematidis
仙灵脾	*xiān líng pí*	12 g	Herba Epimedii
怀牛膝	*huái niú xī*	12 g	Radix et Rhizome Achyranthes
海桐皮	*hǎi tóng pí*	12 g	Cortex Erythrinae

Acupuncture Point Combination:

DU 14 (*dà zhuī*)	DU 9 (*zhì yáng*)	DU 4 (*mìng mén*)
GB 20 (*fēng chí*)	EX-HN 1 (*sì shén cōng*)	GB 34 (*yáng líng quán*)
SP 10 (*xuè hǎi*)	EX-UE 9 (*bā xié*)	SJ 5 (*wài guān*)
EX-LE 4 (*nèi xī yǎn*)	EX-LE 5 (*xī yǎn*)	BL 40 (*wěi zhōng*)

Manipulations: Apply the method and retain the needle for 30 mins for each treatment. The patient received a treatment every other day.

Follow-up Consultations

With a combination treatment of medicinal formulas and acupuncture, the swelling and pain of the ankles were relieved and the patient could walk freely again after a month of treatment. The swelling in the bilateral wrists and interphalangeal joints was resolved, but the morning stiffness and weakness remained. Based on the previous formula, *dǎng shēn* 15 g and *zhì huáng qí* 15 g were added. The acupuncture treatment remained the same. After 2 months of successive treatment, all symptoms resolved, the joint movement was normal and she resumed to a normal life. However, the patient experienced some mild swelling and pain in the ankles during climate changes.

Clinical Analysis

In the acupuncture treatment for *bì* syndrome, Dr. Zhang usually applied a 3-step method on the *du mai* based on the pattern with local acupuncture. The treatment course is generally once every other day, and 1 course of treatment is a month.

At first the treatment method is to strengthen the *du mai* and yang qi, reinforce healthy qi and dispel pathogens, disperse wind and overcome dampness. The points on the *du mai* are used to boost yang, such as DU 14, DU 9 and DU 4. DU 14 is the place where all yang qi converges, so it can boost yang and secure the exterior, dispel wind and overcome dampness. DU 9 is located at the chest level, which is the area of the sea of qi. Hence, this point can tonify the yang of the lung and heart, and benefit qi, nourish blood and dredge the channels. DU 4 is the source of life and can boost the kidney yang, as well as dispel wind and overcome dampness.

The second step of the treatment includes selecting points according to pattern differentiation. For strong pathogenic wind, select GB 20 and DU 16 to dispel wind and overcome dampness, relieve *bì* and strengthen healthy qi. For strong pathogenic cold dampness, select RN 4 and RN 6 to boost primordial yang, dispel cold and overcome dampness. Select GB 34 to unblock channels, warm yang, dispel wind and overcome dampness. For obvious static blood, select SP 10 and SP 8 to unblock channels and invigorate blood. For kidney deficiency, select LV 8 and KI 6 to warm the kidney and boost yang.

The third step is to select local points to the affected areas. For wrist pain, select

SJ 4 to soothe tendons and activate collaterals, disperse masses and relieve pain, SJ 5 to unblock yang, disperse cold and stop pain, and LI 5 to clear heat, disperse wind and stop pain. For pain of interphalangeal joints, use EX-UE 9 to unblock channels, activate blood and stop pain, LI 3 to disperse wind-heat and stop pain, and SI 3 to dredge wind, nourish blood and soften tendons. For knee pain, select EX-LE 4 and EX-LE 5 to dispel wind-dampness and stop pain. ST 36, GB 34 and BL 40 are effective points commonly used for knee pain, all of which can unblock *zang-fu* organs, dredge channels, soothe tendons, activate collaterals and stop pain. ST 34 is especially useful to treat knee pain, which is able to unblock joints, dispel wind and overcome dampness. For toe pain, select LV 3 to purge heat, rectify blood, and stop pain of heat *bì*, SP 4 to rectify the spleen and stomach, and dispel damp turbidity, EX-LE 10 to purge heat and stop pain of heat *bì*, BL 66 to clear heat and stop pain.

COMPREHENSION QUESTIONS

1. How can we differentiate the *bì* syndrome from *wěi* syndrome?
2. What are the key points to pattern differentiation of the *bì* syndrome?
3. Multiple choice questions:

1) The common characteristics of different types of *bì* syndrome are:
A. Different levels of pain with movement inhibition
B. Pain and discomfort in the limbs and joints
C. Body discomfort and heaviness
D. Joint wandering pain
E. Joint pain and numbness

2) The main disease causes of the *bì* syndrome are:
A. Constitutional deficiency
B. Healthy qi weakness
C. Contraction of pathogenic wind, cold, dampness and heat
D. Qi consumption and blood impairment afflicting the *zang-fu* organs
E. All of the above

3) The main formula for treating pain of multiple joints (*lì jié*) is:
A. *Má Xìng Yǐ Gān Tāng* (Ephedra, Apricot Kernel, Gypsum and Licorice Decoction)
B. *Guì Zhī Sháo Yào Zhī Mǔ Tāng* (Cinnamon Twig, Peony and Anemarrhena Decoction)
C. *Wū Tóu Tāng* (Monkshood Root Decoction)
D. *Fáng Jǐ Dì Huáng Tāng* (Stephania Root and Rehmannia Decoction)
E. *Dú Huó Jì Shēng Tāng* (Pubescent Angelica and Mistletoe Decoction)

4) All the following symptoms belong to the symptoms of the *bì* syndrome, except ____.

A. Pain
B. Distressing
C. Heaviness
D. Weakness and lack of strength
E. Numbness

5) If the *bì* syndrome lasts for a long time and the pathogens obstruct the heart and the blood flow becomes inhibited, it often leads to:

A. Convulsive disease
B. Syncope
C. Palpitations
D. Epilepsy
E. None of the above

6) A patient has joint pain, heaviness and swelling of extremities, inhibited movement of the limbs and skin numbness. It belongs to ____ of *bì* syndrome.

A. Migratory *bì* (wind *bì*)
B. Painful *bì* (cold *bì*)
C. Fixed *bì* (dampness *bì*)
D. Heat *bì*
E. Stubborn *bì*

Answers

1. The *wěi* syndrome is a disease characterized by heavy limbs and weak tendons that the patient often lay in bed all day due to weakness. This is a chronic syndrome where the patient can not move and the muscles will atrophy. However, the *bì* syndrome manifests as one or multiple joint pain, swelling and inhibited movement. Only at the later stage of *bì* syndrome, will there also be some withered muscles that is similar to the *wěi* syndrome, but this only happens because of the prolonged stagnation of pathogenic dampness, cold, heat, phlegm and blood stasis.

2. The key points to pattern differentiation of the *bì* syndrome are:

1) Differentiate the pathogenic factors of the *bì* syndrome by observing the different clinical manifestations. The attack of pathogenic wind presents in the symptoms of wondering joint pain. The attack of pathogenic cold presents as a severe joint pain which worsens in the cold weather and slightly resolves in the warmer conditions. The attack of pathogenic dampness features in joint pain and heaviness with some skin numbness. The attack of pathogenic heat is seen as joint redness, swelling and pain.

2) Differentiate the state of the disease evaluating if it is primordially an excess

or deficient pattern by observing the duration and severity of the disease. If the syndrome is acute, the excessive pathogens will be more obvious, while if it is a chronic case, there will be some deficiency and blood stasis and other pathogenic factors.

3) Differentiate if there is a presence of pathogenic phlegm and static blood. These pathogenic factors make the syndrome more severe and difficult to treat. Identifying it early and treating it appropriately will increase the rate of recovery. If the *bì* syndrome lingers for a long time and there are symptoms such as joint swelling, stiffness, deformation, fixed stabbing pain that is relatively moderate in the day and more severe at night, a dark purple tongue with ecchymoses or teeth marks, and a deep, wiry and choppy pulse, it pertains to healthy qi deficiency and lingering pathogens of binding phlegm and static blood. In such a case, it requires to add some herbs that can dredge the phlegm, resolve blood stasis and nourish blood while supplementing the liver and kidney.

3. 1) A, 2) E, 3) C, 4) D, 5) C, 6) C.

4.11 Water Tympanites

Water tympanites is one of the type of tympanites and it is mainly characterized by abdominal distension with thin and tight skin due to the accumulation of water in the abdomen, a pale complexion, difficult urination and bilateral rib-side pain. Most of the patients show a sallow facial complexion, sometimes accompanied by jaundice and the red spider varicose vein on the body. This syndrome is common in clinic and is difficult to be cured.

In Western medicine, it is often associated to cirrhosis ascites, virus hepatitis, schistosomiasis, biliary cirrhosis, tuberculous peritonitis, late stage of intra-abdominal malignant tumors, nephrotic syndrome and malnutrition.

In Chinese medicine, this disease mainly results from liver constraint damaging the spleen, liver failing to govern the free flow of qi, the spleen failing to govern the transportation and transformation causing severe pathogenic water and toxin accumulations in the abdomen. The location of disease is in the liver, spleen, and kidney, and its basic pathomechanism is the disorder of these three organs, leading to qi stagnation, blood stasis, and water retention in the abdomen. Its characteristic pathomechanism is root deficiency and the branch excess with a complex development.

It is important to notice that since this condition is very severe and causes damage of the organ, solemnly expelling the water accumulation from the abdomen will not be sufficient to treat the disease pattern since the deficient root will still exist and cause the disease to reoccur. The pathogenic cold and water damaged the yang qi of the organs and the healthy qi combined with the overuse of cold or cool medicinals will also cause a yang deficiency and water exuberance. Once the pathogenic factors are resolved, it is highly recommended to use supplementing and nourishing medicinals to warm the yang, fortify the spleen, boost the kidney and tonify healthy qi.

CLINICAL PATTERNS DIFFERENTIATION AND TREATMENTS

1. Qi Stagnation and Dampness Retention

Symptoms: Abdominal distension but softness upon palpation, fullness, distension or pain in the hypochondriac region, especially after eating food, decreased ingestion of food, belching and scanty urine, a white and greasy tongue coating and a wiry pulse.

Treatment Principle:

- Soothe the liver and regulate qi

- Strengthen the spleen and resolve dampness

Main Acupuncture Points:

- SP 9 (*yīn líng quán*): To harmonize middle *jiao*, expel dampness and resolve edema
- RN 9 (*shuǐ fēn*): To regulate fluid metabolism and treat edema
- KI 7 (*fù liū*): To treat night sweats and febrile diseases without sweating, regulate fluid passages
- LV 3 (*tài chōng*): *Yuan* point of the liver to relieve chest congestion and irritability
- KI 13 (*qì xué*): To tonify kidney, benefit essence and regulate the water passageway
- ST 40 (*fēng lóng*): To expel phlegm and dampness

Supporting Points:

- ST 36 (*zú sān lǐ*): To tonify spleen, support the correct qi and tonify deficiency
- SP 4 (*gōng sūn*): To invigorate spleen, harmonize middle *jiao* and regulate qi

Recommended Formula: *Chái Hú Shū Gān Sǎn* (柴胡疏肝散, Bupleurum Liver-Soothing Powder) from *The Complete Works of [Zhang] Jing-yue* (*Jǐng Yuè Quán Shū*, 景岳全书) combined with *Wèi Líng Tāng* (胃苓汤, Stomach-Calming Poria Decoction) from the *Teachings of [Zhu] Dan-xi* (*Dān Xī Xīn Fǎ*, 丹溪心法)

Substitute Formula: *Mù Xiāng Shùn Qì Sǎn* (木香顺气散, Costus Root Qi-Balancing Powder)

Patent Formula: *Mù Xiāng Shùn Qì Wán* (木香顺气丸, Costus Root Qi-Balancing Pill)

2. Water Dampness Obstructing the Spleen

Symptoms: Abdominal enlargement, fullness and distension with a sense of water upon palpation, facial puffiness, edema on the lower limbs, gastric or abdominal discomfort or distension that can be alleviated by warmth, mental fatigue, aversion to cold, physical inactivity, scanty urine and loose stools, a white and greasy tongue coating and a slow pulse.

Treatment Principle:

- Warm the middle *jiao* and circulate qi
- Strengthen the spleen and drain dampness
- Promote urination and expel water

Main Acupuncture Points:

- SP 9 (*yīn líng quán*): To harmonize middle *jiao*, expel dampness and resolve edema
- RN 9 (*shuǐ fēn*): To regulate fluid metabolism and treat edema
- KI 7 (*fù liū*): To treat night sweats and febrile diseases without sweating, regulate fluid passages
- SP 6 (*sān yīn jiāo*): To invigorate spleen, liver and kidney, tonify yin and harmonize lower *jiao*
- ST 40 (*fēng lóng*): To expel phlegm and dampness

• BL 20 (*pí shù*): Back-*shu* point of the spleen to regulate middle *jiao* qi, invigorate spleen, resolve hemoptysis

• ST 25 (*tiān shū*): Front-*mu* point of the large intestine to invigorate spleen and stomach, clear damp-heat and resolve dysentery

Supporting Points:

• BL 22 (*sān jiāo shù*): To regulate *san jiao,* resolve dampness, regulate the water passageway, promote urination, benefit original qi, tonify the lumbar region and knees

• ST 27 (*dà jù*): To benefit kidney, nourish essence and treat impotence

Recommended Formula: *Shí Pí Sǎn* (实脾散, Spleen-Strengthening Powder) from the *Categorized Collection of Medical Formulas* (*Yī Fāng Lèi Jù,* 医方类聚)

Substitute Formula: *Zhēn Wǔ Tāng* (真武汤, True Warrior Decoction) plus *Píng Wèi Sǎn* (平胃散, Stomach-Calming Powder)

3. Accumulation of Damp-Heat

Symptoms: Solid abdominal enlargement and fullness, restlessness, a bitter taste in the mouth, thirst with no desire to drink water, dark-yellow urine, constipation or loose stools, might also present with jaundice, a red tongue tip with a yellow, greasy or dark gray coating and a wiry and rapid pulse.

Treatment Principle:

• Clear heat and resolve dampness

• Promote urination and expel water retention

Main Acupuncture Points:

• SP 9 (*yīn líng quán*): To harmonize middle *jiao*, expel dampness and resolve edema

• RN 9 (*shuǐ fēn*): To regulate fluid metabolism and treat edema

• KI 7 (*fù liū*): To treat night sweats and febrile diseases without sweating, regulate fluid passages

• LI 11 (*qū chí*): *He*-sea point of the large intestine to resolve stagnation, expel dampness, alleviate diarrhea and stop pain

• KI 2 (*rán gǔ*): To clear deficient fire

Supporting Points:

• LV 2 (*xíng jiān*): To clear liver fire and spread liver qi

• GB 34 (*yáng líng quán*): To treat lower limb weakness and numbness, relax sinews, benefit joints and stop pain

Recommended Formula: *Zhōng Mǎn Fēn Xiāo Wán* (中满分消丸, Center Fullness Separating and Dispersing Pill) from the *Secrets from the Orchid Chamber* (*Lán Shì Mì Cáng,* 兰室秘藏)

Substitute Formula: *Zhōu Chē Wán* (舟车丸, Vessel and Vehicle Pill)

Patent Formula: *Zhōng Mǎn Fēn Xiāo Wán* (中满分消丸, Center Fullness Separating and Dispersing Pill)

4. Blood Stasis and Water Retention

Symptoms: Firm abdominal enlargement and fullness, exposure of abdominal veins, stabbing pain in the hypochondriac region, a dark complexion, spider varicose veins on the face, neck, chest or arms, palmar erythema, dark purple lips, thirst with an inability to drink water, dark stools, a purplish red tongue and a thready, choppy or hollow pulse.

Treatment Principle:

- Invigorate blood and resolve stasis
- Circulate qi and promote urination

Main Acupuncture Points:

- SP 9 (*yīn líng quán*): To harmonize middle *jiao*, expel dampness and resolve edema
- LV 4 (*zhōng fēng*): Spread liver qi, clear liver and gall bladder heat, activate the channels and relax sinews
- SP 8 (*dì jī*): *Xi*-cleft point of the spleen to resolve dampness and regulate spleen, improve digestion and benefit appetite
- BL 17 (*gé shù*): Influential point of the blood to promote blood circulation and resolve stasis, harmonize blood and stop abdominal pain
- BL 18 (*gān shù*): Back-*shu* point of the liver to spread liver qi, clear liver and gallbladder heat, unbind the chest and promote circulation
- BL 20 (*pí shù*): Back-*shu* point of the spleen to regulate middle *jiao* qi, invigorate spleen, resolve hemoptysis

Supporting Points:

- SP 10 (*xuè hǎi*): To promote blood flow and dispel stasis, invigorate the spleen and cool blood
- ST 25 (*tiān shū*): Front-*mu* point of the large intestine to invigorate spleen and stomach, clear damp-heat and resolve dysentery

Recommended Formula: *Tiáo Yíng Yǐn* (调营饮, Ying Qi-Regulating Beverage) from the *Standards for Diagnosis and Treatment* (*Zhèng Zhì Zhǔn Shéng*, 证治准绳)

Substitute Formula: *Biē Jiǎ Jiān Wán* (鳖甲煎丸, Turtle Shell Decocted Pill)

Patent Formula: *Xuè Fǔ Zhú Yū Wán* (血府逐瘀丸, Blood Stasis Expelling Pill)

5. Water Retention due to Yang Deficiency

Symptoms: Abdominal enlargement, fullness and discomfort which alleviates in the morning and worsens at night, a sallow or bright pale complexion, gastric fullness, a poor appetite, mental fatigue, aversion to cold, cold limbs, edema on the lower limbs, scanty urine, a pale purple and enlarged tongue and a deep, wiry and weak pulse.

Treatment Principle:

- Warm and supplement the spleen and kidney

- Transform qi and promote urination

Main Acupuncture Points:

- SP 9 (*yīn líng quán*): To harmonize middle *jiao*, expel dampness and resolve edema
- KI 5 (*shuǐ quán*): To strengthen the kidney and promote urination
- KI 7 (*fù liū*): To treat night sweats and febrile diseases without sweating, regulate fluid passages
- ST 36 (*zú sān lǐ*): To tonify spleen, support the correct qi and tonify deficiency
- BL 20 (*pí shù*): Back-*shu* point of the spleen to regulate middle *jiao* qi, invigorate spleen, resolve hemoptysis
- BL 23 (*shèn shù*): Back-*shu* point of the kidney to benefit the original qi and kidney yin
- DU 4 (*mìng mén*): To tonify kidney, regulate *du mai*, strengthen lumbar region, treat sexual dysfunction, secure essence and benefit lower limbs

Supporting Points:

- RN 4 (*guān yuán*): To tonify the original qi, nourish kidney, supplement deficiencies and treat general weakness
- DU 20 (*bǎi huì*): To raise clear liver yang, calm the spirit and nourish the sea of marrow

Recommended Formula: *Jì Shēng Shèn Qì Wán* (济生肾气丸, Life-Saving Kidney Qi Pill) from the *Formulas to Aid the Living* (*Jì Shēng Fāng*, 济生方)

Substitute Formulas: *Fù Zǐ Lǐ Zhōng Wán* (附子理中丸, Aconite Center-Regulating Pill) plus *Wǔ Líng Sǎn* (五苓散, Five Substances Powder with Poria)

Patent Formula: *Jì Shēng Shèn Qì Wán* (济生肾气丸, Life-Saving Kidney Qi Pill)

6. Water Retention due to Yin Deficiency

Symptoms: Abdominal enlargement, distention and fullness, exposure of abdominal veins, a grey complexion, purplish lips, dry mouth, restlessness, insomnia, gum or nasal bleeding, scanty urine, a dry and dark red tongue with a wiry, thready and rapid pulse.

Treatment Principle:

- Nourish the kidney and supplement essence
- Soothe the liver and nourish yin
- Promote urination and reduce edema

Main Acupuncture Points:

- SP 9 (*yīn líng quán*): To harmonize middle *jiao*, expel dampness and resolve edema
- KI 5 (*shuǐ quán*): Regulate the kidney and promote urination
- KI 7 (*fù liū*): To treat night sweats and febrile diseases without sweating, regulate fluid passages
- KI 3 (*tài xī*): *Yuan*-source point of kidney to tonify spleen and kidney yin, clear

deficient heat and resolve hemoptysis

- SP 6 (*sān yīn jiāo*): To invigorate spleen, liver and kidney, tonify yin and harmonize lower *jiao*
- BL 18 (*gān shù*): Back-*shu* point of the liver to spread liver qi, clear liver and gallbladder heat, unbind the chest and promote circulation
- BL 23 (*shèn shù*): Back-*shu* point of the kidney to benefit the original qi and kidney yin

Supporting Points:

- ST 36 (*zú sān lǐ*): To tonify spleen, support the correct qi and tonify deficiency
- RN 4 (*guān yuán*): To tonify the original qi, nourish kidney, supplement deficiency and treat weakness

Recommended Formula: *Liù Wèi Dì Huáng Wán* (六味地黄丸, Six Ingredients Rehmannia Pill) from the *Key to Diagnosis and Treatment of Children's Diseases* (*Xiǎo Ér Yào Zhèng Zhí Jué*, 小儿药证直诀) combined with *Yī Guàn Jiān* (一贯煎, Effective Integration Decoction) from the *[Wei] Liu-zhou's Discourse on Medicine* (*Liǔ Zhōu Yī Huà*, 柳州医话)

Substitute Formula: *Mài Wèi Dì Huáng Wán* (麦味地黄丸, Ophiopogon, Magnolivine and Rehmannia Pill)

Patent Formula: *Mài Wèi Dì Huáng Wán* (麦味地黄丸, Ophiopogon, Magnolivine and Rehmannia Pill)

Summary Chart for Water Tympanites

Patterns	Main Points	Supporting Points	Formulae
Qi Stagnation and Dampness Retention	SP 9, RN 9, KI 7, LV 3, KI 13, ST40	ST 36 for nourishing the stomach and spleen function SP 4 for tonifying spleen qi	*Chái Hú Shū Gān Sǎn* with *Wèi Líng Tāng* or *Mù Xiāng Shùn Qì Sǎn*
Water Dampness Obstructing the Spleen	SP 9, RN 9, KI 7, SP 6, ST 40, BL 20, ST 25	BL 22 for expelling excess water accumulation ST 27 to regualte the stools	*Shí Pí Sǎn* or *Zhēn Wǔ Tāng* with *Píng Wèi Sǎn*
Accumulation of Damp-Heat	SP 9, RN 9, KI 7, LI 11, KI 2	LV 2 for clearing heat of the liver GB 34 for clearing damp heat of the liver and gallbladder	*Zhōng Mǎn Fēn Xiāo Wán* or *Zhōu Chē Wán*
Blood Stasis and Water Retention	SP 9, LV 4, SP 8, BL 17, BL 18, BL 20	SP 10 for moving blood and removing stasis ST 25 for moving qi in the abdominal area	*Tiáo Yíng Yǐn* or *Biē Jiǎ Jiān Wán*
Water Retention due to Yang Deficiency	SP 9, KI 5, KI 7, ST 36, BL 20, BL 23 DU 4	RN 4 for fortifying original qi and yang DU 20 for raising yang qi	*Jì Shēng Shèn Qì Wán* or *Fù Zǐ Lǐ Zhōng Wán* with *Wǔ Líng Sǎn*

Continued

Patterns	Main Points	Supporting Points	Formulae
Water Retention due to Yin Deficiency	SP 9, KI 5, KI 7, KI 3, SP 6, BL 18 BL 23	ST 36 for nourishing the stomach and spleen function RN 4 for fortifying original qi and yang	*Liù Wèi Dì Huáng Wán* plus *Yī Guàn Jiān* or *Mài Wèi Dì Huáng Wán*

CASE STUDY 1: Cirrhosis Ascites

Mr. Yang, 42 years old.

Main Complaint: Abdominal distension with ascites for over 2 years and aggravation for a month.

Medical History: The patient started to suffer from abdominal distension 2 years ago. He had been treated before and the diagnosis was cirrhosis. He had taken both Western and Chinese medicines, including *Péng Zhèng Wán* (Tympanites Pill) and *Zhōu Chē Wán* (Vessel and Vehicle Pill). However, his symptoms recurred with the increasing and decreasing of the abdominal swelling. His condition aggravated in the recent month. The patient also had a history of liver cirrhosis without complete recovery.

Presenting Symptoms: fatigue, lack of strength, bilateral rib-side distension, poor digestion, swelling of the scrotum without pain, a red tongue with a yellow and greasy coating and a wiry and slippery pulse.

Physical Examination: Spider varicose veins in the face, bulgy abdomen with borborygmus upon percussion, tympanitic resonance in the upper abdomen and around navel upon percussion. The liver was not palpable and the spleen was enlarged and could be touched below the rib cage at 3 finger width. An X-ray of the oesophagus showed no phlebeurysma.

Liver Function Test: Thymol turbidity 11.3 unit, total protein 63 g/L, albumin 23 g/L, globulin 40 g/L, Van den Bergh test: Direct reaction (−) and indirect reaction (+).

Pattern Differentiation

In this case of water tympanites, the chronic liver cirrhosis caused liver qi stagnation affecting the spleen and causing the spleen and stomach to fail in the transportation and transformation manifesting in the fatigue, lack of strength, bilateral rib-side distension and poor digestion. The red tongue with yellow and greasy coating and the wiry and slippery pulse are symptoms of the pathogenic heat retention. The pathomechanism is the liver qi stagnation and the spleen deficiency with dampness obstruction.

Diagnosis

TCM Diagnosis: Watery tympanites due to liver qi stagnation and spleen deficiency with dampness obstruction

Western Medicine Diagnosis: Cirrhosis ascites

Treatment

This is a chronic case with spleen and stomach weakness with liver qi stagnation causing dampness retention and heat constraint.

Principles:

- Soothe the liver and fortify the spleen
- Promote urination and drain dampness
- Move blood and regulate qi

Formula: Modified *Fù Gān Tāng* (Liver Restoring Decoction)

Ingredients:

黄芪	*huáng qí*	25 g	(raw) Radix et Rhizoma Salviae Miltiorrhizae
丹参	*dān shēn*	25 g	Radix Pseudostellariae
泽泻	*zé xiè*	25 g	Rhizoma Alismatis
山药	*shān yào*	20 g	(raw) Rhizoma Dioscoreae
蚤休	*zǎo xiū*	15 g	Rhizoma Paridis
大腹皮	*dà fù pí*	15 g	Pericarpium Arecae
白术	*bái zhú*	10 g	Rhizoma Atractylodis Macrocephalae (dry-fried)
三棱	*sān léng*	10 g	Rhizoma Sparganii
乳香	*rǔ xiāng*	10 g	Olibanum
广木香	*guǎng mù xiāng*	10 g	Radix Aucklandiae
栀子	*zhī zǐ*	10 g	(raw) Fructus Gardeniae
郁金	*yù jīn*	10 g	Radix Curcumae
牵牛子	*qiān niú zǐ*	6 g	Semen Pharbitidis powder (infused)

Formula Analysis

In this formula, *huáng qí* and *rén shēn* supplement qi and warm yang. *Bái zhú* and *shān yào* supplement the spleen and boost qi. *Dān shēn, yù jīn, guǎng mù xiāng, rǔ xiāng* and *sān léng* serve to soothe the liver, relieve pain, disperse *pǐ* and dissolve stasis. *Zǎo xiū* dissipates masses, alleviates edema, clears heat and resolves toxins. *Zhī zǐ* and *zé xiè* promote urination, percolate dampness and discharge heat. *Dà fù pí* and *qiān niú zǐ* expel water and alleviate edema.

This formula is mainly to supplement and purge simultaneously while supplementing qi, fortifying the spleen, invigorating blood, dissolving stasis, promoting urination, and alleviating edema.

The Chinese patent formula *Xiāo Shuǐ Wán* (Water Dissipating Pill) was also taken orally at 10 g in the morning on an empty stomach, 3 days in a row.

甘遂	*gān suí*	15 g	Radix Kansui (prepared)
广木香	*guǎng mù xiāng*	6 g	Radix Aucklandiae
砂仁	*shā rén*	6 g	Fructus Amomi
黄芩	*huáng qín*	5 g	Radix Scutellariae

Follow-up Consultations

After 3 days of treatment, the patient urinated 7-8 times profusely. After 3 more days, the abdominal distension dissipated greatly, his spirit was clear, physical strength came back, bilateral rib-side distension and fullness resolved and the borborygmus was not severe. According to the changes of pulse and symptoms, the formula was slightly modified, but the main principles remained to soothe the liver and fortify the spleen, invigorate blood and dissolve stasis. Simultaneously, the treatment continued to promote urination and eliminate distension to prevent the recurrence of ascites. After 25 continuous doses of the formula, all symptoms resolved and the liver function was back to normal.

CASE STUDY 2: Chronic Ascites
By Dr. Jiang Chun-hua

Mr. Zeng, 46 years old. 1st consultation on December 30th, 1978.

Main Complaint: Abdominal distention with ascites for over 6 years.

Medical History: The patient suffered from cirrhosis for 6 years and suffered from abdominal distension in the end of 1977. The diagnosis by Western medicine was ascites due to cirrhosis. He was hospitalized twice and was prescribed medicines to promote urination and drain ascitic fluids.

Presenting Symptoms: Abdominal distension with ascites, aversion to cold, cold limbs, low fever, thirst with desire to drink, increased distension after drinking, constipation, scant and dark urine (the urine amount was about 500 ml daily), a pale and bulgy tongue with a yellow and greasy coating and a wiry and deep pulse.

Physical Examination: Enlarged abdomen with extruded navel and exposed veins, spider angioma in the head, neck, chest, and arms. His abdominal circumference is 106 cm.

Laboratory Test: Zinc turbidity test 20 unit, thymol turbidity 20.6 unit, total protein 6.3 g%, albumin 1.65 g%, globulin 4.65 g%, Y globulin 25%.

Diagnosis

TCM Diagnosis: Water tympanites due to yang deficiency leading to water dampness binding transforming to static heat

Western Medicine Diagnosis: Ascites

Treatment

The main pathomechanism of this disease is spleen yang deficiency with water-dampness binding transforming to static heat. If the treatment is to drain the congestion, it will damage the original yang. If the treatment is to supplement deficiency, the pathogens will not be expelled. Therefore, the treatment is to warm yang and promote defecation to simultaneously supplement deficiency and expel pathogens.

Principles:

- Warm yang and promote defecation
- Strengthen the spleen and drain dampness

Ingredients:

红参	*hóng shēn*	6 g	Radix et Rhizoma Ginseng Rubra (decocted separately for drinking like tea)
黄芪	*huáng qí*	60 g	Radix Astragali
白术	*bái zhú*	30 g	Rhizoma Atractylodis Macrocephalae
干姜	*gān jiāng*	3 g	Rhizoma Zingiberis
附子	*fù zǐ*	9 g	Radix Aconiti Lateralis Praeparata(blast-fried)
枳实	*zhǐ shí*	9 g	Fructus Aurantii Immaturus
虫笋	*chóng sǔn*	30 g	worm damaged bamboo shoots
葫芦	*hú lú*	30 g	Fructus Lagenariae
蛰虫	*zhé chóng*	9 g	Eupolyphaga seu Steleophaga
泽泻	*zé xiè*	15 g	Rhizoma Alismatis
大黄	*dà huáng*	9 g	Radix et Rhizoma Rhei
赤芍	*chì sháo*	12 g	Radix Paeoniae Rubra
白茅根	*bái máo gēn*	30 g	Rhizoma Imperatae
茯苓皮	*fú líng pí*	15 g	Cutis Poriae
大腹皮	*dà fù pí*	9 g	Pericarpium Arecae

Follow-up Consultations

After 7 doses of the formula, the volume of urine increased from 500 ml to 1500 ml daily and there were 3 episodes of bowel movements a day. The abdominal distension was relieved quickly and ascites resolved and the appetite returned. After another 7 doses, the patient had 2 bowel movements a day, normal urination and the abdominal circumference reduced to 80 cm. Then, the treatment was adjusted to supplement the center and boost qi while invigorating blood. A follow-up visit 3 years later showed his condition was stable.

Notes

The patient was diagnosed with ascites due to cirrhosis which refers to water tympanites in Chinese medicine. According to the pulse condition and other manifestations, the pathological mechanism of this disease is spleen yang deficiency and internal deficiency of middle *jiao* manifested in the abdominal distension, aversion to cold, cold limbs and pale tongue. On the other hand, there are water retention and binding heat manifesting as exposed veins in the abdomen, spider angioma in the head, neck and chest, low fever, thirst with desire to drink, increased distension after eating, constipation, scanty and dark urine, enlarged tongue with yellow and greasy coating and a wiry pulse. Professor Jiang decided to warm and reinforce spleen yang, strongly supplement original qi, while clearing heat, discharging water, invigorating blood and dissolving stasis. In the formula, he combined *rén shēn, huáng qí, gān jiāng, bái zhú* with *dà huáng, zhé chóng, chóng sǔn, chì sháo* and *bái máo gēn,* which contains both cold and heat medicinals, to supplement and purge simultaneously.

CASE STUDY 3: Chronic Ascites and Tuberculous Peritonitis
By Dr. Xie Xi-liang

Mr. Fei, 13 years old. 1st consultation on December 2nd, 1985.

Main Complaint: Abdominal distension and edema of the body for 3 years.

Medical History: The patient was hospitalized for ascites due to cirrhosis in Xinxiang province in June 1982. Both Chinese medicine and Western medicine treatments were ineffective so he was transferred to a provincial hospital for treatment. The diagnosis was tuberculous peritonitis and ascites due to cirrhosis. The patient was given a large dose of penicillin, streptomycin, and other medicines for tuberculosis for over 2 months, but the medication increased the abdominal distension and the urine amount reduced accompanied with symptoms of systemic edema and inability to walk. He was then transferred to another hospital and given a combination of medicines to protect the liver and inhibit tuberculosis. At that time, the symptoms were slightly relieved. However, his abdominal distension was still severe with a circumference of 86 cm. He then moved to Beijng for treatment in August 1984. After 2 months of treatments, his condition improved. However, due to financial difficulty, he was discharged from the hospital. The patient came for acupuncture treatment on December 2nd, 1985.

Presenting Symptoms: Sallow yellow facial complexion, skinny body with enlarged abdomen and difficult mobility. His abdominal circumference was 86 cm with distending veins. There was dullness upon percussion and the liver edge was unclear, a pale tongue without coating and a thready and rapid pulse.

Diagnosis

TCM Diagnosis: Water tympanites due to spleen and kidney yang deficiency and water retention

Western Medicine Diagnosis: Ascites

Principles:

- Warm and supplement spleen and kidney yang,
- Strengthen qi and move blood
- Expel water and promote urination

Acupuncture Points Combination: RN 9 (*shuǐ fēn*), RN 6 (*qì hǎi*), ST 25 (*tiān shū*)

Manipulations: Apply grain 5 to 7 moxa cones on each point and apply direct moxibustion for once a day. After 2 months of treatment, the symptoms resolved greatly. The abdominal distension gradually relieved and the patient had less difficulty in walk. His family members were asked to apply moxibustion with moxa stick on RN 8 30 minutes daily to strengthen the efficacy. In October 1986, his abdominal distension was alleviated significantly, the spirit improved, and the body weight increased and he was able to go back to work.

Clinical Analysis

This patient was young and weak. He suffered from congenital insufficiency and improper postnatal nourishing which gave rise to spleen and kidney deficiency. As the spleen fails to transport and transform water and food, the production of qi and blood are insufficient and water-dampness is generated and accumulated internally. Spleen and kidney deficiency leads to disturbed qi transformation which fails to warm and remove dampness, causing dampness gatherings, qi and blood stagnation as the water tympanites. Together with binding constraint of liver qi causing blood stasis blocking the collateral, the condition worsened. As the famous doctor, Yu Jia-yan says in the *Precepts for Physicians* (*Yī Mén Fǎ Lǜ*, 医门法律): "distending diseases are merely due to water accumulation, qi stagnation and blood stasis." This case belongs to deficiency in root with pathogenic accumulation, so the treatment is to warm and supplement the spleen and kidney, unblock channels and collaterals by warming, invigorate blood, expel water, regulate the qi and dissipate accumulation. Therefore, RN 9, RN 6 and ST 25 are selected by warming with moxibustion to move qi, dispel blood stasis and expel water. Supplementing the fire of *mìng mén* by applying moxibustion to the RN 8 is able to assist the spleen yang and resume its normal ascending and descending functions of transportation and transformation and smooth the flow of fluids to ensure a favourable effect.

Notes

Water tympanites is a type of tympanites in Chinese medicine. Clinically, it is manifested as abdominal distension like a drum and it mainly results from qi depression damaging the liver, causing blood stasis and obstruction of collaterals and vessels. With time, the liver disease inflicts the spleen, leading to the disorder of transportation and transformation and water-dampness retention. In some cases, it is caused by spleen and kidney yang deficiency which can not be treated by warming and removing the water dampness accumulation. In these cases, the principles are to mainly warm yang and promote urination, supplement the spleen and soothe the liver. Therefore, we can select DU 4 to warm and supplement the kidney yang, and regulate the waterways; BL 20 and ST 36 to fortify the spleen qi and remove water-dampness; RN 12 to soothe the qi in middle *jiao*; and RN 3 to dredge the qi in lower *jiao*; SP 6 to free and regulate the waterways; BL 18 to soothe the liver wood, rectify qi and promote urination. When the liver constraint has been soothed, and the spleen and kidney qi fortified, the dampness will be transformed and water retention will be expelled. Therefore, the swelling and distension will resolve spontaneously.

KEY CLINICAL POINTS

Generally speaking, the clinical differentiation and treatment need a good understanding of root, branch, deficiency and excess. Only by clearly identifying the complexity of the pattern can the treatment be given appropriately. In a pattern mainly due to excess, the principles should be to soothe the liver and rectify the spleen qi, dissolve stasis, and expel the water. In a pattern mainly due to deficiency, the principles are to reinforce healthy qi by warming yang and promoting urination, or nourishing yin and promoting urination depending on the difference of water excess due to yang deficiency and water retention due to yin deficiency. A great emphasis must be given on rectifying the spleen and stomach and fortifying the healthy qi while dispelling pathogens. However, we should never only apply expelling medicinals since it will harm the healthy qi.

Furthermore, following points are noteworthy:

1. Expelling the Accumulation of Water

In short term condition, the healthy qi has not been too damaged with symptoms severe abdominal distension with lingering ascites, scanty urine, constipation, and a strong and forceful pulse, the treatment principles can follow "treating abdominal fullness by elimination" recorded in *Basic Questions: Treatise on Yin-Yang Correspondence to Phenomena* (*Sù Wèn:Yīn-Yáng Yìng Xiàng Dà Lùn*) to expel accumulated water to subdue pain and distension. However, this treatment must be stopped as soon as the syndrome is resolved.

2. Combination of Dispelling and Reinforcing Medicinals

This condition presents with abdominal distension and enlargement resulted from congestion of qi, blood, and water accumulation and should be treated by dispelling pathogen and dispersing distension, moving qi and promoting urination while strengthening healthy qi, recuperating the spleen and stomach functions.

3. Easier to Treat Yang Deficiency than to Treat Yin Deficiency

Water accumulation is a yin type of pathogen, which can be transformed by fortifying yang. Therefore, when the patient with yang deficiency tympanites is treated by yang warming and urination promoting medicinals, the ascites can easily be relieved. When it comes to the yin deficiency type of ascites, warming yang can damage yin, while nourishing yin aggravates the dampness which makes these types more difficult to treat. Clinically, we can choose sweet, cold, bland and percolating medicinals, such as *shā shēn, mài dōng, gān dì huáng, lú gēn, fú líng* and *zé xiè* to enrich yin and promote fluid production without increasing the dampness. Moreover, we can assist the yin enriching medicinals with warming and moving medicinals, such as *guì zhī* or *fù zǐ* to unblock yang and transform qi, as well as avoiding increasing the pathogenic factors.

4. Additional Treatment for Ascites Condition in Remission

After appropriate treatment, the symptoms of ascites may be relieved. However, the healthy qi of the liver and spleen has not fully recovered yet. Thus, qi stagnation and inhibited blood vessels and collaterals still remain, which, if remain untreated, may lead to the recurrence of ascites. At this point, we must modify our treatment to soothe the liver, fortify the spleen, invigorate blood, promote urination, and supplement the healthy qi to prevent reoccurrence of the condition.

5. Using Integrative Chinese and Western Medicine in Critical Water Tympanites

In the late period of cirrhosis, the symptoms of ascites will be severe accompanied by upper gastrointestinal hemorrhage, serious jaundice, infections, or hepatic coma. This is a critical condition which requires careful treatment of the combination of Chinese and Western medicine.

COMPREHENSION QUESTIONS

1. What is the diagnostic criteria of water tympanites?
2. What are the key clinical points to differentiate water tympanites from edema?
3. What are the indications and cautions of using water expelling medicinals?
4. Multiple choice questions:

1) The patient presents with symptoms of abdominal distension with no hardness when pressed, distending fullness or pain below the ribs, poor appetite, belching after having eating, scanty urine, a thin, white and greasy tongue coating and a wiry pulse. The disease pattern is:

A. Accumulation of pathogen and liver qi stagnation

B. Liver constraint and qi stagnation
C. Qi stagnation and blood stasis
D. Qi stagnation and dampness obstruction
E. Accumulation of pathogenic factors with qi stagnation and blood obstruction

2) Mr. Cheng, 71 years old. The patient suffered from cirrhosis for several years with accompanied symptoms of abdominal distending fullness with spider veins, dull facial complexion, cyanosed lips, dry mouth, vexation, insomnia, occasional nose and gum bleeding, scanty urine, a deep red tongue with scanty or peeled coating and a thin, wiry and rapid pulse. The recommended formula is:
A. Modified *Liù Wèi Dì Huáng Tāng* (Six-Ingredient Rehmannia Decoction)
B. Modified *Yī Guàn Jiān* (Effective Integration Decoction)
C. *Zī Shuǐ Qīng Gān Yǐn* (Water Nourishing and Liver Clearing Decoction) combined with modified *Yī Guàn Jiān* (Effective Integration Decoction)
D. *Zuǒ Guī Yǐn* (Left-Restoring Beverage) combined with modified *Yī Guàn Jiān* (Effective Integration Decoction)
E. *Liù Wèi Dì Huáng Tāng* (Six-Ingredient Rehmannia Decoction) combined with modified *Yī Guàn Jiān* (Effective Integration Decoction)

Answers

1. The diagnostic criteria of water tympanites:

In the beginning stage of water tympanites, there is distension in the abdominal cavity which swells as big as a drum with exposed veins on the abdominal wall and protruded umbilicus. It is generally accompanied by lack of strength, poor appetite, jaundice, dark red palm, and bleeding symptoms such as bleeding gums, nosebleed, cutaneous purpura, red streaks, varicose veins on the face, neck, and chest. There is usually a medical history of alcohol drinking, improper diet, or internal damage due to emotional stress.

2. Water tympanites mainly results from the mutual binding of qi, blood, and water in the abdomen due to the damaged liver, spleen, and kidney. There is obvious distension in the abdomen but the swelling in the four limbs is not significant. Edema of the limbs only appear at the later stage, which is often attended with dull and gloomy facial complexion, vascular nevus, red-streak, fullness in the rib-side, and exposed veins in the abdominal wall. The condition of edema is mainly caused by the disorders of the lung, spleen, and kidney which causes an overflow of water-dampness under the skin. Edema often begins at the eyelid, and then spreads to the head and the body, or it begins at the lower limbs and then spread to the whole body, which is often attended with bright pale complexion, soreness of the waist and fatigue.

3. For acute case of water tympanites with a strong constitution, the healthy qi is not excessively consumed and the abdominal distension is severe, accompanied

with scanty urine, constipation, and excess pulse. At this time, treating it according to the principle "treating the fullness of the center by elimination" recorded in *Basic Questions—Treatise on Yin-Yang Correspondence to Phenomena* (*Sù Wèn: Yīn Yáng Yìng Xiàng Dà Lùn*) is appropriate. Hence, treating with water expelling and promoting urination or bowel movement will expel the water-damp encumbering the spleen. As for caution when using these purging and expelling medicinals, we must terminate the treatment as soon as the pattern changes by always observing the condition of the healthy qi. Additionally, this treatment approach is not suitable in chronic cases of water tympanites or in cases of weak healthy qi.

4. 1) D, 2) E.

Part V
Kidney Conditions

5.1 Edema

Edema manifests as body fluid retention flooding at the muscle layer under the skin that can affect any area of the body such as the head, face, eyelids, four limbs, back and abdomen. Edema can be caused by external contraction, irregular diet, or overstrain, leading to failure of the lung to diffuse, descend and regulate qi, weakness of the spleen to transport and transform fluids, and deficiency of the kidney to open and close the water passageway through the bladder. In Western medicine, edema is often related to kidney or heart diseases.

In Chinese medicine, the main etiologies of edema are external contracted pathogenic wind, cold, dampness and heat, water retention and toxin accumulation. The pathomechanism is mainly disorders of the lung, spleen and kidney, the failure of the *sanjiao* to regulate the waterways, and the failure of the bladder to transform qi, bringing forth a fluid retention flooding the muscle and skin layers. The lung, spleen and kidney are interconnected. For example, depleted kidney yang fails to warm the spleen yang causing it to fail in transforming fluid manifesting as edema. In edema induced by external pathogens, the disease location often lies in the lung and spleen. In edema caused by internal injury, the disease location often resides in the spleen and kidney. Furthermore, it is important to notice that edema often becomes a chronic and difficult disease to treat, hence we must always remember to move the static blood and unblock the *san jiao* waterways.

1. Yang Water Retention

A. Wind-Cold Edema

Symptoms: Puffy face and swollen limbs, dysuria, severe aversion to cold with slight fever. Aching pain in the limbs and joints, cough with shortness of breath. Pale red tongue with thin white tongue coating, floating tight or sunken the fine pulse.

Treatment Principle:

- Disperse wind and dissipate cold
- Ventilate lung and promote urination

Main Acupuncture Points:

- BL 13 (*fèi shù*): Back-*shu* point of the lung to nourish lung, descend qi, release exterior, regulate sweating and harmonize breathing
- LI 4 (*hé gǔ*): To release the exterior, clear *yang ming* heat and stop toothache
- SP 9 (*yīn líng quán*): To harmonize middle *jiao*, expel dampness and resolve edema
- BL 22 (*sān jiāo shù*): To regulate *san jiao*, resolve dampness, regulate the fluid passage way and promote urination, benefit original qi, tonify the lumbar region and knees

Supporting Points:

- SJ 5 (*wài guān*): To release the exterior and clear heat
- DU 14 (*dà zhuī*): To clear heat, activate yang qi, treat pain and stiffness of the neck, shoulders and back

Recommended Formula: *Má Huáng Jiā Zhú Tāng* (麻黄加术汤, Ephedra Decoction plus Atractylodes) from the *Essentials from the Golden Cabinet* (*Jīn Guì Yào Lüè*, 金匮要略)

Substitute Formula:

- *Má Huáng Tāng* (麻黄汤, Ephedra Decoction)
- *Má Xìng Wǔ Pí Yǐn* (麻杏五皮饮, Ephedra, Apricot Kernel and Five Kinds of Peels Decoction)

B. Wind-Heat Edema

Symptoms: Puffy face and swollen limbs, inhibited urination, fever with slight aversion to cold, sore throat, dry mouth, a thin yellow tongue coating and a rapid floating pulse.

Treatment Principle:

- Disperse wind and clear heat
- Promote urination and treat edema

Main Acupuncture Points:

- BL 13 (*fèi shù*): Back-*shu* point of the lung to nourish lung, descend qi, release exterior, regulate sweating and harmonize breathing
- LI 4 (*hé gǔ*): To release the exterior, clear *yang ming* heat and stop toothache
- SP 9 (*yīn líng quán*): To harmonize middle *jiao*, expel dampness and resolve edema
- BL 22 (*sān jiāo shù*): To regulate *san jiao*, resolve dampness, regulate the fluid passage way and promote urination, benefit original qi, tonify the lumbar region and knees
- LI 11 (*qū chí*): *He*-sea point of the large intestine to resolve stagnation, expel dampness, alleviate diarrhea and stop pain
- LU 11 (*shào shāng*): To revive consciousness, relieve the surface and clear heat

Supporting Points:

- SJ 5 (*wài guān*): To release the exterior and clear heat

• DU 14 (*dà zhuī*): To clear heat, activate yang qi, treat pain and stiffness of the neck

Recommended Formula: *Yuè Bì Jiā Zhú Tāng* (越婢加术汤, Maidservant From Yue Decoction plus Atractylodis) from the *Essentials from the Golden Cabinet* (*Jīn Guì Yào Lüè*, 金匮要略)

Substitute Formula:

• *Yín Qiào Săn* (银翘散, Lonicera and Forsythia Powder)

Patent Formula: *Shèn Yán Jiě Rè Piàn* (肾炎解热片, Heat-Clearing Tablets for Nephritis)

C. Dampness Toxins Accumulation

Symptoms: Puffy face and swollen limbs, scanty reddish urine, sores and boils on the skin even with cankers, red tongue with a yellow tongue coating and a rapid slippery pulse.

Treatment Principle:

• Ventilate lung and remove toxin

• Promote urination and treat edema

Main Acupuncture Points:

• SP 9 (*yīn líng quán*): To harmonize middle *jiao*, expel dampness and resolve edema

• BL 22 (*sān jiāo shù*): To regulate *sanjiao*, resolve dampness, regulate the fluid passage way, promote urination, benefit original qi, tonify the lumbar region and knees

• LI 11 (*qū chí*): *He*-sea point of the large intestine to resolve stagnation, expel dampness, alleviate diarrhea and stop pain

• LI 4 (*hé gŭ*): To release the exterior, clear *yang ming* heat and stop toothache

• SP 6 (*sān yīn jiāo*): To invigorate spleen, liver and kidney, tonify yin and harmonize lower *jiao*

Supporting Points:

• ST 40 (*fēng lóng*): To expel phlegm and dampness

• ST 36 (*zú sān lǐ*): To tonify spleen, support the correct qi and tonify deficiency

Recommended Formula: *Má Huáng Lián Qiào Chì Xiăo Dòu Tāng* (麻黄连翘赤小豆汤, Ephedra, Forsythia and Rice Bean Decoction) from the *Treatise on Cold Damage* (*Shāng Hán Lùn*, 伤寒论) combined with *Wŭ Wèi Xiāo Dú Yĭn* (五味消毒饮, Five Ingredients Toxin-Removing Beverage) from the *Golden Mirror of the Medical Tradition* (*Yī Zōng Jīn Jiàn*, 医宗金鉴)

Substitute Formula: *Gān Lù Xiāo Dú Dān* (甘露消毒丹, Sweet Dew Toxin-Removing Elixir)

D. Water Dampness Accumulation

Symptoms: Edema with heavy sensation of the body, chest tightness, reduced appetite, nausea with desire to vomit, or vomiting of white foam, a thick white tongue coating and a sunken moderate pulse.

Treatment Principle:

- Reinforce spleen and resolve dampness
- Activate yang and promote urination

Main Acupuncture Points:

- BL 20 (*pí shù*): Back-*shu* point of the spleen to regulate middle *jiao* qi, invigorate spleen, resolve hemoptysis
- ST 36 (*zú sān lǐ*): To tonify spleen, support the correct qi and tonify deficiency
- BL 22 (*sān jiāo shù*): To regulate *san jiao,* resolve dampness, regulate the fluid passage way, promote urination, benefit original qi, tonify the lumbar region and knees
- RN 6 (*qì hǎi*): To support the original qi, tonify kidney and treat general weakness
- RN 9 (*shuǐ fēn*): To regulate fluid metabolism and treat edema

Supporting Points:

- ST 40 (*fēng lóng*): To expel phlegm and dampness
- SP 9 (*yīn líng quán*): To harmonize middle *jiao*, expel dampness and resolve edema

Recommended Formula: *Wèi Líng Tāng* (胃苓汤, Stomach-Calming Poria Decoction) from the *Teachings of [Zhu] Dan-xi* (*Dān Xī Xīn Fǎ*, 丹溪心法)

Substitute Formula:

- *Wǔ Pí Yǐn* (五皮饮, Five-Peel Beverage)
- *Wǔ Líng Sǎn* (五苓散, Five Substances Powder with Poria)

Patent Formula: *Shēn Líng Bái Zhú Sǎn* (参苓白术散, Ginseng, Poria and Atractylodes Macrocephalae Powder)

E. Damp-Heat Retention

Symptoms: Severe generalized edema, reddish or dark yellow urine, bitter taste and sticky sensation in the mouth, abdominal distension and stuffiness, a red tongue with a yellow greasy coating and a rapid slippery pulse.

Treatment Principle:

- Clear heat and drain dampness
- Promote urination and resolve edema

Main Acupuncture Points:

- BL 22 (*sān jiāo shù*): To regulate *san jiao,* resolve dampness, regulate the fluid passage way, promote urination, benefit original qi, tonify the lumbar region and knees
- LI 4 (*hé gǔ*): To release the exterior and clear *yang ming* heat
- SP 9 (*yīn líng quán*): To harmonize middle *jiao*, expel dampness and resolve edema
- RN 9 (*shuǐ fēn*): To regulate fluid metabolism and treat edema

• RN 3 (*zhōng jí*): Front-*mu* point of the bladder to dispel stagnation and harmonize the lower *jiao*, benefit the uterus and regulate menstruation

Supporting Points:

• LI 11 (*qū chí*): *He*-sea point of the large intestine to resolve stagnation, expel dampness, alleviate diarrhea and stop pain

• GB 34 (*yáng líng quán*): To treat lower limb weakness and numbness, relax sinews, benefit joints and stop pain

Recommended Formula: *Shū Záo Yǐn Zǐ* (疏凿饮子, Dredging and Piercing Drink) from the *Formulas to Aid the Living* (*Jì Shēng Fāng*, 济生方)

Substitute Formula:

• *Bì Xiè Fēn Qīng Yǐn* (萆薢分清饮, Hypoglaucae Root Turbidity-Clearing Beverage)

• *Jǐ Jiāo Lì Huáng Wán* (己椒苈黄丸, Tetrandra-Pricklyash-Lepidium-Rhubarb Pill)

Patent Formula: *Bì Xiè Fēn Qīng Wán* (萆薢分清丸, Hypoglaucae Root Turbidity-Clearing Pill)

2. Deficient Type Edema

A. Spleen Yang Deficiency

Symptoms: Edema especially on the lower body, the skin becomes pitted after applying pressure and disappears slowly after releasing the pressure, gastric or abdominal distension, poor appetite, loose stools, sallow complexion, mental fatigue, cold limbs, scanty urine a pale tongue with a white and coating and a deep, slow and weak pulse.

Treatment Principle:

• Warm spleen and tonify yang

• Drain dampness and resolve water retention

Main Acupuncture Points:

• BL 22 (*sān jiāo shù*): To regulate *san jiao*, resolve dampness, regulate the fluid passage way, promote urination, benefit original qi, tonify the lumbar region and knees

• BL 20 (*pí shù*): Back-*shu* point of the spleen to regulate middle *jiao* qi, invigorate spleen, resolve hemoptysis

• ST 36 (*zú sān lǐ*): To tonify spleen, support the correct qi and tonify deficiency

• RN 12 (*zhōng wǎn*): To regulate qi and invigorate spleen

• BL 54 (*zhì biān*): To treat hematuria and bloody stools

• RN 4 (*guān yuán*): To tonify the original qi, nourish kidney, supplement deficiencies and treat general weakness

Supporting Points:

• DU 4 (*mìng mén*): To tonify kidney, regulate *du mai*, strengthen lumbar region, treat sexual dysfunction, secure essence and benefit lower limbs

• RN 10 (*xià wǎn*): To regulate qi, dispel food stagnation and stop abdominal pain

Recommended Formula: *Shí Pí Yǐn* (实脾饮, Spleen-Firming Beverage) from the *Formulas to Aid the Living* (*Jì Shēng Fāng*, 济生方)

Substitute Formula: *Zhēn Wǔ Tāng* (真武汤, True Warrior Decoction) combined with *Wǔ Líng Sǎn* (五苓散, Five Substances Powder with Poria)

B. Kidney Yang Deficiency

Symptoms: Facial puffiness, edema in the lower body with sustained pitting after releasing the pressure, palpitations, panting, a cold, heavy and painful sensation in the lower back, decreased or increased urine output, cold limbs, aversion to cold, mental fatigue, gray or bright, pale complexion, a pale and swollen tongue with a white slippery coating and a deep, slow and weak pulse.

Treatment Principle:

- Warm kidney tonify yang
- Transform qi and resolve water retention

Main Acupuncture Points:

- BL 22 (*sān jiāo shù*): To regulate *san jiao*, resolve dampness, regulate the fluid passage way, promote urination, benefit original qi, tonify the lumbar region and knees
- BL 23 (*shèn shù*): Back-*shu* point of the kidney to benefit the original qi and kidney yin
- RN 6 (*qì hǎi*): To support the original qi, tonify kidney and treat general weakness
- BL 54 (*zhì biān*): To treat hematuria and bloody stools
- ST 28 (*shuǐ dào*): To regulate lower *jiao* qi and resolve constipation
- KI 7 (*fù liū*): To treat night sweats and febrile diseases without sweating, regulate fluid passages

Supporting Points:

- KI 10 (*yīn gǔ*): To tonify kidney and benefit yang, harmonize lower *jiao* and treat sexual dysfunction
- ST 40 (*fēng lóng*): To expel phlegm and dampness

Recommended Formula: *Jì Shēng Shèn Qì Wán* (济生肾气丸, Life-Saving Kidney Qi Pill) from the *Formulas to Aid the Living* (*Jì Shēng Fāng*, 济生方)

Substitute Formula: *Fù Zǐ Lǐ Zhōng Wán* (附子理中丸, Aconite Center-Regulating Pill)

Patent Formula: *Jì Shēng Shèn Qì Wán* (济生肾气丸, Life-Saving Kidney Qi Pill)

Summary Chart for Edema

Patterns	Main Points	Supporting Points	Formulae
Wind-Cold Edema	BL 13, LI 4, SP 9 BL 22	SJ 5 for regulating the *sanjiao* and clearing wind DU 14 for clearing exterior pathogens and raising the clear yang	*Má Huáng Jiā Zhú Tāng* or *Má Huáng Tāng* or *Má Xìng Wǔ Pí Yǐn*

Continued

Patterns	Main Points	Supporting Points	Formulae
Wind-Heat Edema	BL 13, LI 4, SP 9 BL 22, LI 11, LU 11	SJ 5 for regulating the *sanjiao* and clearing wind DU 14 for clearing exterior pathogens and raising the clear yang	*Yuè Bì Jiā Zhú Tāng* or *Yín Qiào Săn*
Dampness Toxins Accumulation	SP 9, BL 22, LI 11, LI 4, SP 6	ST 40 for expelling phlegm and dampness ST 36 for tonifying spleen and regulating qi	*Má Huáng Lián Qiào Chì Xiăo Dòu Tāng* plus *Wŭ Wèi Xiāo Dú Yĭn* or *Gān Lù Xiāo Dú Dān*
Water Dampness Accumulation	BL 20, ST 36, RN 9 BL 22, RN 6,	ST 40 for expelling phlegm and dampness SP 9 for clearing heat and draining dampness	*Wèi Líng Tāng* or *Wŭ Pí Yĭn* or *Wŭ Líng Săn*
Damp-Heat Retention	BL 22, LI 4, SP 9 RN 9, RN 3	LI 11 for clearing heat GB 34 for clearing heat and draining dampness	*Shū Záo Yĭn Zĭ* or *Bì Xiè Fēn Qīng Yĭn* or *Jĭ Jiāo Lì Huáng Wán*
Spleen Yang Deficiency	BL 22, BL 20 ST 36, RN 12 BL 54, RN 4	DU 4 for nourishing original qi and warming the *mingmen* RN 10 for draining water retention	*Shí Pí Yĭn* or *Zhēn Wŭ Tāng* plus *Wŭ Líng Săn*
Kidney Yang Deficiency	BL 22, BL 23 RN 6, BL 54 ST 28, KI 7	KI 10 for draining dampness ST 40 for expelling phlegm and dampness	*Jì Shēng Shèn Qì Wán* or *Fù Zĭ Lĭ Zhōng Wán*

CASE STUDY 1: Chronic Edema

Mr. Yang, 57 years old. 1st consultation 14th May.

Main Complaint: Lower limbs edema and feet numbness for over half a year.

Medical History: The patient suffered from lower limbs edema and feet numbness for over half a year which worsened when standing for long periods of time. He was diagnosed with weakness of the kidney and was hospitalized without any curative effect. On May 9th, he was hospitalized again due to a relapse of lower limbs edema. He was treated by prednisone, albumin and so on. He was discharged after the symptoms resolved. However, the edema occurred again 5 days later and came for treatment. The patient had a history of dilated cardiopathy and cardiac function grade 3. He took digoxin and cordarone daily.

Presenting Symptoms: Mental fatigue, general edema especially in the lower limbs, feet numbness, burning heat sensation in the left sole, dry mouth, scanty and clear urine, a pale dark tongue with teeth marks with a white tongue coating and a deep and thin pulse.

Physical Examination: Pitting edema in the waist and back (+) and in the lower limbs below the knees, dilated heart edge to the left, regular heart beat at 64 bpm. Urine routine test: PRO (++++), UPQ 7.9 g/24 h. Blood biochemical test: TP 32 g/L, ALB 20 g/L, BUN 9.2 mmol/L, Cr 161 μmol/L.

Pattern Differentiation

Nephrotic syndromes pertain to edema in the Chinese medicine, which has a close relationship with the spleen, kidney, lung and *san jiao*. The spleen is the earth organ and the foundation of acquired constitution, while the kidney governs the *mìng mén* fire and is the foundation of congenital constitution. The transformation and transportation functions of the spleen depend on the warmth of kidney yang and in turn, the kidney essence lies on the constant replenishment of food essence transformed and transported by the spleen. Thus, these two organs supplement and promote each other. If the spleen yang is insufficient with weak functions of transformation and transportation then the food essence production will fall short and inevitably lead to kidney essence insufficiency and failure of the spleen to control water manifesting in general edema especially severe in the lower limbs. Feet numbness and burning sensation in the left sole are signs of obstruction due to stasis. The symptoms of dry mouth, a pale dark tongue with teeth marks and a white tongue coating and the deep and thin pulse are signs of obstruction impairing the passage of the body fluid. In this case, the disease location is in the spleen and kidney with a root deficiency and branch excess.

Diagnosis

TCM Diagnosis: Edema due to spleen and kidney deficiency with stasis impairing the body fluid passage way

Western Medicine Diagnosis: Nephrotic edema

Treatment

In this case, the pathomechanism mainly lies in dampness retention due to spleen deficiency causing the stasis obstruction impairing the body fluid passage way. As a result, it manifests as general edema especially severe in the lower limbs, feet numbness and burning sensation on the left sole.

Principles:

- Fortify the spleen to promote urination
- Warm qi to drain dampness
- Dispel stasis and nourish yin

Formula: Modified *Sì Jūn Zǐ Tāng* (Four Gentlemen Decoction) combined with *Zhū Líng Tāng* (Polyporus Decoction) and *Shēng Mài Săn* (Pulse-Engendering Powder)

Ingredients:

黄芪	*huáng qí*	60 g	Radix Astragali
茯苓	*fú líng*	60 g	Poria
党参	*dǎng shēn*	15 g	Radix Codonopsis
白术	*bái zhú*	15 g	Rhizoma Atractylodis Macrocephalae
山药	*shān yào*	30 g	Rhizoma Dioscoreae
猪苓	*zhū líng*	15 g	Polyporus
泽泻	*zé xiè*	15 g	Rhizoma Alismatis
麦冬	*mài dōng*	15 g	Radix Ophiopogonis
滑石	*huá shí*	15 g	Talcum (decocted first)
大腹皮	*dà fù pí*	15 g	Pericarpium Arecae
益母草	*yì mǔ cǎo*	15 g	Herba Leonuri
阿胶	*ē jiāo*	10 g	Colla Corii Asini (melted in decoction)
五味子	*wǔ wèi zǐ*	10 g	Fructus Schisandrae Chinensis
生地	*shēng dì*	10 g	Radix Rehmanniae
甘草	*gān cǎo*	6 g	Radix et Rhizoma Glycyrrhizae

Formula Analysis

This formula combines *Sì Jūn Zǐ Tāng, Zhū Líng Tāng* and *Shēng Mài Sǎn*. It uses large dosages of *huáng qí, fú líng, dǎng shēn, bái zhú* and *shān yào* to fortify the spleen. *Dà fù pí, zhū líng, zé xiè, huá shí* and *yì mǔ cǎo* are used to invigorate blood, promote urination, drain dampness and disperse edema. *Mài dōng, ē jiāo, wǔ wèi zǐ* and *shēng dì* serve to nourish yin and cool blood. *Gān cǎo* harmonizes medicinals.

Follow-up Consultations

All the symptoms resolved after taking the formula for 7 weeks. Physical examination showed mild edema in the lower limbs below the knees (++). Urine routine test: PRO (++), 24 h UPQ 3.1 g Blood biochemical test: TP 46 g/L, ALB 29 g/L, BUN 16.68 mmol/L, Cr 140 μmol/L. The patient was discharged from the hospital on June 30th.

On the second consultation on July 10th the patient had symptoms of mild edema in the lower limbs, relatively scanty urine, a pale dark tongue with white coating and deep and thin pulse.

CASE STUDY 2: Renal Insufficiency Edema

Ms. Liang, 72 years old.

Main Complaint: Renal insufficiency for over 3 years.

Medical History: The patient was diagnosed with renal insufficiency during a physical examination in 2001. She was given *Liù Wèi Dì Huáng Wán* (Six-Ingredient Rehmannia Decoction) for over a year, but the physical examination this year revealed her condition was worsening. The patient also suffered from nausea, no appetite, poor sleep (3 to 4 hrs a night), palpitations, susceptibility to fright, dry mouth, and occasionally acid regurgitation, lumbago, edema of the ankle, aversion to cold and blurry vision. The patient had a history of diabetes for over 30 years, hyperlipemia and hypertension for 20 years as well as rheumatoid arthritis for 12 years.

Presenting Symptoms: poor appetite, nausea, poor sleep, palpitations, susceptibility to fright, lumbago, edema of the ankle, aversion to cold, blurry vision, scanty loose stool 3-4 times a day, normal urine amount, slightly frequent urination, a dark red tongue with a thin, yellow and greasy coating and a weak, wiry and slippery pulse.

Laboratory Test: BUN 14.08 mmol/L, UA 587 μmol/L, Cr 212 μmol/L, TC 6.83 mmol/L, TG 5.15 mmol/L, ESR 32 mm/h, LDL-C 3.49 mmol/L, RF(+).

Pattern Differentiation

This patient had a history of diabetes and hyperlipemia as well as secondary arteriosclerosis of the heart and a damaged vision. As these diseases were chronic they have depleted the healthy qi showing a poor prognosis.

The spleen resides in the middle and is the pivot which transports and transforms water-dampness, raises clear yang and directs the turbid downward. In this case, the spleen is deficient and fails to move the fluids for the stomach, resulting in swelling. As the clear qi fails to ascend and the turbid qi fails to descend, the clear and the turbid are mixed together and the stomach fails to harmonize and descend, manifesting as poor appetite and nausea. If the kidney fails to move the water due to deficiency, the *sanjiao* will be blocked. As a result, stagnation occurs, channels are obstructed and the water seeps into the skin and muscles to become edema manifesting in lumbago, edema of the ankle, aversion to cold, and loose stool. Signs of a dark red tongue with a thin, yellow and greasy coating and a weak, wiry and slippery pulse indicate turbid dampness accumulation. This is a complex pattern of both deficiency of the spleen and kidney with turbid damp accumulation.

Diagnosis

TCM Diagnosis: Edema due to deficiency of the spleen and kidney with turbid dampness accumulation

Western Medicine Diagnosis: Edema

Treatment

In this case, the pathomechanism mainly lies in the spleen and kidney deficiency with turbid damp accumulation

Principles:

- Warm and boost the spleen and kidney

- Harmonize the stomach and redirect the turbid downward
- Promote urination and expel dampness

Formula: Modified *Wèi Líng Tāng* (Stomach-Calming Poria Decoction) combined with *Liù Jūn Zǐ Tāng* (Six Gentlemen Decoction)

Ingredients:

藿香	*huò xiāng*	10 g	Herba Agastachis
紫苏叶	*zǐ sū yè*	10 g	Folium Perillae
黄连	*huáng lián*	3 g	Rhizoma Coptidis
吴茱萸	*wú zhū yú*	3 g	Fructus Evodiae
半夏	*bàn xià*	10 g	Rhizoma Pinelliae
炮姜炭	*páo jiāng tàn*	3 g	charred Rhizoma Zingiberis Praeparatum
苍术	*cāng zhú*	6 g	Rhizoma Atractylodis (dry-fried)
白术	*bái zhú*	10 g	Rhizoma Atractylodis Macrocephalae (dry-fried)
党参	*dǎng shēn*	10 g	Radix Codonopsis
山药	*shān yào*	12 g	Rhizoma Dioscoreae
神曲	*shén qū*	10 g	dry-fried Massa Medicata Fermentata
猪苓	*zhū líng*	12 g	Polyporus
茯苓	*fú líng*	12 g	Poria
泽兰	*zé lán*	12 g	Herba Lycopi
泽泻	*zé xiè*	12 g	Rhizoma Alismatis
淫羊藿	*yín yáng huò*	10 g	Herba Epimedii
巴戟天	*bā jǐ tiān*	10 g	Radix Morindae Officinalis
黄柏	*huáng bǎi*	6 g	Cortex Phellodendri Chinensis
鬼箭羽	*guǐ jiàn yǔ*	15 g	Ramulus Euonymi
菟丝子	*tù sī zǐ*	12 g	Semen Cuscutae
桑寄生	*sāng jì shēng*	15 g	Herba Taxilli
丹参	*dān shēn*	12 g	Radix et Rhizoma Salviae Miltiorrhizae
夜交藤	*yè jiāo téng*	20 g	Caulis Polygoni Multiflori

Formula Analysis

According to symptoms of loose stool, edema of the ankle, lumbago and cold limbs, this formula aims at strengthening the spleen and kidney, dispelling dampness and purging turbidity. *Lián Sū Yǐn* (Coptis and Perilla Decoction) and *Wèi Líng Tāng* (Stomach-Calming Poria Decoction) can harmonize the stomach, purge the turbid and drain dampness, while *Èr Miào Wán* (Two Mysterious Pill) can clear damp-heat in the lower *jiao*. *Liù Jūn Zǐ Tāng* (Six Gentlemen Decoction) can boost the spleen and qi. *Páo jiāng, huáng lián, wú zhū yú* and *bàn xià* are bitter and pungent, which can unblock and purge as well as harmonize the stomach. *Yín yáng huò* and *bā jĭ tiān* warm and boost the kidney. After the spleen qi is recuperated, it will be able to dispel dampness and raise the clear.

This formula can fortify the spleen and boost qi, warm the kidney, harmonize the stomach and purge turbidity to simultaneously treat the root and branch of the disease.

Chinese Patent Medicines: *Zhì Líng Jiāo Náng* (Elixir Capsule), taken 4 capsules, 3 times a day to treat chronic kidney qi deficiency syndrome.

Retention Enema with Herb Decoction: Decoct *dà huáng* 30 g, *mŭ lì* 30 g, and *huái huā* 30 g in water until 150-200 ml remains. Apply the decoction as an enema and retain it for 1-2 hours, 4-6 times a day. This therapy has the function of dredging the bowels, directing the turbid downward, and reducing the nitrogen content in the body.

Follow-up Consultations

After taking 2 months of the formula, the kidney function resumed to normal and laboratory test showed: BUN 6.02 mmol/L, UA 406 μmol/L, Cr 103 μmol/L, TC 5.01 mmol/L, TG 3.85 mmol/L and the blood pressure was 138/82 mmHg. The patient still suffered from uneasiness in the stomach, normal appetite, 2-3 loose stools a day, a slightly dark tongue with thin and yellow coating and thin and slippery pulse. The patient continued taking the same formula with modification for consolidation and the symptoms resolved.

CASE STUDY 3: Chronic General Edema
By Dr. Yang Yuan-de

Mr. Zhang, 21 years old.

Main Complaint: General edema for over a year.

Medical History: The patient suffered from nephritis caused by catching a cold 1 year ago. He received treatment which resolved the symptoms at the time. However, he contracted another external pathogens and the disease relapsed again.

Presenting Symptoms: General pitting edema especially in the lower limbs, scanty urine, loose stools, chest oppression, tasteless in the mouth and poor appetite.

Physical Examination: Urine test: protein (+++), casts (+), WBC (++), RBC (+).

Diagnosis

TCM Diagnosis: Edema due to spleen and kidney yang deficiency

Western Medicine Diagnosis: Edema

Treatment

Principles:

- Fortify the spleen and kidney yang
- Promote urination to drain dampness

Acupuncture Point Combinations:

Group A: RN 9 (*shuǐ fēn*), SP 6 (*sān yīn jiāo*), RN 4 (*guān yuán*), SP 9 (*yīn líng quán*) and SP 6 (*sān yīn jiāo*).

Group B: BL 17 (*gé shù*), BL 20 (*pí shù*), BL 23 (*shèn shù*), BL 32 (*cì liáo*), BL 39 (*wěi yáng*), ST 40 (*fēng lóng*), KI 3 (*tài xī*) and SP 3 (*tài bái*).

Manipulations: Apply acupuncture treatment of the two groups of points alternately. Retain the needles for 40-50 minutes while needling in synchronicity with the respiration for supplementation or even supplementation and drainage, once a day. 10 to 15 treatments is one course of treatment.

Follow-up Consultations

After one course of treatment, the urine volume increased and the edema resolved. The urine routine test showed: protein (+), casts (+−), WBC (+), RBC (−)

The acupuncture treatment continued up to 3 months and the edema and the other symptoms completely resolved while there were no abnormal findings in the urine test.

Notes

Many points can be selected to treat this disease, but the main ones are RN 9, SP 6, RN 4, SP 9, BL 20, BL 23, and KI 3. In this chronic case, the yang qi of the spleen and kidney is impaired causing a blockage of the water flow, distribution and discharge and the water to accumulate in the body manifesting as edema. The treatment is to boost the kidney and warm the spleen. SP 6 is the intersecting point of the three yin channels and a vital point for strengthening the body, which can be applied to treat various diseases caused by the liver, spleen, and kidney, as well as warm yang, activate the spleen, resolve dampness and promote urination. BL 23 serves to warm and boost kidney qi. When the kidney qi is sufficient, *san jiao* can resume its function and so can the bladder. If yang qi of the body is restored, fluids can be transformed. BL 20 and BL 23 together are to warm and boost the spleen and kidney, and dredge the qi of yang channels. RN 4 is to boost original qi, thus helpful to warm and boost the spleen and kidney. RN 9 raises the clear and directs the turbid downward which is a key point in treating edema. SP 6 regulates the qi of three foot yin channels, rectifies the spleen and kidney, and distributes fluids. SP 9 boosts the spleen and drains dampness. Blood converges in BL 17, so it functions to rectify blood and unblock collaterals. BL 23 also has functions of nourishing the liver and kidney, and unblocking the channel qi of the back. KI 3 is the *yuan*-source point of the kidney channel, which can regulate qi, blood, yin and yang of its own channel. All these points together have the effect of warming and boosting the spleen and kidney, promoting urination and expelling dampness.

CASE STUDY 4: Nephritis Edema
By Dr. Zhang Wei-shi

Mr. Li, 36 years old. 1st consultation on June 6th, 2007.

Main Complaint: General edema for a month.

Medical History: The patient was diagnosed with nephritis in August, 2005. At the time, he suddenly suffered from edema of the limbs and face with scanty urination. He was hospitalized twice. The first time, he was administrated prednisone, cyclophosphamide, Chinese medicinals, and so on until the symptoms resolved. However, this time he was hospitalized because the edema reoccured 1 month after the withdrawal of the prednisone.

Presenting Symptoms: General edema, scanty and turbid urine, poor appetite, bitter taste in the mouth, a red tongue with greasy coating and a deep and wiry pulse.

Physical Examination: Face and eyes edema (++), lower limbs edema (++), sign of ascites (+), abdomen circumference 75 cm, blood pressure: 108/82 mmHg. Urine routine test: protein (++), casts (+), WBC (+), pyocyte (++), UPQ 4.06 g/24 h. Serum: cholesterol 7.3 mmol/L, albumin 25 g/L, creatinine 170 mmol/L.

Diagnosis

TCM Diagnosis: Edema due to spleen and kidney yang deficiency

Western Medicine Diagnosis: Edema

Treatment

Principles:

- Fortify the spleen and boost qi
- Warm the kidney to drain dampness

Acupuncture Point Combination:

During the edema stage, apply moxibustion on the RN 9 (*shuǐ fēn*) and RN 6 (*qì hǎi*) to drain, and RN 4 (*guān yuán*) to tonify.

At the non-edema stage, apply nourishing moxibustion on the two groups of points alternately:

Group A: RN 6 (*qì hǎi*), RN 4 (*guān yuán*) and right GB 26 (*dài mài*).

Group B: Bilateral BL 23 (*shèn shù*) and left GB 26 (*dài mài*).

Manipulations: Cut fresh ginger into slices of about 0.1 cm in thickness and 0.8 cm in diameter. Prick 3 to 4 holes in the ginger slices and then place the slices on the selected points. Place some loose moxa onto the middle of the ginger slice and then burn the moxa until it is nearly completely burnt. Remove the moxa cone for drainage and cover with a box for a minute for supplementation. Burn 5 cones on each point, once every other day. One treatment course is 15 treatments and there should be a 5-day rest between two periods. After the moxibustion treatment, place sterilized gauzes with adhesive tape to avoid infections.

Notes

Nephrotic edema syndrome is due to kidney qi deficiency, pathogenic cold and stagnation, which should be treated by tonifying qi, warming cold, raising the sunken, and dispersing stagnation. RN 6 is able to rectify and boost qi, fortify the kidney and consolidate essence. It is a key point for treating all kinds of qi disorder and deficiency. Moxibustion on RN 6 by draining during the edema stage can rectify qi and move the water passageway, while applying the supplementing method during the non-edema stage can boost qi, consolidate essence and fortify the kidney. RN 4 is able to warm the kidney and consolidate essence, boost qi and restore yang. It is the intersecting point of the liver, spleen, kidney channels and *ren mai*. Applying the tonifying method on RN 4 can boost kidney and supplement deficiency.

During the edema stage, applying the drainage method on RN 9 is to strengthen the effect of expelling water, promoting urination and dispersing edema. Medical experts in history had proved that burning moxa cones on the RN 9 has the effect of warming and supplementing the spleen yang, transporting and transforming water dampness and promoting urination. During the non-edema stage, applying the supplementation method on BL 23 and GB 26 can boost healthy qi and supplement deficiency as well as restore kidney functions. The *Yellow Emperor's Inner Classic* (*Huáng Dì Nèi Jīng*, 黄帝内经) records: "For deficiency, supplement", "For cold, warm", and "For the sunken, raise". Moxibustion therapy can achieve curative effects in warming and unblocking channels and collaterals, promoting yang qi, dispelling pathogenic dampness and cold, raising the sunken qi, and invigorating visceral qi transformation functions.

KEY CLINICAL POINTS

Edema is a common disease and its pathological changes mainly lie in the lung, spleen and kidney that interact with each other. As the lung is the mother organ of the kidney, if the lung fails to diffuse and govern the descending function and regulate the waterways, the kidney will lose the function of opening and closing. Then, the body fluids flow into the muscle and skin layers manifesting as edema. The kidney governs water and the spleen manages transportation and transformation. If the spleen is too weak to transport and transform, the water dampness will stagnate and impair yang. If it is treated inappropriately, kidney yang will also be affected and become weak. In turn, weak kidney yang fails to warm the spleen yang which aggravates the edema.

As for the treatment of edema, there are three principles put forward by the *Basic*

Questions—Thick and Sweet Liquors Chapter (*Sù Wèn—Tāng Yè Láo Lǐ Lùn Piān*, 素问·汤液醪醴论篇): "drain prolonged stagnations, open the sweat ducts, and eliminate the bowels." The *Essentials from the Golden Cabinet—Treatment for Edema with Pathological Pulse* (*Jīn Guì Yào Lüè—Shuǐ Qì Bìng Mài Zhèng Bìng Zhì*, 金匮要略·水气病脉证并治) also records: "For edema below the waist, promote urination; for edema above the waist, promote sweating."

In recent years, some scholars based on the theory "Static blood transforms water retention and induces edema. There is a type of edema due to blood stasis and it is called blood edema." recorded in *Treatise on Blood Syndromes* (*Xuè Zhèng Lùn*, 血证论). In this case, it is appropriate to move blood and resolve stasis to improve the curative effect. For patients with high blood pressure due to blood stasis and vessel obstruction, curative effect can be favorable if medicinals that can fortify the spleen qi, invigorate blood and resolve stasis are applied.

In a complex pattern of both excess and deficiency, the focus should be on regulating the middle *jiao* and fortifying the spleen and stomach with formulas such as *Xiāng Shā Liù Jūn Zǐ Tāng* (Costusroot and Amomum Six Gentlemen Decoction), *Xuán Fù Dài Zhě Tāng* (Inula and Hematite Decoction), *Xīn Jiā Huáng Lóng Tāng* (Newly Supplemented Yellow Dragon Decoction) and *Xiǎo Chái Hú Tāng* (Minor Bupleurum Decoction).

For those with obvious kidney qi depletion, kidney boosting medicinals that warm without drying, supplementary without stagnating should be added, such as *xiān líng pí, tù sī zǐ, gǒu qǐ zǐ, chuān xù duàn, nǚ zhēn zǐ, hàn lián cǎo, bā jǐ tiān, sāng piāo xiāo* and *chén xiāng*. Furthermore, following points are worth noticing:

1. In cases of edema due to spleen and kidney yang deficiency, do not overuse yang warming medicinals to prevent harming yin. Medicinals like *gǒu qǐ zǐ, bái sháo* and *shú dì huáng* can be added to seek yang within yin.

2. In the course of edema, attention should be given to severe cases of anuresis, abdominal distension, nausea and vomiting since these patients are in a critical state and need special care. In patients having difficulty taking their medicine, an enema can be used to treat the symptoms. The decoction for enema can be made of *fù zǐ*, raw *dà huáng, mǔ lì, bái mǎ gǔ* and so on.

3. Be cautious when using medicinals with renal toxicity. Recent research shows that medicinals containing aristolochic acid, such as *mǎ dōu líng, guān mù tōng, mù fáng jǐ* and *yì mǔ cǎo* cause renal toxicity and should be refrained from using large dosage or for an extended period of time.

COMPREHENSION QUESTIONS

1. What is the diagnostic criteria of edema?

2. What are the etiology and pathomechanism of chronic renal insufficiency in Chinese medicine?

3. Multiple choice questions:

1) To treat edema, the *Inner Classic* (*Nèi Jīng*, 内经) records: "cleaning the bowels." What does this method refer to?

A. Heat clearing method
B. Sweat promotion
C. Dispersion method
D. Purgation method
E. Harmonization method

2) A patient has suffered from edema for a long time and presents with pitting edema below the waist, aversion to cold, cold limbs, scanty urine, a pale tongue with white and slippery coating, and a deep and weak pulse. What is the appropriate pattern?

A. Overflowing wind edema
B. Damp and toxin retention
C. Water and dampness retention
D. Damp-heat exuberance
E. Weak spleen yang

Answers

1. The clinical manifestations of edema initiating from the eyelids or lower limbs to four limbs and all the body. In a mild case, only the eyelids or tibial edema are present, while in a severe case, edema can present all over the body, with accompanied symptoms of abdominal distension and fullness, panting and inability to lie on the back. In critical cases, there will be anuresis, nausea, vomiting, halitosis, epistaxis, gingival atrophy, headache, spasms, coma, delirium, and so on.

2. Chronic kidney insufficiency has a long disease course and the pathomechanism is complicated with the consumption of healthy qi and obstruction due to pathogenic excess. It is a disease with a deficiency in the root and an excess in the branch. In addition, healthy qi deficiency contains deficiency of qi, blood, yin and yang, while pathogenic excess includes external pathogens of turbid dampness, toxic heat, static blood, stirring wind and phlegm accumulation. The disease locations are mainly in the lung, spleen and kidney. However, other organs such as the liver, heart and stomach are often affected.

The pathomechanism is mainly disorders of the lung, spleen and kidney, the failure of the *san jiao* to regulate the waterways, and the failure of the bladder to transform qi, bringing forth a fluid retention flooding the muscle and skin layers. The lung, spleen and kidney are interconnected. For example, depleted kidney yang fails to warm the spleen yang causing it to fail in transforming fluid manifesting as edema. In edema induced by external pathogens, the disease location often lies in the lung and spleen. In edema caused by internal injury, the disease location often resides in the spleen and kidney. Furthermore, it is important to notice that edema often becomes a chronic and difficult disease to treat, hence, we must always remember to move the static blood and unblock the *san jiao* waterways.

3. 1) C, 2) E.

5.2 Strangury

Strangury is clinically manifested by frequent, urgent, dribbling, difficult and painful urination. The pain before or during urination can radiate to the abdomen, waist and lower back with tightness and pain of the lower abdomen. This disease can present with an acute onset or a chronic course of disease. In some cases of chronic strangury, the symptoms vary in intensity or can come and go according to the level of fatigue and overwork, diet changes, mental or physical stress and so on. In Western medicine, strangury is very similar to some type of urinary tract infection and can be seen as a symptom with other diseases such as pyelonephritis, ureteritis, cystitis, urethritis and so on.

In Chinese medicine, the major etiology of strangury is the stagnation of damp-heat in excess cases and kidney deficiency in deficiency cases. It was recorded as early as in the *Treatise on the Origins and Manifestations of Various Diseases* (*Zhū Bìng Yuán Hòu Lùn*, 诸病源候论) that: "strangury is due to kidney deficiency and heat in the urinary bladder." In some cases there is a concurrent pattern of both excess and deficiency. This disease is located at the kidney and bladder, and it also has some relation to the liver and spleen. The pathomechanism is mainly failure of qi transformation due to kidney deficiency with an accumulation of damp-heat in the urinary bladder. As the kidney and bladder have an interior and exterior relationship, the strength of kidney qi can directly influence the qi transformation and opening of the bladder. If strangury is not cured for a long time, it can easily cause kidney deficiency where the pathogenic heat impairs the kidney yin and the pathogenic dampness injures the kidney yang. Similarly, prolonged kidney deficiency is vulnerable to the invasion of the pathogenic dampness, heat and toxin affecting the bladder causing intermittent relapse of strangury. This disease often begins as an excess pattern and with time, it can become a deficiency pattern.

CLINICAL PATTERNS DIFFERENTIATION AND TREATMENTS

1. Heat Strangury

Symptoms: Frequent and scanty dark yellow urine with a burning sensation and stabbing pain, cramping and distension of the lower abdomen radiating to the lower back, alternating fever and chills, dry throat, bitter taste in the mouth, nausea, vomiting, soreness of the lower back, constipation, a red tongue with a yellow and greasy coating and a slippery and rapid pulse.

Treatment Principle:

- Clear heat and drain dampness
- Promote urination and stop pain

Main Acupuncture Points:

- SP 6 (*sān yīn jiāo*): To invigorate spleen, liver and kidney, tonify yin and harmonize lower *jiao*
- SP 9 (*yīn líng quán*): To harmonize middle *jiao*, expel dampness and resolve edema
- BL 28 (*páng guāng shù*): Back-*shu* point of the bladder to tonify original qi, benefit essence, strengthen lumbus and lower limbs, regulate urination and lower *jiao*
- ST 28 (*shuǐ dào*): To regulate lower *jiao* qi and resolve constipation
- BL 22 (*sān jiāo shù*): To regulate *san jiao*, resolve dampness, regulate the fluid passageway, promote urination, benefit original qi, tonify the lumbar region and knees
- BL 39 (*wěi yáng*): Regulate *san jiao*, regulate urination, activate channel and alleviate pain
- LV 2 (*xíng jiān*): Clear liver fire, spread liver qi, pacify liver wind, relax the sinews, clear heat, calm spirit, cool blood and stop bleeding
- SJ 5 (*wài guān*): To release the exterior and clear heat
- LI 11 (*qū chí*): *He*-sea point of the large intestine to resolve stagnation, expel dampness, alleviate diarrhea and stop pain

Supporting Points:

- RN 3 (*zhōng jí*): Front-*mu* point of the bladder to dispel stagnation and harmonize the lower *jiao*, benefit the uterus and regulate menstruation
- ST 44 (*nèi tíng*): To clear toxic heat and dampness and regulate *yang ming* channels

Recommended Formula: *Bā Zhèng Sǎn* (八正散, Eight Corrections Powder) from the *Beneficial Formulas from the Taiping Imperial Pharmacy* (*Tài Píng Huì Mín Hé Jì Jú Fāng*, 太平惠民和剂局方)

Substitute Formula:

- *Dǎo Chì Sǎn* (导赤散, Red-Guiding Powder)
- *Sān Rén Tāng* (三仁汤, Three Kernels Decoction)

Patent Formula: *Niào Gǎn Níng Kē Lì* (尿感宁颗粒, Niao Gan Ning Granule)

2. Stone Strangury

Symptoms: Patient may experience excretion of sand or stones in the urine, hesitant, interrupted and painful urination, cramping or colic pain in the lower abdomen radiating to the lower back, possible blood in the urine, a red tongue with a thin, yellow coating and a wiry, slippery and rapid pulse.

Treatment Principle:

- Clear heat and drain dampness

- Remove stasis and expel stones

Main Acupuncture Points:

- SP 6 (*sān yīn jiāo*): To invigorate spleen, liver and kidney, tonify yin and harmonize lower *jiao*
- SP 9 (*yīn líng quán*): To harmonize middle *jiao*, expel dampness and resolve edema
- BL 28 (*páng guāng shù*): Back-*shu* point of the bladder to tonify original qi, benefit essence, strengthen lumbus and lower limbs, regulate urination and lower *jiao*
- BL 22 (*sān jiāo shù*): To regulate *san jiao* and resolve dampness, regulate the fluid passageway and promote urination, benefit original qi, tonify the lumbar region and knees
- BL 39 (*wěi yáng*): To regulate *sanjiao*, promote urination, activate channel and alleviate pain
- BL 54 (*zhì biān*): To treat hematuria and bloody stools

Supporting Points:

- RN 3 (*zhōng jí*): Front-*mu* point of the bladder to dispel stagnation and harmonize the lower *jiao*, benefit the uterus and regulate menstruation
- BL 23 (*shèn shù*): Back-*shu* point of the kidney to tonify kidney and fortify yang, supplement qi and strengthen lumbar region

Recommended Formula: *Shí Wěi Săn* (石苇散, Pyrrosia Powder) from the *Arcane Essentials from the Imperial Library* (*Wài Tái Mì Yào*, 外台秘要)

Substitute Formula: *Bā Zhèng Săn* (八正散, Eight Corrections Powder)

Patent Formula: *Pái Shí Kē Lì* (排石颗粒, Stone-Expelling Granule)

3. Blood Strangury

A. Excessive Syndrome

Symptoms: Urgent, hesitant, painful urination with a burning sensation, dark-red urine or blood clots in the urine, intense lower abdominal pain and fullness, restlessness, a red tongue with yellow coating and a slippery and rapid pulse.

Treatment Principle:

- Clear heat and cool blood
- Subdue pain and stop bleeding

Main Acupuncture Points:

- BL 28 (*páng guāng shù*): Back-*shu* point of the bladder to tonify original qi, benefit essence, strengthen lumbus and lower limbs, regulate urination and lower *jiao*
- ST 28 (*shuĭ dào*): To regulate lower *jiao* qi and resolve constipation
- BL 22 (*sān jiāo shù*): To regulate *san jiao* and resolve dampness, regulate the fluid passageway and promote urination, benefit original qi, tonify the lumbar region and knees
- BL 17 (*gé shù*): Influential point of the blood to promote blood circulation and

resolve stasis, harmonize blood and stop abdominal pain

- SP 10 (*xuè hǎi*): To promote blood flow, dispel stasis, invigorate the spleen and cool blood
- KI 2 (*rán gǔ*): To clear deficient fire

Supporting Points:

- ST 25 (*tiān shū*): Front-*mu* point of the large intestine to invigorate spleen and stomach, clear damp-heat and resolve dysentery
- LI 11 (*qū chí*): *He*-sea point of the large intestine to resolve stagnation, expel dampness, alleviate diarrhea and stop pain

Recommended Formula: *Xiǎo Jì Yǐn Zǐ* (小蓟饮子, Field Thistle Decoction) from the *Revised Yan's Prescriptions for Rescuing Lives* (*Chóng Dìng Yán Shì Jì Shēng Fāng* , 重订严氏济生方)

Substitute Formula: *Sān Rén Tāng* (三仁汤, Three Kernels Decoction)

Patent Formula:

- *Fù Fāng Jīn Qián Cǎo Chōng Jì* (复方金钱草冲剂, Compound Herba Lysimachiae Granule)
- *Fù Fāng Huáng Lián Sù Piàn* (复方黄连素片, Compound Berberine Tablet)

B. Deficiency Syndrome

Symptoms: Light-red blood in the urine, slight hesitancy and pain during urination, lower back soreness, fatigue and lassitude, a red tongue with scanty coating and a thready and rapid pulse.

Treatment Principle:

- Nourish kidney yin and qi
- Clear heat and stop bleeding

Main Acupuncture Points:

- BL 28 (*páng guāng shù*): Back-*shu* point of the bladder to tonify original qi, benefit essence, strengthen lumbus and lower limbs, regulate urination and lower *jiao*
- SP 6 (*sān yīn jiāo*): To invigorate spleen, liver and kidney, tonify yin and harmonize lower *jiao*
- SP 9 (*yīn líng quán*): To harmonize middle *jiao*, expel dampness and resolve edema
- KI 5 (*shuǐ quán*): *Xi*-cleft point of the kidney to regulate *chong* and *ren* vessels and treat dysuria
- BL 22 (*sān jiāo shù*): To regulate *san jiao,* resolve dampness, regulate the fluid passageway, promote urination, benefit original qi, and tonify the lumbar region and knees
- BL 17 (*gé shù*): Influential point of the blood to promote blood circulation and resolve stasis, harmonize blood and stop abdominal pain
- BL 20 (*pí shù*): Back-*shu* point of the spleen to invigorate the spleen and resolve dampness

Supporting Points:

- SP 10 (*xuè hǎi*): To promote blood flow and dispel stasis, invigorate the spleen, resolve dampness and cool blood
- SP 1 (*yǐn bái*): To benefit qi and stop bleeding, invigorate the spleen, calm the spirit and restore consciousness

Recommended Formula: *Zhī Bǎi Dì Huáng Tāng* (知柏地黄汤, Anemarrhena-Phellodendron-Rehmannia Decoction) from the *Golden Mirror of the Medical Tradition* (*Yī Zōng Jīn Jiàn*, 医宗金鉴)

Substitute Formula: *Liù Wèi Dì Huáng Wán* (六味地黄丸, Six Ingredients Rehmannia Pill) combined with *Èr Miào Sǎn* (二妙散, Two Mysterious Powder)

Patent Formula: *Zhī Bǎi Dì Huáng Wán* (知柏地黄丸, Anemarrhena, Phellodendron and Rehmannia Pill)

4. Qi Stagnation Strangury

A. Excessive Syndrome

Symptoms: Hesitant, dribbling urination, fullness and distending pain in the rib-side and lower abdomen, a thin and white tongue coating and a deep and wiry pulse.

Treatment Principle:

- Regulate qi and relieve stagnation
- Promote urination and stop pain

Main Acupuncture Points:

- SP 6 (*sān yīn jiāo*): To invigorate spleen, liver and kidney, tonify yin and harmonize lower *jiao*
- BL 18 (*gān shù*): Back-*shu* point of the liver to spread liver qi, clear liver and gallbladder heat, unbind the chest and promote circulation
- SP 9 (*yīn líng quán*): To harmonize middle *jiao*, expel dampness and resolve edema
- BL 28 (*páng guāng shù*): Back-*shu* point of the bladder to tonify original qi, benefit essence, strengthen lumbus and lower limbs, regulate urination and lower *jiao*
- ST 28 (*shuǐ dào*): To regulate lower *jiao* qi and resolve constipation
- LV 3 (*tài chōng*): *Yuan*-source point of the liver to relieve chest congestion and irritability

Supporting Points:

- LV 14 (*qī mén*): Front-*mu* point of the liver to spread liver qi, harmonize liver and stomach
- ST 25 (*tiān shū*): Front-*mu* point of the large intestine to invigorate spleen and stomach, clear damp-heat and resolve dysentery

Recommended formula: *Chén Xiāng Sǎn* (沉香散, Aquilaria Powder) from the *Appendices of the 'Essentials from the Golden Cabinet'* (*Jīn Guì Yì*, 金匮翼)

Substitute Formula:

- *Chái Hú Shū Gān Săn* (柴胡疏肝散, Bupleurum Liver-Soothing Powder)
- *Xiāo Yáo Săn* (逍遥散, Free Wanderer Powder)

Patent Formula: *Xiāo Yáo Wán* (逍遥丸, Free Wanderer Pill)

B. Deficiency Syndrome

Symptoms: Dribbling urination with a heaviness and distension in the lower abdomen, fatigue, poor appetite, pale complexion, a pale tongue and a weak pulse.

Treatment Principle:

- Strengthen the spleen and supplement qi
- Promote urination and stop pain

Main Acupuncture Points:

- BL 28 (*páng guāng shù*): Back-*shu* point of the bladder to tonify original qi, benefit essence, strengthen lumbus and lower limbs, regulate urination and lower *jiao*
- ST 28 (*shuĭ dào*): To regulate lower *jiao* qi and resolve constipation
- BL 22 (*sān jiāo shù*): To regulate *san jiao,* resolve dampness, promote urination, benefit original qi, tonify the lumbar region and knees
- SP 6 (*sān yīn jiāo*): To invigorate spleen, liver and kidney, tonify yin and harmonize lower *jiao*
- SP 9 (*yīn líng quán*): To harmonize middle *jiao*, expel dampness and resolve edema
- BL 23 (*shèn shù*): Back-*shu* point of the kidney to benefit the original qi and kidney yin
- BL 26 (*guān yuán shù*): Tonify original qi and benefit essence, regulate the lower *jiao*, strengthen the lumbar region
- KI 3 (*tài xī*): *Yuan*-source point of kidney to tonify spleen and kidney yin, clear deficient heat and resolve hemoptysis
- KI 13 (*qì xué*): To tonify kidney, benefit essence and regulate the uterus
- ST 36 (*zú sān lĭ*): To tonify spleen, support the correct qi and tonify deficiency

Supporting Points:

- SP 4 (*gōng sūn*): To invigorate spleen, harmonize middle *jiao* and regulate qi
- BL 20 (*pí shù*): Back-*shu* point of the spleen to regulate middle *jiao* qi, invigorate spleen, alleviate diarrhea and stop abdominal pain

Recommended Formula: *Bŭ Zhōng Yì Qì Tāng* (补中益气汤, Center-Supplementing and Qi-Boosting Decoction) from the *Treatise on the Spleen and Stomach* (*Pí Wèi Lùn*, 脾胃论)

Substitute Formula: *Guī Pí Tāng* (归脾汤, Spleen-Restoring Decoction)

Patent Formula: *Bŭ Zhōng Yì Qì Wán* (补中益气丸, Center-Supplementing and Qi-Boosting Pill)

5. Strangury with Chyluria

A. Excessive Syndrome

Symptoms: Turbid, milk-like, oily urination containing clots or blood, coupled with hesitancy and burning sensation, a red tongue with a yellow, greasy coating and a slippery and rapid pulse.

Treatment Principle:

- Clear heat and drain dampness
- Separate clear from the turbidity
- Promote urination and stop pain

Main Acupuncture Points:

- BL 22 (*sān jiāo shù*): To regulate *san jiao,* resolve dampness, regulate the fluid passage way and promote urination, benefit original qi, tonify the lumbar region and knees
- BL 28 (*páng guāng she*): Back-*shu* point of the bladder to tonify original qi, benefit essence, strengthen lumbus and lower limbs, regulate urination and lower *jiao*
- ST 28 (*shuĭ dào*): To regulate lower *jiao* qi and resolve constipation
- SP 9 (*yīn líng quán*): To harmonize middle *jiao*, expel dampness and resolve edema
- ST 40 (*fēng lóng*): To expel phlegm and dampness
- KI 6 (*zhào hăi*): To clear deficient fire and regulate yin motility vessel

Supporting Points:

- LI 11 (*qū chí*): *He*-sea point of the large intestine to resolve stagnation, expel dampness, alleviate diarrhea and stop pain
- GB 44 (*zú qiào yīn*): Clear heat and pacify wind, calm the spirit and alleviate pain

Recommended Formula: *Bì Xiè Fēn Qīng Yĭn* (萆薢分清饮, Hypoglaucae Root Turbidity-Clearing Beverage) from the *Medical Revelations* (*Yī Xué Xīn Wù*, 医学心悟)

Substitute Formula: *Bā Zhèng Săn* (八正散, Eight Corrections Powder)

Patent Formula: *Bì Xiè Fēn Qīng Wán* (萆薢分清丸, Hypoglaucae Root Turbidity-Clearing Pill)

B. Deficiency Syndrome

Symptoms: Chronic oily urine with mild hesitancy and pain, gradual weight loss, dizziness, fatigue and lower back soreness, pale tongue with a greasy coating and a thready and weak pulse.

Treatment Principle:

- Stabilize the kidney
- Restrain the essence

Main Acupuncture Points:

- BL 28 (*páng guāng shù*): Back-*shu* point of the bladder to tonify original qi, benefit essence, strengthen lumbus and lower limbs, regulate urination and lower *jiao*

- ST 28 (*shuǐ dào*): To regulate lower *jiao* qi and resolve constipation
- BL 22 (*sān jiāo shù*): To regulate *san jiao,* resolve dampness, regulate the fluid passageway and promote urination, benefit original qi, tonify the lumbar region and knees
- SP 6 (*sān yīn jiāo*): To invigorate spleen, liver and kidney, tonify yin and harmonize lower *jiao*
- BL 23 (*shèn shù*): Back-*shu* point of the kidney to benefit the original qi and kidney yin
- ST 36 (*zú sān lǐ*): To tonify spleen, support the correct qi and tonify deficiency

Supporting Points:

- KI 3 (*tài xī*): *Yuan*-source point of kidney to tonify kidney yin, clear deficient fire and invigorate spleen
- RN 6 (*qì hǎi*): To support the original qi, tonify kidney and treat general weakness

Recommended Formula: *Gāo Lín Tāng* (膏淋汤, Unctuous Strangury Decoction) from the *Records of Chinese Medicine with Reference to Western Medicine* (*Yī Xué Zhōng Zhōng Cān Xī Lù*, 医学衷中参西录)

Substitute Formula: *Zhī Bǎi Dì Huáng Tāng* (知柏地黄汤, Anemarrhena-Phellodendron-Rehmannia Decoction)

Patent Formula: *Zhī Bǎi Dì Huáng Wán* (知柏地黄丸, Anemarrhena-Phellodendron-Rehmannia Pill)

6. Strangury due to Overstrain

Symptoms: Chronic, intermittent dribbling urination that worsens with exertion, lower back soreness, knee weakness, lassitude and fatigue, a pale tongue and a weak pulse.

Treatment Principle:

- Strengthen the spleen
- Tonify the kidney

Main Acupuncture Points:

- BL 28 (*páng guāng shù*): Back-*shu* point of the bladder to tonify original qi, benefit essence, strengthen lumbus and lower limbs, regulate urination and lower *jiao*
- ST 28 (*shuǐ dào*): To regulate lower *jiao* qi and resolve constipation
- BL 22 (*sān jiāo shù*): To regulate *san jiao,* resolve dampness, regulate the fluid passageway and promote urination, benefit original qi, tonify the lumbar region and knees
- ST 36 (*zú sān lǐ*): To tonify spleen, support the correct qi and tonify deficiency
- BL 23 (*shèn shù*): Back-*shu* point of the kidney to benefit the original qi and kidney yin
- BL 24 (*qì hǎi shù*): Tonify kidney and fortify yang, tonify the lumbar region and

lower limbs, regulate the blood and qi

- KI 3 (*tài xī*): *Yuan*-source point of kidney to tonify kidney yin, clear deficient fire and invigorate spleen

Supporting Points:

- BL 20 (*pí shù*): Back-*shu* point of the spleen to regulate middle *jiao* qi, invigorate spleen, alleviate diarrhea and stop abdominal pain
- SP 4 (*gōng sūn*): To invigorate spleen, harmonize middle *jiao* and regulate qi

Recommended Formula: *Wú Bĭ Shān Yào Wán* (无比山药丸, Matchless Dioscorea Pill) from the *Important Formulas Worth a Thousand Gold Pieces for Emergency* (*Bèi Jí Qiān Jīn Yào Fāng*, 备急千金要方)

Substitute Formula: *Yòu Guī Wán* (右归丸, Right-Restoring Pill)

Patent Formula: *Jì Shēng Shèn Qì Wán* (济生肾气丸, Life-Saving Kidney Qi Pill)

Summary Chart for Strangury

Patterns	Main Points	Supporting Points	Formulae
Heat Strangury	SP 6, SP 9, BL 28 ST 28, BL 22 BL 39 , LV 2, SJ 5 LI 11	RN 3 for dispelling stagnation and promoting urination ST 44 for clearing toxic heat and draining dampness	*Bā Zhèng Săn* or *Dăo Chì Săn* or *Sān Rén Tāng*
Stone Strangury	SP 6, SP 9, BL 28 BL 22, BL39, BL 54	RN 3 for dispelling stagnation and promoting urination BL 23 for fortifying the kidney and regulating qi	*Shí Wěi Săn* or *Bā Zhèng Săn*
Excessive Blood Strangury	BL 28, ST 28 BL 22, BL 17, SP 10 KI 2	ST 25 for removing stagnation and clearing damp heat LI 11 for clearing heat and expelling stagnation	*Xiăo Jì Yĭn Zĭ* or *Sān Rén Tāng*
Deficiency Blood Strangury	BL 28, SP 6, SP 9 KI 5, BL 22, BL 17 BL 20	SP 10 for nourishing and cooling blood SP 1 for stopping bleeding and fortifying the spleen qi	*Zhī Băi Dì Huáng Tāng* or *Liù Wèi Dì Huáng Wán* plus *Èr Miào Săn*
Excessive Qi Stagnation Strangury	SP 6, BL 18, SP 9 BL 28, ST 28, LV 3	LV 14 for regulating liver qi and treating rib side pain ST 25 for removing stagnation and clearing damp heat	*Chén Xiāng Săn* or *Chái Hú Shū Gān Săn* or *Xiāo Yáo Săn*
Deficiency Qi Stagnation Strangury	BL 28, ST 28, BL 22 SP 6, SP 9, BL 23 BL 26, KI 3, KI 13 ST 36	SP 4 for tonifying spleen qi and regulating the water BL 20 for strengthening the spleen qi	*Bŭ Zhōng Yì Qì Tāng* or *Guī Pí Tāng*
Excessive Strangury with Chyluria	BL 22, BL 28 ST 28, SP 9, ST 40 KI 6	LI 11 for clearing heat and resolving stagnation GB 44 for clearing heat and calming the spirit	*Bì Xiè Fēn Qīng Yĭn* or *Bā Zhèng Săn*

Continued

Patterns	Main Points	Supporting Points	Formulae
Deficiency Strangury with Chyluria	BL 28, ST 28 BL 22, SP 6, BL 23 ST 36	KI 3 for tonifying kidney qi and clearing empty fire RN 6 for supporting original qi and treating general weakness	*Gāo Lín Tāng* or *Zhī Bǎi Dì Huáng Tāng*
Strangury due to Overstrain	BL 28, ST 28 BL 22, ST 36 BL 23, BL 24 KI 3	BL 20 for strengthening the spleen qi SP 4 for tonifying spleen qi and regulating the water	*Wú Bǐ Shān Yào Wán* or *Yòu Guī Wán*

CASE STUDY 1: Acute Strangury

Ms. Jiao, 41 years old.

Main Complaint: Frequent, urgent and painful urination with blood for a day.

Medical History: The patient suffered from aversion to cold and fever with frequent, urgent and painful urination after having bath and washing clothes at 2 o'clock in the afternoon the day prior. She had the urge to urinate with interruption every 10 minutes and there were streaks of blood in the urine.

Presenting Symptoms: Aversion to cold, no sweating, vexation, bitter taste in the mouth, belching, poor appetite, vomiting of a scant amount of bitter liquid in the morning, heaviness in the lower abdomen, frequent urination once every half hour, urgent and bloody urination, painful and cutting like feeling upon urination, a pale tongue with a white greasy coating and a wiry and rapid pulse.

Physical Examination: Temperature: 38.2 ℃, pulse: 96 bpm, respiration: 24 bpm, blood pressure: 118/78 mmHg. Urine routine test: WBC 9360, neutrophil 82; protein (+), RBC (+++).

Pattern Differentiation

Strangury is the result of kidney deficiency and heat in the urinary bladder. The kidney and bladder are interiorly and exteriorly related, both of which are in charge of water management. It is recorded in the classical medical texts: "Kidney deficiency results in frequent urination and heat in the urinary bladder produces difficult urination. Urination that is frequent and difficult is seen as dribbling and inhibited." This patient had urgent, frequent, painful and bloody urine which implies it is a case of "extreme heat retention causing blood strangury". This patient had an excess retention of dampness in the body which made her prone to contract exterior pathogenic dampness which transformed into heat and moved into the blood layer causing blood stangury.

Diagnosis

TCM Diagnosis: Stangury due to damp-heat retention and blood stasis
Western Medicine Diagnosis: Acute urinary track infection

Treatment

Principles:

- Harmonize *shao yang* and soothe *san jiao*
- Clear heat and remove dampness
- Promote urination and stop bleeding

Formula: Modified *Xiǎo Chái Hú Tāng* (Minor Bupleurum Decoction) combined with *Wŭ Líng Săn* (Five Substances Powder with Poria).

Ingredients:

柴胡	*chái hú*	30 g	Radix Bupleuri
黄芩	*huáng qín*	12 g	Radix Scutellariae
法半夏	*fă bàn xià*	10 g	Rhizoma Pinelliae Praeparatum
猪苓	*zhū líng*	12 g	Polyporus
茯苓	*fú líng*	12 g	Poria
泽泻	*zé xiè*	15 g	Rhizoma Alismatis
滑石	*huá shí*	25 g	Talcum
甘草	*gān căo*	3 g	Radix et Rhizoma Glycyrrhizae
银花藤	*yín huā téng*	30 g	Caulis Lonicerae
车前草	*chē qián căo*	30 g	Herba Plantaginis
白茅根	*bái máo gēn*	30 g	Rhizoma Imperatae
黄连	*huáng lián*	3 g	Rhizoma Coptidis
黄柏	*huáng băi*	12 g	Cortex Phellodendri Chinensis

Formula Analysis

This formula is modified according to Zhang Zhong-jing's *Xiăo Chái Hú Tāng* to soothe qi movement and harmonize *shao yang* together with *Wŭ Líng Săn* to drain dampness by fortifying the spleen and moving water by transforming qi.

In this formula, *chái hú*, bitter and neutral can soothe qi movement and disperse pathogenic heat harassing *shao yang* and *san jiao*, while *huáng qín* is accompanied to clear and discharge heat constraint. *Fă bàn xià* checks adverse flow of qi and stops vomiting. *Gān căo* clears heat, harmonizes the middle and is able to disperse pathogenic factors outside from the skin and sweat pores. *Fú líng*, *zhū líng* and *zé xiè* can transform qi, eliminate dampness, and promote urination, which are further accompanied with sweet and cold *chē qián căo* for assisting percolating dampness, purging heat, and promoting urination. *Yín huā téng* clears heat, purges fire and removes toxins. *Bái máo gēn* cools, promotes urination and stops bleeding. *Huá shí* and *gān cǎo* implify the functions of *Liù Yī Sǎn* (Six-to-One Powder). With the property of bland, cold and heavy, *huá shí* can drain dampness, clear heat, purge fire, descend and benefit urethra.

Chinese Patent Medicines:

1) *Zhī Bǎi Dì Huáng Wán* (Anemarrhena, Phellodendron and Rehmannia Pill)

The basis of *Zhī Bǎi Dì Huáng Wán* (Anemarrhena, Phellodendron and Rehmannia Pill) is the well known *Liù Wèi Dì Huáng Wán* (Six-Ingredient Rehmannia Pill) with the addition of *zhī mǔ* and *huáng bǎi*. *Zhī mǔ* and *huáng bǎi* are added to strengthen the effect of nourishing kidney yin and clearing pathogenic fire. It is usually effective to treat stangury due to excessive pathogenic fire with yin deficiency such as in cases of blood strangury. It is often combined with *Èr Zhì Wán* (Double Supreme Pill), which consists of *nǚ zhēn zǐ* and *hàn lián cǎo*. Take 6 g in honey pill form, 9 g in small honey pill form, and 1 pill in big honey pill form, twice a day.

2) *Niào Gǎn Níng Chōng Jì* (Peaceful Pee Soluble Granules)

This formula can clear heat, remove toxins, relieve strangury and promote urination. It is indicated for frequent, urgent and painful urination in acute urinary tract infection, acute cystitis, acute pyelonephritis, chronic cystitis, and chronic pyelonephritis. Infuse 15 g with water, 3 to 4 times a day.

Follow-up Consultations

After 3 days of taking the formula, the body temperature was 36.8 ℃ and urination was normal but the appetite was poor. Based on the previous formula, *huáng lián* and *huáng bǎi* were removed, while *nán shā shēn* 25 g and dry-fried *gǔ yá* 12 g and *mài yá* 12 g were added to resume stomach qi for improving appetite. After one month in the hospital, she was in good spirit, and appetite and urine were normal. Urine test confirmed there were no abnormalities. The formula was substituted by patent formula *Zhī Bǎi Dì Huáng Tāng* (Anemarrhena, Phellodendron and Rehmannia Decoction) for 5 days until she was discharged from the hospital. After her discharge, she was asked to take 9 g of *Zhī Bǎi Dì Huáng Wán* in the morning and 9 g of *Bǔ Zhōng Yì Qì Wán* (Center-Supplementing and Qi-Boosting Decoction) in the evening. There was no relapse in one-year follow-up visits.

CASE STUDY2: Acute Strangury
By Dr. Zhang Ou & Han Hong

Ms. Liu, 50 years old.

Main Complaint: Frequent, urgent and painful urination for a week with aggravation for two days.

Medical History: The patient felt pulling pain, distension and fullness in the lower abdomen which was followed by frequent urination up to 20 times a day. The symptoms were relieved a little after she took erythrocin. In recent 2 days, the symptoms were aggravated and she felt burning pain in the external opening of urinary tract.

Presenting Symptoms: Lumbago, painful, burning and urgent urination and fever.

Urine routine test: RBC (++), WBC (++), pyocyte (++).

Diagnosis

TCM Diagnosis: Strangury due to heat retention

Western Medicine Diagnosis: Acute urinary track infection

Treatment

Principles:

- Unblock qi and soothe *san jiao*
- Clear heat and promote urination

Acupuncture Point Combination: RN 5 (*shí mén*)

Manipulations: Insert a 2 *cùn* long needle quickly into RN 5 with a depth of 1.5 *cùn*. The needling sensation should radiate to the external genitalia. If there is no needling sensation, lift the needle to the subcutaneous area and insert the needle again by changing the needling direction. Retain the needle for 20 minutes and treat once a day.

Follow-up Consultations

After one treatment, the symptoms of pulling pain, urgent and frequent urination were relieved and she urinated 10 times that day. All the symptoms were resolved after 5 treatments of the same method. The patient continued 5 more treatments to consolidate the treatment.

Notes

Acupuncture can be effective in the treatment of acute strangury to relieve pain and treat the syndrome especially in the acute phase. RN 5 is the key point of lower abdomen and the front-*mu* point of the *san jiao* which is responsible to regulate the waterways. Therefore, needling RN 5 can relieve strangury and soothe qi movement of the *san jiao*. Remember to advise your patient to empty the bladder before the acupuncture treatment.

KEY CLINICAL POINTS

1. In Urgent Conditions, Treat the Branch; in Moderate Conditions, Treat the Root.

When treating strangury with complex patterns, we need to evaluate if it is an urgent case or not. In the case where the pain is very severe with danger to the patient's life, we will need to treat the branch by expelling the pathogenic factors to stop the pain. In more moderate cases or with recurring cases of strangury with mild symptoms, we need to treat the root of the pattern and tonify deficiency to prevent the syndrome from manifesting again. Also it is important to remember that after clearing damp-heat in an acute case, it is important to reinforce healthy qi.

2. Avoid Promoting Sweating and Supplementing.

It is recorded in ancient medical texts that the treatment of promoting sweating and supplementing should be avoided in the syndrome of strangury. For example, *Essentials from the Golden Cabinet-Wasting-thirst, Inhibited Urine and Strangury Chapter* (*Jīn Guì Yào Lüè-Xiāo Kě Xiǎo Biàn Bú Lì Lín Bìng Piān*, 金匮要略・消渴小便不利淋病篇) records: "Do not apply sweating for strangury." *Teachings of [Zhu] Dan-xi-Strangury* (*Dān Xī Xīn Fǎ-Lín*, 丹溪心法・淋) states: "The last treatment approach to be used is qi reinforcing, as by supplementating the qi, it will cause more distending and heat." However, it is not necessarily true in every clinical case.

Strangury often comes with fever, but it is not due to attack of exogenous pathogens. It is the result of damp-heat steaming and the binding of the pathogen and healthy qi. In these cases, to promote sweating is certainly inappropriate. Strangury usually lies in heat in the bladder with the depletion of the body fluid, hence applying sweat promoting medicinals would further deplete the body fluids and aggravate the symptoms. However, if the strangury syndrome is induced by external contraction of pathogens in the exterior layer with aversion to cold or wind and heat sensation, then we can promote the sweat and release the exterior to remove the pathogen from the exterior layer.

Applying the supplementing or tonifying approach in strangury in the pattern of excessive heat or excessive dampness would only increase the pressure and aggravate the symptoms. It is best to remove the pathogens by clearing heat and draining dampness and only when the pathogens are resolved, can we supplement the kidney qi and essence and fortify the spleen qi.

3. Treating Stone Strangury

When treating stone strangury, use medicinals that can promote urination, relieve strangury and eliminate stones. Some clinical studies show that medicinals such as *chuān shān jiǎ, wáng bù liú xíng, dāng guī* and *táo rén* can soften stones and *dà huáng, chuān xiōng* and *niú xī* can promote the peristalsis of the urethra and the discharge of stones. Therefore, for patients with chronic or acute stone strangury, we can add qi rectifying, blood invigorating and stasis resolving medicinals on the basis of *Shí Wěi Tāng* (Talcum and Phragmites Powder).

COMPREHENSION QUESTIONS

1. How can we differentiate blood in the urine and blood strangury?
2. How do we different the types of strangury and treatment principles?
3. Multiple choice questions:

1) The optimal formula for blood strangury of deficiency pattern is:

A. *Xiǎo Jì Yǐn Zǐ* (Field Thistle Drink)

B. *Zhī Bǎi Dì Huáng Wán* (Anemarrhena, Phellodendron and Rehmannia Pill)

C. *Dǎo Chì Sǎn* (Red-Guiding Powder)

D. *Qiàn Gēn Sǎn* (Madder Root Powder)

E. *Èr Zhì Wán* (Double Supreme Pill)

2) The Chinese medical classical text stating that "Strangury is due to kidney deficiency and heat in the urinary bladder" is:

A. *Nèi Jīng* (*Inner Classic*)

B. *Jīn Guì Yào Lüè* (*Essentials from the Golden Cabinet*)

C. *Zhōng Zàng Jīng* (*Central Treasury Classic*)

D. *Zhū Bìng Yuán Hòu Lùn* (*Treatise on the Origins and Manifestations of Various Diseases*)

E. *Bèi Jí Qiān Jīn Yào Fāng* (*Important Formulas Worth a Thousand Gold Pieces for Emergency*)

Answers

1. Bloody urine and blood strangury both have the main symptom of having blood in the urine manifesting as red colored urine of light or darker colours. The key characteristic to differentiate them is the presence or absence of pain during urination. Bloody urine often has no manifestation of pain, though mild distending pain may be experienced in bloody urine; while the level of pain in blood strangury is much more severe.

2. There are three steps to treat strangury on the basis of pattern differentiation:

1) Differentiate the categories of strangury.

There are six types of strangury which have different pathological mechanisms and manifesting symptoms. It is important to distinguish which type of strangury is presenting to be able to treat it accordingly. Heat strangury has an acute onset with symptoms of fever, burning, painful, frequent and scanty urination. Stony strangury has the presence of small or sand like pebbles in the urine causing severe pain during urination or causing sudden interruption of urine flow and colic pain in the waist and abdomen due to the blockage in ureter and kidney. Qi strangury manifests as obvious abdominal distension, difficult, painful urination, and dribbling after urination. Blood strangury manifests as having traces of blood or blood clots in the urine accompanied by severe pain. Chylous strangury manifests as turbid and cloudy urine or slippery and greasy urine. The feature of strangury due to overstrain is chronic or recurring strangury with dribbling after urination which relapses due to overstrain.

2) Differentiate excess and deficiency patterns.

Once the appropriate type of strangury is identified, we must recognize if it is an excess or deficiency pattern on basis of its manifestations. Generally speaking, excess patterns have an acute onset with severe symptoms and are usually caused by damp-heat in the bladder, stone accumulation, and qi stagnation. Deficient patterns often have a chronic course of disease with recurring symptoms of mild pain during urination and are usually due to kidney and spleen qi deficiency. Qi strangury, blood strangury, and chylous strangury all have patterns of deficiency, excess and combination of excess and deficiency.

3) Differentiate the urgency of the root and branch.

Different types of the strangury can co-exist and transform into each other, so we should differentiate the urgency of the symptoms in pattern differentiation. The general guideline for determining the root or the branch needs to be the priority in the treatment principle of strangury. When the symptom of pain is severe and the patient's life is threatened as in stone strangury, the branch is more important to treat immediately. When the symptoms are acute and the pathogenic factors are more severe with a strong healthy qi or a strong root, the treatment will also be removing the pathogenic factors first and once they have resolved, the treatment will change to nourish the healthy qi. In cases where there are no pathogenic factors and the symptoms are mild due to a deficiency, the treatment will automatically fortify the root to reinstate the function of the kidney and spleen.

3. 1) B, 2) D.

5.3 Dementia

Dementia is caused by declined brain marrow mass causing the dysfunction of mental activities such as lack of short and long term memory as well as primary bodily functions. In mild cases, there are symptoms such as indifferent facial expression, reluctance to speak, slow reactions and forgetfulness. In serious cases, the manifestations are saying nothing at all, staying alone at home, muttering nonsense, or acting abnormally with sudden weeping and laughing, no appetite or food intake for several days.

In Chinese medicine, the syndrome of dementia mainly results from internal injury due to qi stagnation and blood stasis clouding the clear orifices, or prolonged illness causing blood deficiency and brain marrow depletion, or kidney essence deficiency gradually resulting in brain marrow depletion and malnourishment. The basic pathogenesis of dementia is the decline of marrow and brain mass causing the dysfunction of mental activities. The location of this syndrome is in brain and it is closely related to the dysfunction of the heart, liver, spleen and kidney. The syndrome is characterized by qi, blood and kidney essence deficiency as the root with excess pathogens of turbid phlegm and static blood as the root. The commonly encountered syndrome in clinic is the deficiency and excess complex syndrome. This syndrome is commonly seen in diseases such as senile dementia, vascular dementia, mixed dementia, brain atrophy, hydrocephalus with normal brain pressure, cerebral amyloid angiopathy (CAA), metabolic encephalopathy and toxic encephalopathy.

CLINICAL PATTERNS DIFFERENTIATION AND TREATMENTS

1. Qi Stagnation and Blood Stasis

Symptoms: Dull expression, slow reactions, inhibited speech, forgetfulness, timidity, chest stuffiness, frequent sighing, distending epigastric pain, belching, rough and scaly skin, dark complexion, dry mouth with no desire to drink, a dark tongue with ecchymosis or purpuras with a thin white coating and a wiry and thin pulse.

Treatment Principle:

- Promote blood circulation to resolve stasis
- Open the orifices and awaken the mind

Main Acupuncture Points:

- DU 20 (*bǎi huì*): To open the orifices, awaken the mind, calm the spirit and nourish the sea of marrow

- EX-HN 1 (*sì shén cōng*): To benefit the brain, calm the spirit and awaken the mind
- GB 12 (*wán gǔ*): Main point for treating mental disorders
- ST 36 (*zú sān lǐ*): To promote qi and blood circulation
- BL 17 (*gé shù*): Influential point of the blood to activate blood circulation, dispel stasis and unbind the chest
- SP 10 (*xuè hǎi*): To promote blood flow and dispel blood stasis and calm the spirit

Supporting Points:

- LV 14 (*qī mén*): Front-*mu* point of the spleen to spread liver and regulate qi, harmonize liver and spleen
- RN 17 (*dàn zhōng*): Front-*mu* point of the pericardium and sea of qi to promote pectoral qi and blood circulation and unbind the chest

Recommended Formula: *Tōng Qiào Huó Xuè Tāng* (通窍活血汤, Orifice-Soothing Blood-Activating Decoction) from the *Correction of Errors in Medical Works* (*Yī Lín Gǎi Cuò*, 医林改错)

Substitute Formula: *Xuè Fǔ Zhú Yū Tāng* (血府逐瘀汤, Blood Stasis Expelling Decoction)

Patent Formula: *Xuè Fǔ Zhú Yū Wán* (血府逐瘀丸, Blood Stasis Expelling Pill)

2. Turbid Phlegm Heat Obstructing Orifices

Symptoms: Red face and eyes, sudden violent anger, staring angrily without speaking, erratic movement and language, paranoia, insomnia, depression, epigastric and abdominal fullness and distension, self inflicted harm, constipation, turbid urine, a thick yellow greasy tongue coating and a deep and slippery or rapid and forceful pulse.

Treatment Principle:

- Strengthen spleen and expel phlegm
- Soothe the liver and regulate qi
- Open the orifices and move the stools

Main Acupuncture Points:

- LV 3 (*tài chōng*): *Yuan*-source point of the liver to spread liver qi, clear heat, promote circulation, soothe emotional outbursts and calm the mind
- BL 18 (*gān shù*): Back-*shu* point of the liver to regulate and smoothen qi flow, resolve depression and harmonize the liver
- ST 40 (*fēng lóng*): To expel phlegm and dampness
- SP 9 (*yīn líng quán*): To invigorate spleen, harmonize middle *jiao* and expel dampness
- LI 11 (*qū chí*): To clear intestinal heat and calm the mind
- DU 23 (*shàng xīng*) and DU 24 (*shén tíng*): To clear the head and open the orifices

- EX-HN 1 (*sì shén cōng*): To benefit the brain and open the orifices

Supporting Points:

- GB 13 (*běn shén*) and GB 20 (*fēng chí*): To treat extreme cases of manic psychosis
- ST 44 (*nèi tíng*): To clear stomach fire with damp-heat obstructing the orifices
- EX-UE 11 (*shí xuān*): To revive consciousness and open the senses

Recommended Formula: *Xǐ Xīn Tāng* (洗心汤, Heart-Clearing Decoction) from the *Records of Pattern Differentiations* (*Biàn Zhèng Lù*, 辨证录)

Substitute Formula: *Dí Tán Tāng* (涤痰汤, Phlegm-Flushing Decoction)

Patent Formula:

- *Sū Hé Xiāng Wán* (苏合香丸, Storax Pill)
- *Xīn Nǎo Jiàn Jiāo Náng* (心脑健胶囊, Capsule for Heart and Brain)

3. Marrow Depletion

Symptoms: Dull expression, palpitations, forgetfulness, lethargy, vertigo, tinnitus, poor appetite, pale lips, nails and tongue, pale complexion, thin loose stools, a pale and enlarged tongue with white or lacking coating and a thin and weak pulse.

Treatment Principle:

- Tonify qi and nourish blood
- Invigorate brain and awaken the mind

Main Acupuncture Points:

- DU 20 (*bǎi huì*): To open the orifices and awaken the mind, calm the spirit and nourish the sea of marrow
- EX-HN 1 (*sì shén cōng*): To benefit the brain and open the orifices
- ST 36 (*zú sān lǐ*): To promote qi blood circulation
- GB 39 (*xuán zhōng*): Influential point of marrow to nourish marrow, benefit bones and sinews, treat vertigo and tinnitus
- DU 16 (*fēng fǔ*): To nourish the sea of marrow and calm the mind
- BL 17 (*gé shù*): Influential point of the blood to activate blood circulation, dispel stasis and unbind the chest

Supporting Points:

- EX-HN 24 (*ān mián*): To calm the spirit, treat insomnia, vertigo and mental disorders
- HT 7 (*shén mén*): *Yuan*-source point of the heart to regulate and tonify heart qi, calm the spirit and treat amnesia

Recommended Formula: *Bā Zhēn Tāng* (八珍汤, Eight Gem Decoction) from the *Categorized Synopsis of the Whole* (*Zhèng Tǐ Lèi Yào*, 正体类要)

Substitute Formula:

- *Qī Fú Yǐn* (七福饮, Beverage with Seven Drugs)
- *Rén Shēn Yǎng Róng Tāng* (人参养荣汤, Ginseng Supporting and Nourishing Decoction)

Patent Formula: *Hé Chē Dà Zào Wán* (河车大造丸, Placenta Great Pill)

4. Liver Blood and Kidney Yin Deficiency

Symptoms: Low spirit, apathy, anxiety, dizziness, tinnitus, despair, fatigue, frequent sobbing, low concentration ability, poor memory, suspicion, night sweats, painful and sore lower back and knees, impotence, seminal emission, diarrhea, a pale red tongue with white coating and a thin and wiry pulse.

Treatment Principle:

- Tonify kidney yin and liver blood
- Nourish kidney essence and marrow

Main Acupuncture Points:

- KI 3 (*tài xī*): *Yuan*-source point of the kidney to nourish kidney yin and strengthen the lumbus
- SP 6 (*sān yīn jiāo*): To tonify liver and kidney yin, improve circulation and astringe lower fluid passages
- BL 18 (*gān shù*): Back-*shu* point of the liver to clear liver and gallbladder fire, regulate and smoothen the qi flow, resolve depression and harmonize the liver
- BL 23 (*shèn shù*): Back-*shu* point of the kidney to benefit the original qi and kidney yin
- BL 52 (*zhì shì*): To tonify kidney essence
- DU 20 (*bǎi huì*): To nourish the sea of marrow and calm the spirit

Supporting Points:

- KI 7 (*fù liū*): To nourish kidney yin and treat night sweating with edema
- KI 12 (*dà hè*): To treat kidney essence deficiency

Recommended Formula: *Zhī Bǎi Dì Huáng Wán* (知柏地黄丸, Anemarrhena, Phellodendron and Rehmannia Pill) from the *Golden Mirror of the Medical Tradition* (*Yī Zōng Jīn Jiàn*, 医宗金鉴)

Substitute Formula: *Zuǒ Guī Yǐn* (左归饮, Left-Restoring Beverage)

Patent Formula: *Qǐ Jú Dì Huáng Wán* (杞菊地黄丸, Lycium Berry, Chrysanthemum and Rehmannia Pill)

5. Spleen and Kidney Yang Deficiency

Symptoms: Dull expression, forgetfulness, lethargy, lower back and knees soreness and pain, limb coldness, heaviness and weakness, poor appetite, frequent night urination or incontinence, sticky and loose stools, a pale and enlarged tongue with teeth marks with a greasy or clear slippery coating and a deep and thin pulse.

Treatment Principle:

- Tonify kidney yang and secure essence
- Invigorate spleen and tonify qi

Main Acupuncture Points:

- SP 6 (*sān yīn jiāo*): To invigorate spleen and kidney, improve circulation, astringe lower fluid passages, benefit lower limbs and stop diarrhea

- KI 3 (*tài xī*): *Yuan*-source point of kidney to tonify kidney and benefit spleen, regulate menstruation and treat lower limb disorders
- RN 12 (*zhōng wǎn*): Front-*mu* point of the stomach to invigorate spleen and stomach, harmonize middle *jiao* and regulate qi
- DU 4 (*mìng mén*): To tonify kidney, regulate *du mai*, strengthen lumbar region, secure essence and benefit lower limbs
- RN 4 (*guān yuán*): Front-*mu* point of the small intestine to benefit the uterus, tonify original qi, supplement deficiencies, treat diarrhea and regulate menstruation
- BL 52 (*zhì shì*): To tonify kidney essence

Supporting Points:

- EX-CA 5 (*wèi shàng*): To tonify and raise the middle qi
- ST 27 (*dà jù*): To nourish essence

Recommended Formula: *Huán Shào Dān* (还少丹, Rejuvenation Elixir) from the *Collected Prescriptions* (*Jí Yàn Fāng*, 集验方)

Substitute Formula: *Jīn Guì Shèn Qì Wán* (金匮肾气丸, Golden Cabinet's Kidney Qi Pill)

Patent Formula: *Huán Shào Dān* (还少丹, Rejuvenation Elixir)

Summary Chart for Dementia

Patterns	Main Points	Supporting Points	Formulae
Qi Stagnation and Blood Stasis	DU 20, EX-HN 1, GB 12, ST 36, BL 17, SP 10	LV 14 for liver and spleen disharmony RN 17 for chest impediment	*Tōng Qiào Huó Xuè Tāng* or *Xuè Fǔ Zhú Yū Tāng*
Turbid Phlegm Heat Obstructing Orifices	LV 3, BL 18, ST 40, SP 9, DU 23, LI 11, DU 24, EX-HN 1	GB 13 plus GB 20 for manic psychosis ST 44 for stomach fire EX-UE 11 for loss of consciousness	*Xǐ Xīn Tāng* or *Dí Tán Tāng*
Marrow Depletion	DU 20, EX-HN 1, ST 36, GB 39, DU 16, BL 17	EX-HN 24 for insomnia and vertigo HT 7 for amnesia	*Bā Zhèn Tāng* or *Qī Fú Yǐn* or *Rén Shēn Yǎng Róng Tāng*
Liver Blood and Kidney Yin Deficiency	KI 3, SP 6, BL 18, BL 23, BL 52, DU 20	KI 7 for night sweats and edema KI 12 for essence deficiency	*Zhī Bǎi Dì Huáng Wán* or *Zuǒ Guī Yǐn*
Spleen and Kidney Yang Deficiency	SP 6, KI 3, RN 12, DU 4, RN 4, BL 52	EX-CA 5 for middle qi sinking ST 27 for essence deficiency	*Huán Shào Dān* or *Jīn Guì Shèn Qì Wán*

CASE STUDY 1: Dementia

Mr. Li, 58 years old.

Main Complaint: Apathetic facial expression and slow reaction for 7 years with aggravation for 3 months.

Medical History: About 7 years ago, the patient gradually developed apathetic facial expression, was slow in reacting to conversations and events with discontinuous dizziness and forgetfulness. The patient did not pay attention to the symptoms and received no systemic diagnosis and treatment, so the symptoms aggravated. In the recent 3 months, symptoms became more severe, and since the onset of the disease, his mental state and sleep were poor with an aversion to cold. The patient also suffered from hyperlipemia (HLP) for 15 years, and discontinuously took simvastatin and *Xuě Zhī Kāng Jiāo Náng* (Healthy Blood Fat Capsule) orally to stabilize it in a normal range.

Presenting Symptoms: slow in reaction, apathetic facial expression, declined capacity to calculate, low consciousness, poor spirit, slight obesity, frequent urination and stools, reluctance to speak to others, a red tongue with a scanty coating and a thready and rapid pulse.

Physical Examination: Temperature: 36.5℃, pulse: 75 bpm, respiration: 20 bpm, blood pressure: 125/75 mmHg. The patient walked independently into the ward and was cooperative. He spoke clearly and the answers were slow. Nervous system examination showed cranial nerves (−), the strength of the muscle was normal. Cerebral CT confirmed an encephalatrophy. Examination for fundus oculi confirmed a retinal arteriosclerosis Grade II.

Pattern Differentiation

The patient was over fifty years old and due to malnourishment and overwork the spleen and stomach were weak causing an accumulation of turbid phlegm which clouded the clear orifices and led to the brain impairment. As the qi of brain is disconnected from the *zang* qi, the brain marrow declines causing symptoms of apathetic facial expression, slow reaction and forgetfulness. The location of the disease is in the brain and it is closely related to the dysfunction of the heart, liver, spleen and kidney. This case pertains to a deficient root and an excess branch.

Diagnosis

TCM Diagnosis: Dementia due to turbid phlegm clouding the orifices

Western Medicine Diagnosis: Dementia

Treatment

The pathogenesis of this case is malnourishment with spleen and stomach deficiency engendering turbid phlegm clouding the orifices and obstructing the brain leading to the declined brain marrow and mental activities.

Principles:

- Fortify the spleen and remove dampness
- Eliminate phlegm and open the orifices

Formula: Modified *Wēn Dǎn Tāng* (Gallbladder Warming Decoction)

Ingredients:

陈皮	*chén pí*	10 g	Pericarpium Citri Reticulatae
半夏	*bàn xià*	8 g	Rhizoma Pinelliae
茯苓	*fú líng*	10 g	Poria
枳实	*zhǐ shí*	10 g	Fructus Aurantii Immaturus
竹茹	*zhú rú*	10 g	Caulis Bambusae in Taenia
瓜蒌	*guā lóu*	10 g	Fructus Trichosanthis
菖蒲	*chāng pú*	10 g	Rhizoma Acori Tatarinowii
远志	*yuǎn zhì*	8 g	Radix Polygalae
丹参	*dān shēn*	15 g	Radix et Rhizoma Salviae Miltiorrhizae
麝香	*shè xiāng*	3 g	Moschus (infused)
炙甘草	*zhì gān cǎo*	5 g	Radix et Rhizoma Glycyrrhizae Praeparata cum Melle

Formula Analysis

This formula equally reinforces healthy qi and removes phlegm. Reinforcing healthy qi is to fortify the spleen and generate qi. Removing phlegm is to remove turbid pathogen that harasses the heart and the mind. To fortify the spleen and remove the phlegm, *fú líng* is combined with *chén pí, bàn xià, zhú rú* and *guā lóu* to also treat symptoms such as heaviness of the head, sudden weeping and laughing, muttering to himself and foaming at the mouth. *Shè xiāng* was infused and taken orally to open orifices. *Dān shēn* invigorates blood and dissolves stasis to unblock the brain orifice. These ingredients achieves the effect of fortifying the spleen and removing turbidity as well as eliminating phlegm to open the orifices.

Follow-up Consultations

After 20 doses of the formula, the facial expression of the patient became more rich than before. He was able to communicate with others, his memory and orientation improved, and he could live partially independently. After taking the formula for 2 months, the spirit of patient improved greatly and he could fully live on his own.

CASE STUDY 2: Paralysis and Dementia

Mr. Zhang, 85 years old. 1st consultation on August 2nd, 2012.

Main Complaint: Paralysis of the extremities for 10 years, slow reaction for 4 years and fever for 1 day.

Medical History: The patient suffered from paralysis of the left extremities 10 years ago due to a cerebral infarction which resolved after treatment. About 4 years ago, the patient started becoming slower at responding with involuntary tremors of the upper limbs especially in stillness. He felt dizzy with paroxysmal flusteredness, chest oppression and shortness of breath. At the time, the patient received treatment for Parkinson's disease and the symptoms were sometimes mild and sometimes severe. About 1 year ago, the patient had a relapse of the left-sided paralysis of the extremities, unclear speech and inability to walk by himself. A CT scan of the head indicated subcortical arteriosclerotic encephalopathy. The symptoms were not significantly relieved after treatment. From then on, he could not get out of bed, and was unable to straighten his lower limbs with urinary and fecal incontinence. One day ago, he suffered from a fever with loose nasal discharge, and expectoration of white and thin phlegm. The body temperature was not taken at that time. The temperature gradually dropped by taking *Sù Xiào Shāng Fēng Jiāo Náng* (Quick-Acting Cold Capsule), but there were still a runny nose. The patient also suffered from poor sleep, dry stools once every few days and urinary incontinence.

Physical Examination: Temperature: 36.2 ℃, pulse: 74 bpm, respiration: 20 bpm, blood pressure: 120/80 mmHg. There was some trembling of the upper limbs and some lack of muscle strength on both upper limbs with normal strength on the lower limbs.

Pattern Differentiation

This case of dementia was caused by deficiency of five *zang*-organs, especially the liver and kidney with essence and blood insufficiency, which damaged the sea of marrow manifesting in the dysfunction of mental activities. The deficiency of the spleen also generated phlegm turbidity which clouded the clear orifices.

Diagnosis

TCM Diagnosis: Dementia due to wind harassing the upper body with liver blood and kidney yin deficiency

Western Medicine Diagnosis: Dementia and paralysis

Treatment

Principle:

- Enrich yin and subdue yang
- Extinguish wind and unblock the collaterals

Acupuncture Point Combination: DU 20 (*bǎi huì*), EX-HN 1 (*sì shén cōng*), DU 24 (*shén tíng*), GB 13 (*běn shén*), EX-HN 3 (*yìn táng*), GB 20 (*fēng chí*), ST 36 (*zú sān lǐ*), ST 40 (*fēng lóng*), SP 6 (*sān yīn jiāo*), KI 3 (*tài xī*) and LV 3 (*tài chōng*).

Manipulations: The acupuncture points on the head are applied to awaken the brain and regulate spirit, and ST 36 (*zú sān lǐ*), SP 6 (*sān yīn jiāo*) and LV 3 (*tài chōng*) were used to unblock channels and collaterals, achieving the effect of gathering spirit and resuming intelligence. Needle the acupuncture points mentioned and retain the needles for 30 minutes. Ten treatments makes one course and give three to five courses consecutively.

Chinese Patent Medicines: *Dān Qí Piān Tān Jiāo Náng* (Salvia and Astragalus Capsule), *Yì Shèn Yǎng Gān Hé Jì* (Kidney-Boosting and Liver-Nourishing Preparation) and *Huà Yū Tōng Mài Zhù Shè Yè* (Stasis-Resolving and Vessel-Unblocking Injection) were given to boost qi, invigorate blood, nourish the kidney and soothe the liver.

BRIEF SUMMARY

According to the "Four-Spiritual Acupuncture" (DU 20, EX-HN 1), "Intelligence-Three Acupuncture" (DU 24, GB 13), "Awaken Spirit-Three Acupuncture" (DU 20, DU 24, EX-HN 3) are applied to awaken and regulate spirits. ST 36 and ST 40 are used to dissolve phlegm and expel stasis. SP 6, KI 3 and LV 3 are applied to nourish and enrich the liver and kidney and unblock channels and collaterals.

KEY CLINICAL POINTS

1. In clinic, it is important to differentiate the deficiency and excess syndromes, and decide which *zang*-organs are responsible for the dementia. As most cases are a combination of excess and deficiency, it is also important to distinguish which is the priority.

2. Apart from the five commonly seen patterns of dementia mentioned above, there are also some other patterns which should be treated by modifying the corresponding formulas.

3. Dementia is a chronic and degenerative disorder; hence, persistent treatment is necessary for the patient to achieve results. Meanwhile, it is important to cultivate the mind, stimulate the body and train the memory to prevent the progression of the illness.

COMPREHENSION QUESTIONS

1. What is the etiology and basic pathogenesis of dementia?

2. What are the key points for syndrome differentiation and treatment of dementia?

3. Multiple choice questions:

1) The basic pathogenesis of dementia is:

A. Qi deficiency and essence depletion with turbid phlegm clouding the orifices

B. Depletion of the sea of marrow causing the dysfunction of mental activity

C. Phlegm and blood obstructing collaterals with depletion of the sea of marrow

D. Spleen and kidney deficiency with phlegm and blood obstructing collaterals

E. Dysfunction of mental activity due to turbid phlegm clouding the orifices

2) All the patterns below are the representative patterns of dementia, except:

A. Depletion of the sea of marrow

B. Spleen and kidney deficiency

C. Phlegm turbidity clouding the orifices

D. Internal obstruction of static blood

E. Exterior cold and interior heat

3) For dementia with clinical manifestations of apathetic facial expression, reluctance to speak, loss of mental function, normal appetite, drooling from the mouth, a pale tongue with a greasy coating and a slippery pulse. This syndrome is due to:

A. Depletion of sea of marrow

B. Spleen and kidney yang deficiency

C. Phlegm and blood stasis obstruction

D. Internal obstruction of static blood

E. Phlegm turbidity clouding the orifices

4) For dementia with clinical manifestations of apathetic facial expression, declined memory, soreness and weakness of the lumbar and knees, flushed cheeks, night sweating, tinnitus, a thin and reddish tongue with a scanty tongue coating and a deep, wiry, thready and rapid pulse. The recommended formula is:

A. *Huán Shào Dān* (Back to Young Pill)

B. *Qī Fú Yǐn* (Seven Blessings Decoction)

C. *Zhī Bǎi Dì Huáng Wán* (Anemarrhena, Phellodendron and Rehmannia Pill)

D. *Zhuǎn Dāi Tāng* (Being Intelligent Decoction)

E. *Jīn Guì Shèn Qì Wán* (Golden Cabinet's Kidney Qi Pill)

Answers

1. Many causes can contribute to dementia and the major ones with their pathogeneses are listed below.

A. Physical and mental weakness due to old age

The brain is the sea of marrow and house of the original spirit. It is in charge of all mental and physical activities. When we reach old age, the functions of *zang-fu* organs decrease due to both liver blood and kidney yin deficiency, or essence depletion, which contribute to the lack of marrow production leading to the decreased brain marrow and reduced mental activities manifesting as the syndrome of dementia. As the classical text *Correction of Errors in Medical Works* (*Yī Lín Gǎi Cuò*, 医林改错) states: "the elderly with poor memory is a manifestation of the gradual depletion of the brain marrow." Besides, the qi and blood circulation in elderly people is slower and tends to be stagnated leading to obstruction of the collaterals resulting in dysfunction of mental activities and dementia.

B. Impairment due to excessive emotions

Being constantly dissatisfied, depressed and angry damage the liver qi and cause stagnation leading to binding of liver qi attacking the spleen which fails to transport nutrients resulting in gathering of dampness and phlegm clouding the clear orifices. The dampness and phlegm may also transform into heat and fire, harassing the spirit and leading to emotional disorder and sudden weeping and laughing.

Excessive thinking damages the spleen and heart. As the heart yin and blood are consumed and spleen is deficient, there is a lack of qi and blood production depriving the brain from nourishment of the marrow leading to mental disorder.

Sudden or chronic fright and fear will damage the kidney essence leading to the depletion of the sea of marrow where the brain will be malnourished resulting in dementia.

C. Consumption of prolonged illness

Prolonged illness of wind stroke, vertigo or other diseases affecting the brain gradually impair the healthy qi, deplete the yin, yang, essence, qi and blood of the kidney, heart, liver and spleen, further causing a lack of nourishment to the brain.

2. Key points of the syndrome differentiation:

Dementia pertains to a root deficiency and branch excess while the commonly seen syndrome in clinic is a deficiency-excess complex.

For dementia due to a deficiency syndrome, it mainly manifests as lack of spirit, lusterless complexion, emaciation, reluctance to speak and weak movements. There are three patterns including depletion of the sea of marrow, liver blood and kidney yin depletion and spleen and kidney yang deficiency.

For dementia due to an excess syndrome, it mainly manifests as lack of mental ability, dull facial expression, slow mental and physical reaction, and sudden changes of emotion demonstrating the pathogenic factors such as turbid phlegm, static blood and wind fire clouding the spirit and harassing the orifices.

Treatment principles:

Treating such a complex and debilitating disease as dementia has a long course of treatment where nourishing the healthy qi, yin and yang and replenishing the essence is required, while simultaneously unblocking channels, removing obstruction and expelling phlegm and draining fire.

3. 1) B, 2) E, 3) E, 4) A.

Index by Disease Names and Symptoms

Index by Formulas

Notes

Notes

Notes

图书在版编目（CIP）数据

内科学 =Internal medicine/ 刘柏炎，（加）苏璇，叶晓主编．—北京：人民卫生出版社，2014
（英文版中医病案教育系列）
ISBN 978-7-117-20003-5

Ⅰ.①内… Ⅱ.①刘…②苏…③叶… Ⅲ.①中医内科学－英文 Ⅳ.①R25

中国版本图书馆 CIP 数据核字（2014）第 262500 号

中医病案教育系列：内科学（英文版）

主　　编：刘柏炎　Suzanne Robidoux　叶晓
出版发行：人民卫生出版社（中继线 010-59780011）
地　　址：中国北京市朝阳区潘家园南里 19 号
世界医药图书大厦 B 座
邮　　编：100021
网　　址：http://www.pmph.com
E - mail：pmph @ pmph.com
购书热线：010-59787592　010-59787584　010-65264830
开　　本：787 × 1092　1/16
版　　次：2014 年 12 月第 1 版　2014 年 12 月第 1 版第 1 次印刷
标准书号：ISBN 978-7-117-20003-5/R · 20004